Statistical Design, Monitoring, and Analysis of Clinical Trials

Chapman & Hall/CRC
Biostatistics Series

RECENTLY PUBLISHED TITLES

Statistical Design, Monitoring, and Analysis of Clinical Trials

Principles and Methods

Second Edition

Weichung Joe Shih
Rutgers University
Piscataway, New Jersey, USA

Joseph Aisner
Rutgers Cancer Institute of New Jersey
New Brunswick, New Jersey, USA

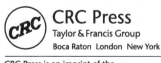

CRC Press
Taylor & Francis Group
Boca Raton London New York

CRC Press is an imprint of the
Taylor & Francis Group, an **informa** business
A CHAPMAN & HALL BOOK

Second edition published 2022
by CRC Press
6000 Broken Sound Parkway NW, Suite 300, Boca Raton, FL 33487-2742

and by CRC Press
2 Park Square, Milton Park, Abingdon, Oxon, OX14 4RN

© 2022 Weichung Joe Shih and Joseph Aisner

First edition published by CRC Press 2015

CRC Press is an imprint of Taylor & Francis Group, LLC

Library of Congress Cataloging-in-Publication Data
Names: Shih, Weichung Joe, author. | Aisner, Joseph, author.
Title: Statistical design, monitoring, and analysis of clinical trials :
principles and methods / Weichung Joe Shih, Rutgers University Piscataway, New Jersey, USA, Joseph Aisner, Rutgers Cancer Institute of New Jersey New Brunswick, New Jersey, USA.
Description: Second edition. | Boca Raton : CRC Press, 2022. | Series:
Chapman & Hall/CRC biostatistics series | Includes bibliographical references and index.
Identifiers: LCCN 2021022345 (print) | LCCN 2021022346 (ebook) |
ISBN 9780367772444 (hardback) | ISBN 9781032009599 (paperback) | ISBN 9781003176527 (ebook)
Subjects: LCSH: Clinical trials—Statistical methods.
Classification: LCC R853.C55 S48 2022 (print) | LCC R853.C55 (ebook) | DDC 610.72/7—dc23
LC record available at https://lccn.loc.gov/2021022345
LC ebook record available at https://lccn.loc.gov/2021022346

ISBN: 9780367772444 (hbk)
ISBN: 9781032009599 (pbk)
ISBN: 9781003176527 (ebk)

DOI: 10.1201/9781003176527

Typeset in Palatino
by codeMantra

Contents

Preface

The second edition of this book was written largely during the winter of 2020–2021, a few months after my retirement, which started a year earlier as a gradual retirement plan offered by the university for tenured faculty. More remarkably, it was a time when the world was witnessing the centurial crisis—the novel coronavirus Covid-19. Nations and cities were shut down, business halted, schools and public places closed, people locked indoors, and millions lost their lives.

As the world fought the Covid-19 pandemic, the public was attuned eagerly to the daily news on drug and vaccine developments. Health officials, physicians, and policy leaders were frequently interviewed by media, reporting and commenting on the progress and key preliminary results from ongoing observational studies and clinical trials. Vivid debates on data quality and strength of evidence were broadcasted. More and more people became keen in understanding at least some of the concepts of clinical trials such as sample size, control group, incidence rate, diagnostic testing, efficacy and safety, treatment versus prevention, interim analysis, and even "independent data monitoring committees." I sensed a mission for the book amid the emergent crisis.

This new edition includes several references to Covid-19. A new section in Chapter 5, for example, is added on logistic regression analysis, which contains a dataset from the first placebo-controlled, double-blind trial of remdesivir conducted in China, for which I was privileged to serve on its data and safety monitoring board.

In response to comments from reviewers on the previous edition, a new Chapter 6 on survival data analyses is added, which expands the fundamental material in Appendix 4.1 to full discussions on Cox regression and non-proportional hazards. It immediately follows Chapter 5 where the analysis of covariance for continuous endpoints and logistic regression analysis for binary endpoints are presented.

Also, in response to requests from readers, more discussions on sample size reestimation methods and other modern adaptive designs, especially with predictive biomarkers, are added. When engaging in adaptive designs, a thorough understanding of the multiple hypotheses is necessary. Thus, several new chapters are added, including a chapter on the multiplicity issue and methods to control the familywise error rate, a chapter on the different aims of popular biomarker-based trials, and a chapter on seamless Phase II/III trials. The new material on sample size reestimation and adaptive design reflects the recently updated guidance issued by the international health authorities as well as my practice in consulting activities in these areas.

The American Statistical Association recently, after long discussions, outlined six principles on the widely used p-values. For the interest of many applied statisticians and clinical trialists, an illustrative discussion to elaborate these principles is featured in Chapter 14.

Finally, there was another important guidance update from international health authorities, that is, regarding the missing data problem. We retain the discussion on the missing data last—in Chapter 15. However, the topic has been expanded to defining "estimand" and strategies of handling "intercurrent events."

Obviously, the new additions of sections and chapters have expanded the book to a new dimension beyond the first edition, which is mainly for teaching second-year students in graduate schools at an introductory level. Although teachers may still select proper chapters to fit in their course contents, the new material may be more suitable for an advanced level course or consulted as references for working professionals in clinical trials. More computer software or codes are included for practitioners to use. Either way, I hope the readers find the second edition helpful and an enjoyable read.

On closing, I would like to express my deep gratitude to my dear family, friends, students, and colleagues for your continuing support and companionship during my nearly 40-year career and semi-retirement life so far. Tomorrow, as we celebrate the Easter of 2021, winning the war against the vicious pandemic is near, may God protect and bless you all.

Weichung Joe Shih
Piscataway, New Jersey
April 3, 2021

Preface (First Edition)

Clinical trials, as an enterprise, reflect the work of many participants and the expertise they bring to bear: biologists, toxicologists, pharmacologists, medical investigators, research nurses, project managers, computer programmers, database specialists, medical writers, health authority regulators, and, of course, biostatisticians. One needs only attend an annual conference of the Society for Clinical Trials to discover a network of participants from many different disciplinary areas who all contribute to clinical trials. This book, however, concentrates on the biostatistics component of the enterprise.

Most of this book is based on the teaching material that we used for public health and medical students, residents, and fellows over the past 15 years. In addition to our academic experience, we also worked on clinical trials sponsored by pharmaceutical companies and governmental health organizations. We benefited from the experience of working with teams on a wide variety of clinical development projects, and we found that the biostatistics component of clinical trials is truly an integration of many fundamental scientific principles and statistical methods. Chapter 1 is an overview, which begins with ethical and safety principles, criteria for quality studies, and classification of different types of clinical trials. Chapters 2 and 3 cover core trial design concepts. Many design issues in clinical trials stem from the fact that a clinical trial needs to balance the two aspects of its nature: scientific experiment and clinical practice. For a scientific experiment, validity (Chapter 2) and efficiency (Chapter 3) are the main considerations. Students using this book need some basic knowledge in hypothesis testing and confidence intervals to learn, in Chapter 4, the principles and methods of sample size and power calculation. Thus, the fundamental principles of probability and inferential statistics are prerequisites for using this book. Regarding analytical methods, students must learn regression, analysis of variance and covariance, analysis of categorical data, longitudinal data, and survival data. However, a one-semester course in clinical trials is neither just an overview of statistical methods, nor can it cover these methods in depth. We cover the fundamental analysis of covariance and stratified analysis in Chapter 5 and leave many other topics of methods in the appendices of other related chapters. Almost all modern clinical trials involve data monitoring and interim analyses. We devoted Chapters 6–8 to sequential designs and methods, from two-stage Phase II cancer trials to Phase III group sequential trials, including monitoring safety, futility, and efficacy. Following the sequential trials and interim analyses, a more recent topic is the monitoring and modification of the maximum information in the middle of a clinical trial. In Chapter 9, we discuss the development of sample size reestimation and adaptive group sequential procedures, but only briefly, because this subject remains an open research area. We end the book with a discussion of missing data in Chapter 10. Missing data is not totally avoidable, but it should and can be minimized by proper trial design and responsible trial conduct. Missing data is an old issue, but a recent report from the National Research Council has brought the importance of this issue again into the spotlight. In Chapter 10, we discuss some matured methods and one newly developed method under different assumptions regarding the nature of the missing data. The sequence of the chapters is based on our view of a logical progression of concepts and technical levels as taught in our courses. We move from design concepts, sample size calculation, to analytical methods including ANCOVA, then to trial monitoring with sequential designs, interim analyses, adaptive midcourse modification, and finally we give special attention to the ubiquitous problem of missing data. Some instructors may rearrange the sequence or supplement with other topics according to individual preference. In all chapters, in-class discussions and exercises are held for the students to practice. Many examples are from trials published in medical journals or our consulting projects. Where computation is required, we provide instructions for acquiring and using an online software program; we also introduce simple commands using R functions or SAS® procedures for some techniques, although some homework assignments also train students to carry out computer simulations.

Our training and work experience in both academia and industry, as well as in consulting to governmental health authorities, allow us to present teaching material that reflects different aspects of clinical trials that may be oriented to academic research, commercial development, or public health. However, finding the proper level and coverage was a challenge. Because this course was taught in a public health and medical school environment, it is interesting to observe that some concepts such as control of confounding and bias were relatively easy to grasp for students from epidemiology, whereas the essence and calculation of critical values and study power were relatively comprehensible for students from the biostatistics program. Hence, to provide a balanced set of homework assignments, in-class exercises, and examinations for the whole class was a concern for us. In addition to having different disciplinary backgrounds, students were often at different stages of their academic or career pursuits. For example, in the same class, we saw students who were about to finish their master's degrees and were searching for jobs in the pharmaceutical or biotech industries, mixed with students who had already acquired Master of Science or Master of Public Health degrees and were in the second or third years of their doctoral programs. In some semesters, the course also attracted pharmacy students or physicians in their residency or fellowship programs from the medical schools or the university cancer centers. They cerainly extended the classroom discussions to another dimension, especially for review and critique of the medical literature, which we often excerpted as part of the teaching material.

Input from students and colleagues allowed us to develop and focus the course material. The result, we believe, spans the spectrum of those who deal with clinical trials directly and those who read and interpret the material. For the student of statistics, we believe this work places in context the specific principles and methods applicable to clinical trials, and the mathematical exercises illustrate the process. For the clinicians who engaged in the course, we further believe that, even if the formulae and their derivation seemed daunting, the course helped to focus their understanding of how clinical data are collected, monitored, and analyzed. Importantly, the study of biostatistics of clinical trials helps us develop vital collaborators to the team of investigators. In addition, the study of biostatistics helps the clinical investigator understand what the statistical methods can provide. Educated consumers of biostatistics make better investigators and furthermore develop their critical reading skills. To that end, statistical critiques are now often included in the Oncology Fellows' Journal Club presentations at the Rutgers Cancer Institute of New Jersey.

Because this book is based on our teaching material over the years, our primary goal for the book is to serve as a text for colleagues teaching clinical trials in a similar academic setting. As a text for a one-semester course, there are certainly materials that we chose to omit in this first edition, such as subgroup analysis and multiple tests and comparisons. Thus, we leave plenty of opportunity in this book for other colleagues to fill in and improve upon.

To students, we hope that you find this book an enjoyable read and that you learn from it. To fellow teachers, we hope that you find this book a useful text for your class.

Acknowledgments (First Edition)

We sincerely thank the many students and colleagues who participated in our teaching and working experience in clinical trials. We are grateful for the opportunity developed in the setting of the Rutgers University School of Public Health and the Rutgers Cancer Institute of New Jersey, which provided the setting, support, colleagues, and students from whom we learned so much. In particular, we would like to thank our colleagues Irving K. Hwang, Gordon K. K. Lan, Dirk F. Moore, Yong Lin, Yujun Wu, and Pamela Ohman-Strickland, who have lectured with us at one time or another. We would also like to acknowledge Tina Chang Young, a student of this course (Spring 2013) and now a Doctor of Public Health candidate at the Rutgers School of Public Health, who read the initial and final drafts and provided numerous suggestions that improved the clarity of this book.

Weichung Joe Shih
Department of Biostatistics
Rutgers School of Public Health & Rutgers Cancer Institute of New Jersey
Rutgers, The State University of New Jersey

Joseph Aisner
Medical Oncology
Robert Wood Johnson Medical School & Rutgers Cancer Institute of New Jersey
Rutgers, The State University of New Jersey
July 2015

Authors

Weichung Joe Shih, PhD, has been tenured professor and chair of the Department of Biostatistics, Rutgers School of Public Health, Rutgers University, New Brunswick, NJ, and director of Biometrics Division at the Rutgers Cancer Institute of New Jersey, New Brunswick, NJ. He is an elected fellow of the American Statistical Association (1996) and an elected member of the International Statistical Institute (2001). Prior to joining academia, he spent his formative years (1982–1999) at Merck Research Laboratories, Rahway, NJ. He served on the Advisory Board of the US FDA for reviewing new drug applications and was an associate editor of professional journals, including *Statistics in Medicine, Controlled Clinical Trials, Clinical Cancer Research, Statistics in Biopharmaceutical Research,* and *Statistics in Bioscience.* He pioneered in the field of sample size reestimation for clinical trials, which has evolved into the field of adaptive designs. He also first advocated the use of consistency criterion for international bridging studies, which is now adopted by the ICH guidance for global multiregional clinical trials. He has collaborated extensively with physicians in various therapeutic areas and authored numerous papers in statistical methodology in clinical trials. His research interests include adaptive designs and missing data issues. He has been honored as professor emeritus of Rutgers University since July 2019.

Joseph Aisner, MD, is a professor of medicine and a professor of environmental and occupational medicine at the Robert Wood Johnson Medical School of Rutgers University, New Brunswick, NJ, director of Medical Oncology Unit at the Robert Wood Johnson University Hospital, New Brunswick, NJ, and co-leader of the Clinical Investigations Program at the Rutgers Cancer Institute of New Jersey. He has published extensively and has served on the editorial boards of multiple journals, including *Journal of Clinical Oncology, Cancer Therapeutics, Medical Oncology, Clinical Cancer Research,* and *Hematology-Oncology Today.* He is a fellow of the American College of Physicians and the American Society of Clinical Oncology. He serves on and chairs several National Data Monitoring Committees, has served on multiple National Institutes of Health (NIH) Study Sections, and has headed two National Cooperative Cancer Study Groups. His research interests include cancer clinical trials and evaluation of therapeutic interventions.

1

Overview

Before we start, consider these two questions:

- Who was the pioneering British clinician who established the link between smoking and lung cancer?
- Who was the principal investigator who first used a randomized, controlled clinical trial to test streptomycin in the treatment of pulmonary tuberculosis in 1940?

1.1 What is a Clinical Trial?

In this book, we define *clinical trial* as "an experiment that studies the relationship between a disease or condition and a medical intervention for prevention, diagnosis, or treatment using human subjects." The ultimate goal of a clinical trial should be to advance medical knowledge and to improve medical practice to benefit the patients.

To better appreciate this definition, we will first answer the two questions posed above: The correct answer to both is *Sir Austin Bradford Hill* (1897–1991), Dean of the London School of Hygiene and Tropical Medicine (1955–1957). Hill conducted two types of clinical studies, both involving human subjects; however, the first study, linking smoking and lung cancer (1950), was based on observational investigations, and the second, prospectively testing streptomycin in the treatment of pulmonary tuberculosis, was an experiment, that is, a clinical trial.

Clinical studies conducted in medical schools include retrospective surveys of clinical data or accumulated case reports, which are often cross-sectional, as well as *clinical trials*, which are always prospective and thus require both a baseline and a follow-up period. Not all clinical studies are clinical trials, but all clinical trials are also clinical studies.

In Hill's article on statistical methods "General Summary and Conclusions" (1937), he states that "in both clinical and preventive medicine, and in much laboratory work, we cannot escape from the conclusion that... many of the problems we wish to solve are statistical and that there is no way of dealing with them except by the statistical method." This statement highlights the critical role of statistics in the medical sciences. In other words, biostatistical methods have become one of the fundamental tools in the evaluation of medical information.

Many, but not all, statistical principles and methods used in clinical trials are also applicable to other types of clinical studies. A statistician or an epidemiologist should distinguish the nature of the study, in order to properly interpret the result. The statistical analysis is thus the tool for understanding results and meanings in all forms of clinical studies. Statisticians, epidemiologists, and even clinical trialists need to understand the statistical tools that they rely on for interpreting the data, much like a carpenter needs to understand what a hammer can or cannot do.

Our definition of clinical trials is in line with that discussed in the ICMJE (International Committee of Medical Journal Editors) guidelines. Some authors have defined a clinical trial as "a prospective study comparing the effect and value of interventions against a control in human beings" (Friedman, Furberg, and DeMets 1996). In our opinion, this describes a requirement for a *good* clinical trial, but it is a restrictive definition that excludes a large portion of clinical trials that are conducted without *concurrent controls*. We certainly are interested in good clinical trials. In fact, to understand what constitutes a good clinical trial is a central objective of this book. Many investigators certainly would object if we said that a single-arm dose-finding study in cancer patients was not a clinical trial. As an example of a clinical study that led to medical knowledge and defined the standard of care in a noncontrolled setting, consider the Papanicolaou test for cervical cancer, which reduced the disease-specific mortality from cervical cancer by nearly 70% from early 1930 to 1974 (Cramer 1974, Michael 1999). The path to medical knowledge is a process in which different levels of evidence are developed by different types of clinical studies, as summarized in Table 1.1. Randomized, controlled trials (RCTs) are certainly at the highest level in the hierarchy of evidence.

1.2 Requirements for a Good Experiment

An experiment should always be conducted by the primary investigator under an initial set of well-defined conditions and procedures. For a clinical trial, this set of conditions and procedures should be documented in a protocol. The trial protocol also serves as the operational manual for all participating investigators and staff to follow. This system is akin to an operational method in any laboratory experiment.

1.2.1 An Ancient Story for Example

Read the following excerpt from the Book of Daniel 1: 1–16 (606 BC), which may be the earliest mention of a clinical study with dietary intervention in ancient history.

TABLE 1.1

Hierarchy of Evidence for Intervention Studies

Type of Evidence	Level of Evidence	Description
Systematic review of RCTs or meta-analysis	1 (highest)	A synthesis of evidence from all relevant RCTs with homogeneity
Individual RCT	2	An experiment in which subjects are randomly assigned to a treatment group or control group
Individual cohort study or a clinical trial without randomization or without control group	3	Cohort study: a follow-up observational study of a group(s)/cohort(s) to determine the development of an outcome(s) such as a disease, or an experiment in which subjects are not randomly assigned to a treatment group or control group
Case–control	4	Case–control study: a retrospective comparison of subjects with a condition or event (case) with those who do not have the condition or event (control) to determine characteristics (such as a treatment exposure) that might predict or alter the condition
Systematic review of qualitative or descriptive studies of series of cases	5	A synthesis of evidence from qualitative or descriptive studies to answer a clinical question
Expert opinion without explicit critical appraisal or consensus	6 (lowest)	Authoritative opinion of expert committee

Source: Bums PB, et al., *Plastic and Reconstructive Surgery* 128: 305–310, 2011; Melnyk BM and Fineout-Overholt E, *Evidence-Based Practice in Nursing and Healthcare: A Guide to Best Practice.* Lippincott, Williams & Wilkins, 2010.

In the third year of the reign of Jehoiakim king of Judah, Nebuchadnezzar king of Babylon came to Jerusalem and besieged it… Then the king (of Babylon) ordered Ashpenaz, chief of his court officials, to bring into the king's service some of the Israelites from the royal family and the nobility—young men without any physical defect, handsome, showing aptitude for every kind of learning, well informed, quick to understand, and qualified to serve in the king's palace. He was to teach them the language and literature of the Babylonians. The king assigned them a daily amount of food and wine from the king's table. They were to be trained for three years, and after that they were to enter the king's service.

Among those who were chosen were some from Judah: Daniel, Hananiah, Mishael, and Azariah.

But Daniel resolved not to defile himself with the royal food and wine, and he asked the chief official for permission not to defile himself this way. Now God had caused the official to show favor and compassion to Daniel, but the official told Daniel, "I am afraid of my lord the king, who has assigned your food and drink. Why should he see you looking worse than the other young men your age? The king would then have my head because of you."

Daniel then said to the guard whom the chief official had appointed over Daniel, Hananiah, Mishael, and Azariah, "Please test your servants for ten days: Give us nothing but vegetables to eat and water to drink. Then compare our appearance with that of the young men who eat the royal food, and treat your servants in accordance with what you see." So he agreed to this and tested them for ten days.

At the end of the ten days, they looked healthier and better nourished than any of the young men who ate the royal food. So the guard took away their choice food and the wine they were to drink and gave them vegetables instead.

In-Class Discussion: Could this story be viewed as a clinical study—and as a clinical trial? What information can you provide to support your answer? In your opinion, was it a "good" clinical trial? Why or why not?

1.2.2 Essential Steps of a Clinical Trial

More details will be discussed in later chapters, but the following outlines the essential steps of a clinical trial:

- Idea inception: The idea of a trial comes from a scientific rationale and a medical need to address. Investigators also have to catch the window of opportunity for conducting a clinical trial: public awareness of the disease burden, which is related to generating adequate interest for the study. If untested procedures are already accepted as the standard practice, it may be too late to propose a clinical trial. In proposing a clinical trial, some funding agencies may require the investigator to submit a short *letter of intent* (LOI), which is a brief outline of the essential elements of a trial protocol including rationale, objectives, participants, methods, and initial estimates of sample size and study duration. (See Homework 1.1 for sample LOI excerpts.)

- Planning: Planning includes preparing the study protocol, calculating the sample size, arranging study sites, and contracting personnel. It also includes having appropriate regulatory paperwork approved, such as the Investigational New Drug (IND) application by the US Food and Drug Administration (FDA) or the European Medicines Agency (EMA), obtaining local institutional review board (IRB) review and approval, ensuring medical supplies and equipment, budgeting, case report form (CRF) preparation, and assessment of feasibility in subject numbers and other resources for initiating and conducting the trial.

- Conduct and monitoring: This step includes screening, enrolling, scheduling, and administering study intervention to subjects. It also involves data collection, completing the CRFs, and database management. Monitoring ongoing clinical trials is necessary because trials are very expensive in monetary costs and human resources, and thus careful monitoring is critical to ensure the trial's quality and ethics.

- Data analysis: Data analysis actually starts at the study planning stage when sample size and statistical methodologies are prepared, as well as during the ongoing trial monitoring. Upon completion of the trial, statistical analyses will yield study results for interpretation.

- Report writing and publication: There is a popular saying that "a job is never finished until all the paperwork is done." For industry-sponsored trials, a clinical study report (CSR) is written by the trial sponsor and submitted to health agencies for commercial license approval. Journal publications help to inform the medical community of the results; these publications also often serve as a marketing vehicle for manufacturers. For trials sponsored by research grants from government organizations and foundations such as the National Institutes of Health (NIH), Department of Veterans Affairs, Department of Defense, and National Science Foundation, the study report and journal publication are documentation for grant accounting. In other words, these publications serve as the "deliverables" of the grant.

- Next phase trial: Trials sponsored by industry often involve a series of steps in the strategy of New Drug Application (NDA) or Biologic License Application (BLA) in the USA, or Marketing Authorization Application (MAA) in Europe. A trial's outcome likely affects other related trials in the NDA, BLA, or MAA package. Completed academic trials can often result in new or revised hypotheses. In either case, scientific knowledge is advanced by clinical trials. The ultimate goal of all clinical trials should thus be to advance medical knowledge and to improve medical practice to benefit the patients.

Statisticians need to participate in each of these steps. The statistician in a clinical trial needs to be more than a consultant. In fact, he or she should be a full-fledged member of the investigative team and must take responsibility for the scientific integrity of the study, as well as make assessments of its safety, efficacy, and futility. As Ederer (1979) noted, a statistician engaged in a clinical trial should be prepared to become both a student of the science and a teacher for the use of statistics during the course of the study. This process entails studying and learning in detail the clinical subject matter and, often, teaching fundamental statistical and research concepts to collaborators.

1.2.3 Essential Sections of a Clinical Trial Protocol

The protocol for the trial is the central document that guides the study throughout the course of the work and serves as the roadmap. It is also an operations manual and must therefore be written in excruciating detail, especially for multicenter trials, in order to ensure consistency across sites where any ambiguity may lead to differences in interpretation. A complete protocol usually contains the following sections (details of some topics are discussed in later sections or chapters):

- Introduction: Includes rationale and purpose of the trial (i.e., background and significance).
- Objectives and endpoints: Includes scientific hypotheses (primary and secondary) to test and specific aims to accomplish.
- Design: Includes randomization, blinding, control treatment, sample size, and study duration.
- Patient eligibility: Includes inclusion and exclusion criteria, used to define the subject population. These criteria will impact, in part, the future generalizability of the trial results.
- Conduct procedures and visit schedule: Includes dose and dose adjustment, laboratory and clinical examination schedule, patient withdrawal guidance, and trial flowcharts for more complex trials.
- Measurements: Includes assessment criteria for clinical and laboratory findings to measure the outcomes in efficacy and safety.
- Statistical considerations: Includes sample size justification, randomization process (if pertinent), study monitoring and interim analysis (if applicable), and methodology for statistical analyses and handling of missing data.
- Quality control and assurance procedures.
- Appendices: Include informed consent form, references or medical criteria/definition of response, and quality-of-life or other questionnaires if applicable.

1.2.4 Definition of a Well-Designed Study and Guidance for Evaluating a Protocol

Baumgardner (1997) summarized the fundamental requirements for a well-designed clinical trial as follows:

- Clear, definable, and relevant goals are sought.
- Adequate controls are in place.
- Samples are selected randomly.

- Measurements are made blindly and without bias.
- Appropriate statistical analysis is applied.

Following these guidelines, we can develop a checklist for reviewing a trial protocol:

Overall:

- Statement of objective(s).
- Statement of hypotheses in relation to the objectives.

    (It is important to clearly convey the two items above; otherwise, the results of the research would be regarded as exploratory, hypothesis generating, or a "fishing expedition.")

- Background, often presented as a literature review.
- Rationale for the trial that defines its significance.

    (Explain why the research question follows logically from previous research in the literature. Identify specific gaps that the clinical trial is intended to fill.)

- Pharmaceutical information, including source of agents, in the event that agents are to be used.

Design Aspects:

- Type of control, randomization, stratification, and degree of blinding.
- Patient eligibility criteria. Must include the disease risk and relevant population characteristics, disease stage, medical history, and prior and concomitant therapies for inclusion and exclusion.
- Sample size requirement and justification. Projection of recruitment period and location of centers require realistic expectations of accrual, effect size, and feasibility.
- Endpoint specification.

    (Prioritize the primary, secondary, and other endpoints. They should correspond to the hypotheses and must address the objectives.)

- Diagnostic criteria.

    (This element relates the disease, condition, or risk and its stage/ severity under study. Every study should use the current diagnostic methodology available to all the investigators.)

- Measurement reliability.

    (Measurement reliability helps with the interpretation of the study results. The meaningful effect of a treatment needs to be judged against the measurement error.)

- Quality control or quality assurance procedures.

    (Operational procedures for assuring the quality and consistency of the data are important and particularly important to a multicenter trial.)

Conduct Aspects:

- Define timeline for pretreatment evaluation (screening), start of study (baseline), follow-up visits, and end of study.

  (The length of follow-up should consider disease severity, assumptions of intervention effect on disease, and time necessary for treatment to work or reach the specified endpoint. These considerations should be balanced with the chance of subjects' withdrawal if the study is too long and the chance that the concept under study will become outdated.)
- Study parameters, laboratory tests, and patient monitoring.
- Frequency, timing, and types of contact with the patient and provisions for long-term follow-up if pertinent to study questions or aims.

  (Examples include periodic clinic visits, patients' diary entries or interviews with caretakers, and phone calls.)
- Instructions for treatment administration, dose modification, interruption, rescue medication, and discontinuation of study treatment in case of toxicity or intolerability as determined by patient or by the clinician acting in the best interests of patient safety.
- Toxicity monitoring and adverse event reporting.
- Treatment evaluation and criteria.
- Data collection, record keeping, and data processing.

  (For multicenter studies, it is advantageous to have a central laboratory facility for newer tests and methods, to avoid inter-laboratory variation and to standardize normal ranges.)
- Statistical methods.

  (Include proper control of type I error/false-positive rate, adequate power for primary and key secondary endpoints, considerations of subgroups, trial monitoring, interim assessments, and missing data issue.)
- Human subject protection.

  (Approval by an IRB and with ongoing approvals as required.)
- Bibliography.
- Appendix.

  (Includes informed consent form, endpoint evaluation criteria, toxicity criteria, and other procedure references.)

When reviewing a published clinical trial report, in addition to the items listed above, we should pay attention to the following:

- Any exclusions after randomization.
- Comparability of baseline characteristics among treatment or comparator groups.
- Compliance or adherence to the treatment course.

- Appropriate statistical analyses.
- Appropriate data summaries and graphical displays.
- Major findings in efficacy and safety.
- Clear statement of conclusions.
- Complete discussion, including possible limitations of the study and suggestions for future research.
- In the case of "negative" results, an assessment of alternative hypotheses or obstacles (pitfalls) in the conduct of the study.

1.3 Ethics and Safety First

Because clinical trials involve experimentation on human subjects, they prompt ethical and safety concerns. At the beginning of this textbook, students are required to complete an online training program on studies involving human subjects and to obtain a certificate as their first homework exercise; many use the CITI training program. CITI stands for Collaborative Institutional Training Initiative (https://www.citiprogram.org/). This program consists of a series of topics that provide up-to-date regulatory requirements for the protection of human subjects in research (Homework 1.2). These regulatory requirements are the natural outgrowth of historical clinical studies that are today considered unethical, inappropriate, or abusive in their disregard of basic human rights and justice. Consider the problems posed by the blood "transfusion" by mouth to Pope Innocent VIII in the fifteenth century or, in modern times, the human experimentation on prisoners (and racial "undesirables") by the Nazis, the Tuskegee experiments on the natural behavior of syphilis (in minorities), and the Willowbrook experiments on the transmission of hepatitis in children with intellectual disabilities. As an exercise, pose the rationale for these studies and state why they were inappropriate. These and other such experiments led to several documents to define conduct in clinical studies. In the following sections, we briefly review the important points of some of the historical documents that led into the current regulations for conducting clinical trials.

1.3.1 Nuremberg Code (1947) and Helsinki Declaration (1964)

The Nuremberg Code was established after World War II. Later, the World Medical Association (WMA) published the Helsinki Declaration, which is currently being followed and updated by the WMA. These documents together specify the following ethical principles and guidelines for clinical trials:

- Competent and voluntary consent must be obtained from all participants.
- There should be no reasonable alternative to conducting the experiment (to show the effect of the intervention).
- Study should have a basis in biological knowledge and animal studies.
- Unnecessary suffering and injury must be avoided.
- Participants should have no expectation for death or disability (as a result of participation in the study).
- Any risk should be consistent with the humanitarian importance of the study.
- Study must be conducted by qualified individuals.
- Participants can withdraw, at will, at any time.
- Investigator is under obligation to terminate the experiment if injury seems likely.

1.3.2 Belmont Report (1976)

The Belmont Report provides a more modern perspective to the ethical principles and guidelines.

Respect for Persons

As an application of the principle of respect for persons, IRBs composed of representatives from the fields of science, statistics, ethics, and law, as well as a lay person, are formed to provide ethical oversight of clinical studies at the site of individual investigators. An IRB must approve each protocol before any study can be conducted in that institution. All participants' privacy should be respected and protected.

Beneficence

As an application of the principle of beneficence, the researcher should maximize benefits and minimize risks for trial participants and should make participants cognizant of the potential risks and benefits.

Justice

As an application of the principle of justice, participants should be selected equitably, without exploitation of vulnerable populations. Direct or indirect coercion should be avoided.

1.3.3 Informed Consent

The US FDA has issued a draft guidance titled *Informed Consent Information Sheet*.[1] This guidance describes the basic and additional elements of informed

---

[1] US Department of Health and Human Services, Food and Drug Administration, OGCP, CDER, CBER, CDRH (2014). "Informed Consent Information Sheet: Guidance for IRBs, Clinical Investigators, and Sponsors" available from http://www.fda.gov/RegulatoryInformation/Guidances/ucm404975.htm (accessed on July 21, 2014).

consent and includes topics such as review of patient records, children as subjects, and subject participation in more than one study.

A list of mandatory topics to be included in an informed consent form is given in Appendix 1.1.

1.3.4 Discussion

"Subject," "participant," "patient," and "volunteer" are common nomenclatures that are often used interchangeably in clinical trials to refer to an individual enrolled in the study. It is interesting to read the ethical principles in the Belmont Report, in which the participants of clinical trials are considered volunteers, and participation in clinical trials is considered a human right that needs to be equitably offered to all eligible persons. First, it is important to recognize that any medical practice based on unproven treatments is likely not ethical. A clinical trial is ethical when there is adequate collective doubt about the value of the new therapy (Fredrickson 1968) or a suggestion that another treatment or approach may be superior. Therefore, a clinical trial is a necessary step as an investigation for advancing medical practice in both efficacy and safety. In some parts of the world, newspapers occasionally have shocking headlines such as "Drug Testing on Our School Children," "Deaths and Injuries in Drug Trial," and "Patients Treated with Sugar Pills." Without understanding the details, readers often gain a misleading picture of clinical trials from these eye-catching titles. Those who study the doctrines of appropriate clinical trial design and conduct will hopefully be inspired to educate others, whenever there is an opportunity to do so, about the correct concept and method of clinical trials. Secondly, as citizens of the society and also consumers of medical products, the public needs to understand the FDA, EMA, and other regulatory agencies' responsibility to approve medicines and devices to protect the public health.

Ethical considerations also have a strong impact on such aspects of study design as randomization, blinding, placebo control, sequential design for monitoring safety and efficacy, and early stopping procedures. Subjects' right to withdraw and investigators' obligation to remove any endangered subject from participation in a trial have also led to the ubiquitous problem of missing data in clinical trials. Chapter 15 is devoted to dealing with the issue of missing data.

In summary, all fundamental issues in clinical trials can be viewed as arising from the need to balance rigorous scientific experimentation with ethical medical practice. For a good scientific experiment, we expect the clinical trial to provide valid and efficient answers to the hypothesis being tested. On the other hand, we also require that the clinical trial be designed and conducted realistically to follow good medical practice. The feasibility of conducting a clinical trial is the key to its success. Statistics provides scientific validity and efficiency, whereas laws, rules, regulations, and oversight uphold ethics.

1.4 Classifications of Clinical Trials

In the study and discussion of clinical trials, we often come across different descriptions for trials in the literature. Because different types of trials may lead to different issues and require different methods for analysis, it is useful to make classifications as follows.

1.4.1 By Medical Intervention

For example:

- Drug
- Biologic (e.g., vaccine)
- Surgical, radiological procedures
- Medical device
- Screening approaches and technologies
- Behavior modification to achieve health goals
- Biomarker assessments.

Note that the US FDA's different branches (CDER, CBER, CDRH) are set up to review these interventions.[2]

1.4.2 By Disease or Therapeutic Area

For example:

- Oncology
- Cardiovascular—heart, lung, blood
- Infectious diseases (e.g., HIV/AIDS)
- Neurological, psychological disorders
- Endocrine diseases (e.g., diabetes, osteoporosis)
- Renal and metabolic disorders
- Mental health disorders.

Note that each of these areas corresponds to an area of research at one of the institutes at the NIH.

---

[2] CDER—Center for Drug Evaluation and Research; CBER—Center for Biologics Evaluation and Research; CDRH—Center for Devices and Radiological Health.

1.4.3 By the Phase of Drug Development as the Stage of the Experiment

Most of the clinical trials on drugs are classified according to whether they take place before (Phases 0^3, I, II, and III) or after (Phases IV and V) an NDA or MAA is filed. The trial phases are sequentially numbered from early to late phases in the development of therapeutic agents. In many ways, the earlier the trial phase, the closer the design approaches an ideal experiment in that experimental conditions, such as objectives, participants, and doses, are more restrictive and well controlled. The study duration is relatively shorter, and the goals of the study can be accomplished with a smaller sample (enrolled subject) size. Objective measurements are often the endpoints, and safety is the driving concern. By contrast, the later phase studies often recruit a study population closer to a generalized target population reflecting medical practice with realistic complications, resulting in less restriction on the study design. The sample size is relatively larger, and the study duration is usually much longer. Subjective clinical endpoints are often preferred. For example, survival duration is a well-defined and measurable endpoint used in many later phase studies (and considered the "gold standard"). The early phases, as weighing more on scientific experiments, tend to be exploratory in nature and often confirm biological principles. The later phases are confirmatory for defined endpoints of clinical benefit for regulatory approval of the efficacy and still, to a certain extent, an expansion of the safety profile of the drug under investigation. Phase III trials are usually considered a high level of evidence and thus are often pivotal to regulatory approval to market the medical product. A recent development, further discussed later, is the accelerated approval process from earlier phase studies when clinical efficacy is seen in an area with a paucity of treatments (unmet medical need), but these approvals often come with a commitment to complete an appropriate later (Phase III) trial. Pharmaceutical and biotech companies usually prepare a comprehensive medical study plan that includes all trials to be conducted in their drug development process with target timelines. This scheme may not be appropriate for trials conducted in an academic setting.

It should be noted that the scheme for oncology trials is very different from that above. Because cancer is a devastating disease, patients participated in Phase I oncology trials are usually those who have received previous treatments and exhausted potentially effective options. An exception would be for an individual with a cancer for which there is no known effective therapy. The main aims of such trials are to define the optimal dose for further testing, defining safety and toxicity, and exploration of the pharmacokinetics (what the body does to the drug) and pharmacodynamics (what the drug does to the body). With recent advances in biomarker research as exemplified in genomic research, cancer therapies for specific targets have become popular

---

[3] For definition of Phase 0 trial, see Coloma PM (2013) and CDER (2006).

Scheme of Phases of Clinical Trials in Drug Development Process (Non-Oncology)

Ideal Experiment (With Restrictive Conditions)		Real-Life Practice (With Complications)	
Phase I	Phase II	Phase III	Phase IV
Subjects Condition:			
Healthy	Mild disease	Moderate to severe disease	All stages
Main Goals:			
Dose finding; Safety response	Early efficacy and safety	Confirmatory efficacy and limited safety	Long-term follow-up safety and efficacy
Bioavailability (absorption, distribution, metabolism, and elimination); Clinical pharmacology			
Major Design:			
Crossover design		Parallel-group design	
Sample Size Range:			
$n = 20–40$		n in the hundreds per group	

in clinical trials. These trials involve screening and diagnosis of particular groups of cancer patients carrying specific gene mutations. Phase I trials that match a target gene mutation with the targeting agent for that mutation have shown considerable promise, as illustrated by Tsimberidou et al. (2012). Phase II cancer trials, designed to better calibrate clinical benefit, are often completed in a shorter timeframe and include a smaller sample size compared to Phase III studies. Usually, cancer *objective response rate* (ORR) is used as the primary endpoint and *progression-free survival* (PFS) as the secondary endpoint. Phase III cancer trials often use PFS or ideally, the *overall survival* (OS), that is, counting deaths from all causes as events, as the primary endpoint. However, as noted above, other less objectively measured endpoints have entered into this arena of trials.

Considering the rising cost of drug development in terms of economical parameters and human suffering from disease, many investigators, trial sponsors, and regulatory agencies are pursuing strategies for shortening the development process. For example, modifying study design to seamlessly combine some of the trial phases might eliminate the time needed for recruiting new centers and initiating another round of grant reviews, contracts, and IRB approvals. Whether this approach actually saves any of the time or cost of drug development remains to be seen, but related statistical issues in these trials, especially in controlling the overall type I error rate, have already been and are currently being investigated by many researchers. We will discuss the seamless Phase II/III trial design and analysis in more detail in a later chapter.

For the regulatory authority to expedite the NDA review process, two important documents are the 1997 FDA Modernization Act, Section 112, entitled *Expediting Study and Approval of Fast Track Drugs* ("the Act") and the FDA's *Guidance for Industry: Fast Track Drug Development Programs* (FTDDP), FDA (2014). The purpose of the FTDDP is to facilitate the development and expedite the review of new drugs that are intended to treat serious or life-threatening conditions and that demonstrate the potential to address unmet medical needs. The Act states that an application for approval of a fast-track product may be approved if it is determined that "the product has an effect on a clinical endpoint or on a surrogate endpoint that is reasonably likely to predict clinical benefit." However, the Act also puts limitations on accelerated approval: The sponsor must conduct appropriate post-approval (Phase III or IV) studies to validate the surrogate endpoint or otherwise confirm the effect on the clinical endpoint. The FDA may also withdraw the approval of a fast-track product using expedited procedures if, among other concerns such as safety issues, the sponsor fails to conduct the required study or if a post-approval study of the fast-track product fails to verify the clinical benefit of the product. For example, IRESSA™ (gefitinib tablets 250 mg) was approved under the accelerated approval regulation as monotherapy for the treatment of patients with locally advanced or metastatic non-small cell lung cancer (NSCLC) after the failure of both platinum-based and docetaxel chemotherapies in May 2003. The effectiveness of IRESSA was initially based on ORR. Subsequent studies intended to demonstrate an increase in survival have been unsuccessful. IRESSA's claim for NSCLC treatment was removed in June 2005 (Drugs@FDA, 2005).

Another example is Makena. In 2011, the FDA approved Makena for the prevention of recurrent preterm birth in women with a singleton pregnancy and a previous spontaneous singleton preterm birth. This approval was based on findings from a trial that showed that hydroxyprogesterone caproate, Makena's active ingredient, reduced the risk of recurrent preterm birth. However, that trial did not show significant difference between Makena and placebo in the composite endpoint for neonatal outcomes. Although 3 of 15 evaluated measures of neonatal complications showed statistically significant improvements with Makena, none of the analyses adjusted for multiple statistical testing, a shortcoming that increases the probability of false-positive findings, and they may not reflect true treatment effects. Nevertheless, for a serious condition without approved treatments, FDA granted accelerated approval based on the drug's effect on a surrogate endpoint that was reasonably likely to predict clinical benefit, but requested a post-approval study to confirm clinical benefit. Later, the required post-approval confirmatory trial did not demonstrate an effect of Makena on the surrogate endpoint of preterm birth, contradicting the findings from the previous trial, nor did it show an effect on neonatal outcomes. In October 2019, concurring with an advisory committee's recommendation, and on the basis of the totality of evidence, CDER concluded that withdrawal of Makena is warranted (Chang et al. 2020).

The third example is KEYTRUDA™ (pembrolizumab) on the metastatic small cell lung cancer (SCLC) indication. The accelerated approval for KEYTRUDA on this indication was granted in June 2019 based on tumor response rate and durability of response data from KEYNOTE-158 (cohort G) and KEYNOTE-028 (cohort C1). Continued approval for this indication was contingent upon completion of the post-marketing requirement establishing superiority of KEYTRUDA as determined by overall survival (OS). As announced in January 2020, KEYNOTE-604, the confirmatory Phase III trial for this indication, met one of its dual primary endpoints of progression-free survival, but did not reach statistical significance for the other primary endpoint of OS. After consultation with the FDA, Merck announced withdrawal from the US indication for KEYTRUDA on March 1, 2021. The announcement stated that Merck's consultation with the FDA on this withdrawal is part of an industry-wide evaluation of indications based on accelerated approvals that have not yet met their post-marketing requirements..

Thus, accelerated approval is only conditional approval for a drug. Nevertheless, the prospect of early availability on the market of a drug has broad implications for patients as well as for the drug manufacturer. A recent study (Moore and Furberg 2013) reported that eight drugs approved in 2008 under FTDDP took a median of 5.1 years of clinical development time to gain approval, compared with 7.5 years for 12 drugs under standard review. A striking example of this accelerated approval is seen in the drug Xalkori® (crizotinib capsules), where conditional, accelerated approval was granted in August 2011 based on durable ORR in two single-arm open-label studies (NCI, 2013). In November 2013, the FDA granted regular approval for crizotinib for the treatment of patients with metastatic NSCLC based on an open-label active-controlled multinational randomized trial (with 347 patients enrolled). In this trial, crizotinib demonstrated superior PFS and ORR in patients with anaplastic lymphoma kinase (ALK)-positive NSCLC whose disease progressed after platinum-based doublet chemotherapy. Accelerated approval has also stimulated the pharmaceutical industry to explore other approaches to improve trial efficiency. However, because fewer patients are studied as part of the expedited drug approval process, such drugs may reach the market with significant safety questions unanswered. The statistical issues surrounding two kinds of type I errors, namely, the "conditional approval" and "final approval" type I errors, are discussed in the study by Shih et al. (2003).

In addition to the major phases in the above scheme, there are Phase 0 and V clinical trials. Phase 0 trials are exploratory IND studies that involve very limited human exposure and usually have no therapeutic or diagnostic intent. Phase 0 trials bridge the gap between traditional preclinical testing and clinical studies; these trials are intended to provide a better understanding of a new compound's pharmacokinetics (PKs), pharmacodynamics (PDs), organ penetration, and effect on the putative target of the intervention before the initiation of Phase I trials. These Phase 0 trials often compare preoperative biopsies with surgically excised tissue following short exposure to the agent in question and thus pose unique statistical and ethical questions. Phase V trials are studies conducted following NDA/BLA approval in order to seek additional marketing claims for new indications, sometimes with new formulations or combinations with other approved compounds. Because the compound was already approved for another indication earlier, some previous safety, PK, PD, and dose-ranging information might be used and may not need to be repeated for the new claim application.

1.4.4 By Disease Present (Remedial/Therapeutic Trials) or Absent (Prevention Trials)

Prevention trials can further be classified into *primary* or *secondary prevention*. Primary prevention seeks to intervene in the processes that induce the disease either by lifestyle modifications (changing destructive habits) or by therapeutic agents of very low toxicity intended to disrupt the carcinogenic process. For example, vaccine trials are often primary prevention as are smoking cessation trials, which typify a lifestyle behavior modification approach. Secondary prevention trials often appear as early diagnosis trials (such as screening studies) or as intervention trials since the objective is to prevent recurrence or postpone further progression of the disease. For example, the National Lung Screening Trial (NLST) was a secondary prevention trial that compared chest X-rays (previously shown as not especially helpful) with low-dose CT scans, the latter of which reduced lung cancer-specific mortality by nearly 20% in an at-risk population by finding disease at an earlier stage (National Lung Screening Trial Research Team 2011). The landmark Scandinavian Simvastatin Survival Study (also known as the 4S study) was a secondary prevention study that was designed to evaluate the effect of a cholesterol-lowering drug called simvastatin on mortality and morbidity in patients with coronary heart disease.

In general, all prevention trials are held to much higher safety standards by the IRB and other regulatory agencies because participants are either healthy or have lower disease severity. In addition, prevention trials often require longer study time and larger sample sizes, especially when the incidence rate of the primary clinical endpoint is low for relatively healthier participants.

The possibility of using surrogate endpoints (e.g., antibody counts in vaccine trials) is an important design consideration, and the identification of appropriate biomarkers is a strong necessity.

Further reading regarding the design of prevention trials can be found in Shih and Wang (1991) (Homework 1.3).

1.4.5 By Design Feature

- Single site or multicenter
- Placebo, concurrent active control, or historical control
- Crossover or parallel groups
- Fixed dose or titrated dose
- Fixed sample size or group sequential design
- Open label or blind (single-, double-, or triple-blind)
- Number of arms
- Geographical extent (local, regional, or global).

1.4.6 By Hypothesis and Statistical Inference

- Exploratory (hypothesis-generating) trial
- Superiority trial
- Proof of comparability (equivalence or noninferiority trial).

1.5 Multidisciplinary Teamwork in Clinical Trials

To conclude this chapter, we emphasize that clinical trials, as an enterprise, require organization and teamwork. All members of the team must recognize the specialties of the team members and their contributions to the study to facilitate collaboration and thus a successful trial. Functional personnel in a clinical trial team may consist of the following:

- Scientists, including biochemists, biologists, toxicologists, pharmacologists, and biomarker specialists
- Medical monitor and project coordinator
- Clinical investigators and pharmacists at hospitals and medical centers
- Specialists in data management, quality assurance, and computer technology
- Statistician and epidemiologist
- Regulatory affairs staff
- Chemical engineer and drug-supply manager

- Marketing personnel
- Bioethicist, patient advocate, and voluntary participants.

Appendix 1.1: Elements of Informed Consent

The informed consent discussion, written informed consent form, and any other written information to be provided to participants of a trial should include explanations of the following mandatory topics:

1. That the study involves research.
2. The purpose of the study and approximate number of subjects involved in the study.
3. The expected duration of the subject's participation in the study.
4. The study treatment(s) and the probability for random assignment to each treatment.
5. The study procedures to be followed, including all invasive procedures.
6. Those aspects of the study that are experimental.
7. The reasonably foreseeable risks or inconveniences to the subject and, when applicable, to an embryo, fetus, or nursing infant.
8. The reasonably expected benefits. When there is no intended clinical benefit to the subject, the subject should be made aware of this.
9. The alternative procedure(s) or course(s) of treatment that may be available to the subject and their important potential benefits and risks.
10. That the records identifying the subject will be kept confidential and, to the extent permitted by the applicable laws and/or regulations, will not be made publicly available. If the results of the study are published, the subject's identity will remain confidential.
11. That the study sponsor, monitor, and/or their representative, the IRB/IEC,[4] and the regulatory authority(ies) will be granted direct access to the subject's original medical records for the verification of clinical study procedures and/or data, without violating the confidentiality of the subject, to the extent permitted by the applicable laws and regulations, and that, by signing and dating a written informed consent form, the subject or the subject's legally acceptable representative is authorizing such access.
12. The subject's responsibilities.

---

[4] Institutional ethics committee.

13. The compensation and/or treatment available to the subject in the event of study-related injury.

14. The anticipated prorated payment, if any, to the subject for participating in the study.

15. The person(s) to contact for further information regarding the study and the rights of study subjects and whom to contact in the event of study-related injury.

16. That the subject's participation in the trial is voluntary and that the subject may refuse to participate or withdraw from the study, at any time, without penalty or loss of benefits to which the subject is otherwise entitled.

17. The foreseeable circumstances and/or reasons under which the subject's participation in the study may be terminated.

18. The anticipated expenses, if any, that subject will incur as a result of participation in the study.

19. The consequences of a subject's decision to withdraw from the research and procedures for orderly termination of participation by the subject.

20. That the subject or the subject's legally acceptable representative will be informed in a timely manner if information becomes available that may be relevant to the subject's willingness to continue participation in the study.

21. Any element(s) required by local regulations (e.g., FDA, other non-US health authorities).

The following additional topics are mandatory for inclusion in the informed consent of studies enrolling women of childbearing potential (WOCBP):

1. General Statement

   The subject must not be pregnant and should not become pregnant during exposure to the investigational product unless that is the endpoint of the study. Subjects should be instructed to contact the investigator if they plan to change their contraception method or if they need to take any prescription drug or other medication not prescribed by investigator. Sexually active subjects must use an effective method of contraception during the course of the study, in a manner such that risk of failure is minimized. The informed consent must indicate that information on pregnancy prevention for WOCBP has been reviewed with the subject by the investigator or study designee.

2. Laboratory and Animal Reproductive Toxicology

   The consent should include a statement addressing what is known about the investigational product from laboratory and animal reproductive toxicity studies concerning possible mutagenic and/or teratogenic effects. The consent should indicate that this information has limited predictive value for humans.

3. Unforeseeable Risks

The consent must indicate that exposure to the investigational product may involve currently unforeseeable risks to the subject (or embryo or fetus, if the subject is or may become pregnant).

4. Occurrence of Pregnancy or Suspected Pregnancy

The informed consent must include study contact name(s) and telephone number(s) for the subject to call if she becomes pregnant or suspects pregnancy, has missed her period or it is late, or if she has a change in her usual menstrual cycle (e.g., heavier bleeding during her period or bleeding between periods).

5. Discontinuation from the Study

Any subject who becomes pregnant during the course of the study will be immediately withdrawn (unless allowed or stated differently in the protocol) and referred for obstetrical care. All financial aspects of obstetrical, child, or related care are the responsibility of the subject.

6. Pregnancy Follow-Up

If a subject becomes pregnant, the investigator will seek access to the subject's and/or infant's clinic/hospital records through the pregnancy, and for a minimum of 8 weeks following delivery.

7. Use of a Study-Prohibited Contraceptive Method

When applicable, the informed consent should clearly indicate if a contraceptive method is prohibited (e.g., when hormonal contraceptive interaction with the investigational product(s) is known or suspected). In this situation, a study participant should be instructed to notify the investigator or study designee if a prohibited contraceptive method is initiated during the course of the study so that additional precautions can be taken, or the subject discontinued from the study.

8. Noninvestigational Product Interactions with Hormonal Contraceptives

Women using a hormonal method of contraceptive (e.g., oral contraceptives or implantable or injectable agents) must be instructed to notify the investigator or study designee of the need to take any prescription drug or other medication not prescribed by the investigator. The purpose of this statement is to identify any potential noninvestigational product interaction with the contraceptive that might reduce the effectiveness of the contraceptive method.

Sources: Protocol under US IND number and/or non-IND: 40710 (Feb-05–1999). A multi-center, double-blind, placebo-controlled, randomized fixed-dose study of nefazodone ER in the treatment of depressed patients.

HOMEWORK 1.1

The following are excerpts from three LOIs produced by a university cancer center in a training course. Suppose that you are a reviewer and have been asked to provide critiques and constructive suggestions to the researchers. Based on your learning of the course so far, comment on each of them regarding the following aspects: (a) Is the proposed study a clinical trial? Why or why not? (b) Are the study objective(s) clearly stated? (c) Does the design (including the endpoints and statistical consideration) match the objective? If not, provide suggestion(s).

LOI-1

Use of the Memorial Symptom Assessment Scale in Patients with Cervical Cancer

Objective
To determine the intensity of symptoms and the distress those symptoms cause in patients with cervical cancer.

The Rationale for Performing the Trial
There is currently a lack of literature regarding the use of the Memorial Symptom Assessment Scale in cervical cancer. Determining the symptoms experienced by women who have cervical cancer will be helpful in the further elucidation of interventions to alleviate these symptoms. Further study would also assist in determining the impact of these symptoms on patients' quality of life and their ability to function as women.

Design Would Be Used to Accomplish the Main Objectives of the Trial
Use of questionnaires and description of independent variables with correlation statistics to determine significance.

LOI-2

Study of Safety and Effectiveness of the Use of Gemcitabine and Irinotecan in Women with Refractory Ovarian Cancer

Objectives
   1. The primary objective is to determine toxicity and response to combination therapy with irinotecan and gemcitabine in refractory ovarian cancer.

2. Secondary objectives are to estimate the time to progression and median survival time.

3. An exploratory objective is to assess whether there is a correlation between response and P-gp and CD44 expression in the original tumor and/or recurrent tumor.

Rationale

Irinotecan and gemcitabine are well-tolerated single agents, each with ovarian cancer antitumor activity. Combining the two agents is appealing because each has a potentially distinct mechanism of action. Irinotecan inhibits topoisomerase I, and gemcitabine inhibits DNA polymerases by competing with dCTP for the enzymes. Gemcitabine also serves as a substrate for polymerases by competing with dCTP for the enzymes and as a substrate for polymerase ε and polymerase α by further inhibiting DNA synthesis. Furthermore, irinotecan stabilizes DNA strands that offer sites for the insertion of gemcitabine triphosphate during relegation of DNA. Preclinical data suggest dose-dependent synergistic interactions for the two drugs in lung small cell cancer, breast cancer, and HL-60 leukemia cell lines. Maximum tolerated dose for the gemcitabine/irinotecan combination was determined in a Phase I study. This study was followed by a Phase II trial testing this combination in pancreatic cancer and showed some efficacy. Although combination regimens using gemcitabine have been explored in the treatment of ovarian cancer, the gemcitabine/irinotecan combination has never been tested.

In ovarian cancer, second-line regimens usually involve single-drug therapy. These regimens have only limited response (17%–30%) of short duration (median response 4 months). Better regimens using drug combination are needed.

Our laboratory has data that suggest a possible correlation between ovarian cancer expression of CD44 and drug resistance. We also have preliminary data correlating CD44 expression and P-gp expression in resistant ovarian cancer cells. There are also published data correlating CD44 expression in breast cancer with P-gp expression. Dr. Smith's laboratory published observations indicating that leukemic cells with high P-gp protein content become more metastatic in vivo when treated with P-gp substrate drugs. These observations suggest that P-gp and CD44 may interact and convey an invasive chemo-resistant phenotype to cancer cells. We are interested in determining the level of expression of these two membrane proteins in recurrent ovarian tumors and correlating these findings with treatment outcome.

If this drug regimen improves 6-month survival, we will then compare this regimen with standard therapy in a Phase III trial.

Study Design
This is a Phase II study of combination therapy with gemcitabine 1000 mg/m² (Days 1 and 8) and irinotecan 100 mg/m² (Days 1 and 8) every three weeks. Patients diagnosed with recurrent ovarian carcinoma resistant to platinum and good performance status will be eligible. Patients who have received two prior chemotherapy regimens will be eligible. The primary endpoint will be 6-month survival. Secondary endpoints are to estimate time to progression and determine whether there is a correlation between clinical response and tumor CD44 and P-gp levels.

LOI-3

Ovarian Preservation in Women Undergoing Cancer Therapy

Background
Although cancer therapy has led to marked improvements in disease-free intervals and OS in patients with malignancies, quality-of-life issues have become a major concern for patients and the physicians caring for them. Many of our therapies lead to ovarian failure in our younger patients due to either high-dose chemotherapy or radiation therapy, leading to the development of menopausal symptoms and loss of fertility. Reproductive endocrinologic techniques are improving, and we can now consider offering our patients ovarian transplantation in a research setting as an alternative to ovarian failure, thus providing the possibility of reestablishing reproductive potential in the future and hopefully leading to an improvement in patients' quality of life.

As in vitro fertilization (IVF) techniques have improved, embryo cryopreservation has become a safe and accepted method of storing the fertilized gamete. The development of technology to cryopreserve unfertilized female gametes has been less successful. There have only been a few pregnancies that have resulted from frozen gametes; this low fertilization rate is a result of hardening of the zona pellucida, an increased incidence of aneuploidy, and damage to the cytoskeleton, leading to significant changes in the organization and trafficking of molecules and organelles. Ovarian cryopreservation has therefore been considered a viable alternative to the cryopreservation of oocytes. Cryopreservation of primordial follicles found in ovarian tissue has met with greater success, because these follicles are less differentiated, possess fewer organelles, and lack a zona pellucida.

Primordial follicles have successfully been harvested from mice, cryopreserved, and transplanted back into oophorectomized animals. Estrogenic activity and live-born young have been reported after continuous culture of mouse follicles from the primordial stage (1, 2)[5].

---

[5] Four citations and a treatment schema in the original LOI are omitted here.

Oktay reported on two patients who underwent ovarian transplantation prior to undergoing surgery or radiation therapy for benign ovarian cysts and Stage IIIB squamous cell carcinoma of the cervix, respectively (3)[5]. In both patients, menopause was confirmed after transplantation by measuring serum follicle-stimulating hormone. In both patients, restoration of estradiol levels confirmed that the ovaries were functioning, and the patient who underwent surgery for benign ovarian cysts resumed spontaneous ovarian function after transplantation was performed (4)[5]. Three of the four patients had evidence of resumption of ovarian function, although short-lived. The women involved in the study were 46–49 years old, which most likely impacted the reported outcomes. These two case reports provide evidence that this is a viable treatment option we can begin to offer our patients in a research setting.

Trial Design
This will be a prospective trial consisting of several tiers. Eligibility criteria will include the following:

1. Age of diagnosis (less than 40)
2. Menstrual status (premenopausal) based on markers including follicle-stimulating hormone (FSH), estradiol, and inhibin, as well as a transvaginal ultrasound
3. Desire to preserve ovarian function for fertility reasons or to prevent the development of menopause
4. Treatment regimen consisting of chemotherapy, radiation therapy, or a combination that will most likely render the patient sterile at the completion of their treatment.

When a patient is identified, she will be approached to determine if she is interested in ovarian transplantation. If she declines, she will be asked to participate in our quality-of-life questionnaire to determine if there is an improvement in the quality of life of the patients receiving ovarian transplantation versus the patients who do not.

Patients who agree to participate will then enter the treatment portion of the trial, which will consist of trying to prevent ovarian failure through the use of GnRH agonists or antagonists prior to chemotherapy or radiation therapy. Women whose normal ovarian function is maintained will enter the quality-of-life component of the study and be followed regarding future pregnancy outcomes and the development of menopause. Women who unfortunately develop ovarian failure will undergo transplantation of ovarian tissue. These patients will be followed for resumption of menstrual function and pregnancy outcomes. A treatment schema is attached.

Objectives

1. Successful transplantation of ovarian tissue with resumption of ovarian function, reversal of menopausal symptoms, and restoration of reproductive function

2. To determine whether GnRH agonists or GnRH antagonists are better at preserving ovarian function in women receiving chemotherapy or radiation therapy

3. To determine if the quality of life of patients participating in the clinical trial is improved compared to that of patients who decline to participate

4. To determine prognostic factors of ovarian recovery in women receiving chemotherapy (both epidemiologic and molecular markers).

HOMEWORK 1.2

Log in to https://www.citiprogram.org/ and complete the in-depth training on the protection of human subjects in research. Obtain a certificate of completion for the CITI program.

HOMEWORK 1.3

Reading: "Overview of Some Important Issues in Designing Clinical Trials for Prevention of Chronic Diseases" (Shih, W. J., and Wang, C., *Pharmaceutical Medicine* 1991, 5: 87–96).

References

Baumgardner KR. (1997). A review of key research design and statistical analysis issues. *Journal of Oral Surgery, Oral Medicine, Oral Pathology, Oral Radiology, and Endodontics* 84: 550–556.

Burns PB, Rohrich RJ, and Chung KC. (2011). The levels of evidence and their role in evidence-based medicine. *Plastic and Reconstructive Surgery* 128: 305–310.

CDER (Center for Drug Evaluation and Research). Guidance for Industry, Investigators, and Reviewers: Exploratory IND Studies (2006). http://www.fda.gov/downloads/Drugs/GuidanceComplianceRegulatoryInfomration/Guidance//ucm078933.pdf (accessed April 5, 2014).

Chang CY, Nguyen CP, Wesley B, Guo J, Johnson LL, Joffe HV. (2020). Withdrawing approval of Makena — A proposal from the FDA Center for Drug Evaluation and Research. *New England Journal of Medicine* 2020; 383: e131. doi: 10.1056/NEJMp2031055.

Coloma PM. (2013). Phase 0 clinical trials: Theoretical and practical implications in oncologic drug development. *Open Access Journal of Clinical Trials* 5: 119–126.

Cramer DW. (1974). The role of cervical cytology in the declining morbidity and mortality of cervical cancer. *Cancer* 34: 2018–2027.

Ederer F. (1979). The statistician's role in developing a protocol for a clinical trial. *The American Statistician* 33:116–119.

FDA (US Food and Drug Administration). (2004). Challenge and Opportunity on the Critical Path to New Medical Products, http://www.fda.gov/downloads/ScienceResearch/SpecialTopics/ClinicalPathInitiative/CriticalPathOpportunitiesReports/ucml13411.pdf (accessed April 5, 2014).

FDA (US Food and Drug Administration). Speeding Access to Important New Therapies: Fast Track, Accelerated Approval and Priority Review, www.fda.gov/forconsumers/byaudience/forpatientadvocates/speedingaccesstoimportantnewtherapies/ucml28291.htm (accessed April 5, 2014).

FDA. Code for Federal Regulations, Title 21, Part 50. Protection of Human Subjects. http://www.accessdata.fda.gov/scripts/cdrh/cfdocs/cfcfr/CFRsearch.cfm?CFRPart=50 (accessed April 5, 2014).

Fredrickson DS. (1968). The field trial: Some thoughts on the independent ordeal. *Bulletin of the New York Academy of Medicine* 44: 985–993.

Friedman LM, Furberg CD, and DeMets DL. (1996). *Fundamentals of Clinical Trials.* New York: Springer.

Hill AB. (1937). General summary and conclusions. *Lancet* I: 883–885.

ICMJE (International Committee of Medical Journal Editors). http://icmje.org/recommendations/browse/publishing-and-editorial-issues/clinical-trial-registration.html. (Accessed February 12, 2021).

Melnyk BM and Fineout-Overholt E. (2010). *Evidence-Based Practice in Nursing and Healthcare: A Guide to Best Practice.* Lippincott, Philadelphia, Williams & Wilkins.

Merck (2021). https://s2.q4cdn.com/584635680/files/doc_news/Merck-Provides-Update-on-KEYTRUDA-pembrolizumab-Indication-in-Metastatic-Small-Cell-Lung-Cancer-in-the-US-2021.pdf (accessed on 3/1/2021).

Michael CW. (1999). The Papanicolaou smear and the obstetric patient: A simple test with great benefits. *Diagnostic Cytopathology* 21(1): 1–3.

Moore TJ and Furberg CD. (2013). Development times, clinical testing, postmarket follow-up, and safety risks for the new drugs approved by the US Food and Drug Administration: The class of 2008. *JAMA Internal Medicine* 174: 90–95. doi:10.1001/jamainternmed.2013.11813.

National Cancer Institute. (2013). Cancer Drug Information: FDA Approval for Crizotinib. http://www.cancer.gov/cancertopics/druginfo/fda-crizotinib (accessed April 5, 2014).

National Lung Screening Trial Research Team. (2011). The National Lung Screening Trial: Overview and study design. *Radiology* 258 (1): 243–253. doi:10.1148/radiol.10091808.

Shih WJ and Wang C. (1991). Overview of some important issues in designing clinical trials for prevention of chronic diseases. *Pharmaceutical Medicine* 5: 87–96.

Shih WJ, Ouyang P, Quan H, Lin Y, Michiels B, and Bijnens L. (2003). Controlling type I error rate for fast-track drug development programs. *Statistics in Medicine* 22: 665–675.

Tsimberidou AM, Iskander NG, Hong DS, Wheler JJ, Falchook GS, and Fu S. (2012). Personalized medicine in a phase I clinical trials program: the MD Anderson Cancer Center initiative. *Clinical Cancer Research* 18 (22): 6373–6383.

2

Concepts and Methods of Statistical Designs

As we mentioned in Chapter 1, most fundamental design issues in clinical trials arise from the need to strike a balance between scientific experiment and good clinical practice in a trial. Whereas laws and regulations guard the ethical aspects of trial design, statistics addresses scientific validity and efficiency, which, in turn, enhance the medical ethics and practice. Although many design issues surface in the development of a clinical trial, in this chapter we focus on the major concerns for trial validity, and we discuss the concerns for trial efficiency in Chapter 3. First, we consider the various types of validity: external validity, internal validity, and repeatability. We then explore the phenomenon of regression toward the mean to illustrate a kind of bias, which can be accounted for when there is a concurrent control group in the design. Logically, we need to consider at least two observations per subject in a clinical trial, one as the baseline and the other as a follow-up measurement. In this two-dimensional setting, we review the notion of bivariate normal distribution and the expression of simple linear regression as we discuss the topic of regression toward the mean. Finally, we conclude this chapter by discussing several methods of randomization and blinding that are commonly used in clinical trials to make the control group fully functional for achieving internal validity.

2.1 External Validity

External validity is the validity of inferences as they pertain to the generalizability to future subjects rather than the specific trial participants (Rothwell, 2005). It implies the applicability of the study results to general medical practice. Richard Horton (2000), past editor of *The Lancet*, once commented that "the issues of external validity are the most important that face clinical research today and that the failure to resolve them is largely responsible for the indifference doctors world-wide show toward research evidence." Many agree that this is what *evidence-based medicine* represents: getting research evidence into practice (Evidence-Based Medicine Working Group, 1992). Within the framework of a clinical trial protocol, the characteristics of patients, treatment and procedures, outcome measures, and follow-up in the trial protocol together define the generalizability and applicability of the trial results. For any New Drug Application (NDA), these data are the basis for the information contained in the drug package insert and will greatly influence the "labeled" indications for use and thus the marketing implications for the drug manufacturer. Manufacturers would like to make the product available to the widest possible population; hence, they would prefer the eligibility criteria (defined by the "inclusion/exclusion criteria" section of the trial protocol) to be as loose as possible. By contrast, clinical scientists would like to control the heterogeneity of trial participants to isolate the signal from the noise; thus, they would prefer a set of more focused inclusion and exclusion criteria. Because the trial has a better chance of fulfilling its scientific aim when these criteria are more focused, balancing these two needs is a very important consideration in the trial design.

When we consider the patient population included and data generated in a trial, we should recognize that the participants in a clinical trial, at least in concept, represent a sample of all potential participants defined by the inclusion and exclusion criteria of the study protocol. This representativeness allows generalization to future recipients and users of the medical product under investigation. When the study is finished, we can thus assume that the baseline characteristics of the participants in the trial reflect the patient population as defined by the eligibility criteria in the study design. On the other hand, we might also find out that intercurrent events occurred, which could cause incomplete information. The path from the target population to which the medical product is to be applied to the actual data samples used for analyses is a *sampling process*. The reverse direction, where we use data analyses to derive conclusions from the sample data for application to the target population, is an *inferential process* (Figure 2.1). Inferences are made based on observed data, statistical methods, and certain assumptions. One such assumption is that the data generated in the trial are derived from a *random* sample of the target population. The extent of the generalizability or applicability of the trial results, that is, the external validity of the trial, depends on how closely this assumption approaches reality.

To illustrate this concept further, let us consider the lipid-lowering treatment for prevention of coronary heart disease (CHD) as an example. The Coronary Drug Project (1973) studied a cholesterol-lowering therapy (cholestyramine) in men between the ages of 30 and 64 who had experienced at least one myocardial infarction (MI), that is, heart attack. The criteria involving the specific gender, age, and baseline condition (such as prior MIs) of patients limited the generalizability of cholestyramine's efficacy to a larger population. Almost 20 years later, the 4S study (Scandinavian Simvastatin Survival Study 1994) tested Zocor® and reported a reduction in major coronary events for both sexes, aged 60 or more. This was an astonishing medical advancement in cholesterol-lowering therapy for older individuals of both genders. Nevertheless, the efficacy was indicated only for patients with hypercholesterolemia. Finally, a primary prevention study of acute coronary events tested Mevacor® in men and women with average cholesterol levels (Downs et al. 1998)

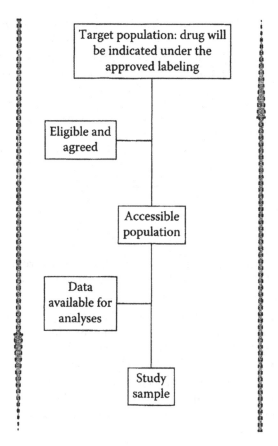

FIGURE 2.1
Sampling path (from top to bottom) and inferential path (reverse direction) for external validity of a clinical trial.

and fully extended the efficacy for the class of cholesterol-lowering medicines (HMG-CoA reductase inhibitors) to the general public. Subsequent studies with various HMG-CoA inhibitors resulted in differential FDA labeling (e.g., Crestor®) for MI prevention based on the protocol's patient inclusion and exclusion criteria and endpoints.

In addition to the eligibility criteria, the investigator's medical practice site can also be a factor for the external validity of a clinical trial. In this regard, to extend generalizability, the later phases of a clinical trial should be conducted by multiple investigators in a variety of medical settings, including university teaching hospitals, community medical centers, and private clinics, as well as in various geographical regions that may have different environmental and practice conventions. A discrete example of this problem is illustrated by the case of the Serostim® NDA for the treatment of short bowel syndrome. In June of 2003, the FDA Gastrointestinal Drugs Advisory Committee rejected the manufacturer's NDA primarily because of the lack of generalizability of the pivotal study: The study had included only two centers, one of which accrued the vast majority of patients. Only after the manufacturer conducted a further study in more and diverse centers, as requested by the FDA, was the medicine approved for open use and marketing.

Despite the examples above, assessment of external validity can be very complex and usually requires more clinical than statistical expertise. There are no accepted guidelines on how the external validity of randomized controlled trials (RCTs) should be assessed. However, Horton (2000) made a summary of questions asked by Julian and Pocock (1997) as a helpful checklist:

Patients Studied

1. Were the patients included in the trial adequately representative of the patients to be encountered in normal clinical practice? Were the eligibility criteria too narrow or too broad?
2. Were adequate steps taken to ensure that a high proportion of eligible patients was randomized? In particular, was a log kept of all patients with the appropriate condition, and how do randomized patients compare with those not randomized (both eligible and ineligible)?
3. Was the setting of the trial and the manner of patient selection appropriate? Were the eligibility criteria too narrow or too broad? Have the [investigators] inappropriately extrapolated their findings to types of patients that were not adequately represented?

Treatments

1. Was the treatment under comparison, including dose schedule, duration of treatment, noncompliance, and the control regimens (placebo or standard treatment), appropriate for normal clinical practice and determining future treatment policy in such patients?
2. Were all aspects of current good clinical practice (for example, ancillary care) adequately taken into account?

Outcome Measures and Follow-up

1. Were the outcome measures (endpoints, indicators of patient response) appropriate for reaching overall conclusions about the treatments under investigation?
2. Was too much evidence given to surrogate markers of response (for example, physiological indicators) rather than to more major

indicators of overall prognosis (for example, mortality, major clinical events)?

3. Was the duration of treatment and length of patient follow-up sufficiently reliable to assess the efficacy and safety of treatment?

4. Were adequate steps taken to elicit all relevant adverse events and side effects of treatment?

Balanced Discussion and Conclusion

1. Have the authors given adequate considerations to the limitations of their study in all the above respects?

2. Have the authors given a balanced account of evidence from other related studies or have they given undue weight to their own findings?

Source: Horton, R., *Statistics in Medicine*, 19: 3149–3164, 2000. With permission.

2.2 Internal Validity

Internal validity is the reasonable representation of the treatment effects within the study population. Internal validity is a prerequisite for external validity. The primary concerns for internal validity are as follows:

- If differences in the treatment groups are observed, are the differences due to patient characteristics, the treatments, or chance?
  (Logically, the goal for validity here is to rule out patients and chance as causes of the effect.)

- If no differences are observed in the treatment groups, is this fact due to misconduct, lack of precision (study power), or true equivalence?
  (In this case, the goal for validity is to rule out misconduct or lack of power.)

The fundamental idea for supporting internal validity is to design trials that include comparable groups such that the outcomes, whether different or the same, measure only the effect of the treatment, and nothing else. To accomplish this goal, we should adhere to the methodologies below to avoid or minimize bias in the following areas:

- treatment allocation—by use of randomization and stratification

- assessing treatment effects—by use of a concurrent control group and by masking the treatment group assignment

- study monitoring and data analysis—by use of ongoing review by disciplined investigators and expert statisticians
- fishing expeditions—by setting predefined hypotheses and endpoints in the protocol.

Single-arm trials have also been useful in obtaining regulatory approvals for treating rare, serious, and chronic diseases with no approved treatments. For a single-arm trial, the burden of "Demonstrating Substantial Evidence of Effectiveness for Human Drug and Biologic Products" as described in the FDA guidance (FDA 2019) relies on the natural history of the disease and the associated endpoint under study to ensure that the subject responses are impossible to occur by chance in such a way that the magnitude and duration of response are clinically and statistically meaningful.

2.3 Repeatability

The basic philosophy for repeatability of clinical trials is that scientific experiments should be verified by replication. The FDA and EMA usually favor applications with two or more pivotal trials for the approval of an NDA, BLA, or MAA. These trials may vary somewhat in the patient population or control agent used. Therefore, they are usually not strictly exact replicates. In certain situations, however, a single large trial with different centers showing consistent results may also be acceptable, especially for studies with mortality or serious morbidity endpoints, because these types of trials are hard to repeat, especially in the setting of positive results. Showing consistency among centers and predefined subgroups is essential for demonstrating repeatability in the case of a single large trial.

2.4 The Phenomenon of Regression toward the Mean and Importance of a Concurrent Control Group

In Chapter 1, we noted that Friedman, Furberg, and DeMets (1996) restrict their definition of clinical trials to those that are compared against a control group. Although this definition excludes many single-arm early-phase trials in oncology funded by NIH and usually conducted by the designated cancer centers or the cancer cooperative groups (unless their definition also meant to include *historical control* or *self-baseline control*), it highlights the importance of a *concurrent control group* for the internal validity of a clinical trial. We further illustrate this point here by examining the phenomenon of regression toward the mean. We raise this topic in this early chapter because we also want the readers to review the basic method of regression, which is a prerequisite for the level of this book. Regression methodology is used throughout this book, from the study design stage to data monitoring and analysis later. The material in Chapter 5 ("Analysis of Covariance and Stratified Analysis") requires the readers to be familiar with the regression method.

2.4.1 Regression toward the Mean: Definition and Example

Regression toward the mean is a phenomenon that occurs when a second measurement is made only for those individuals with an "extreme" initial measurement. On average, the second measurement tends to be less extreme than the first, even in the absence of any medical intervention. It came from the phrase *regression towards mediocrity*, which was originally coined by Sir Francis Galton (1886) to characterize the tendency for tall parents to produce shorter offspring and vice versa (Bland and Altman 1994). We should recognize this phenomenon because it often occurs in clinical trials when we include patients with high or low measurements at baseline. For example, we study antihypertensive treatments on patients with high blood pressures, cholesterol-lowering therapies on patients with hyperlipidemia, and bone-strengthening medicines on postmenopausal osteoporotic women with low bone-mineral density.

In-Class Discussion: Figure 2.2a and b shows two illustrations clipped from the article "Effects of Oral Alendronate and Intranasal Salmon Calcitonin on Bone Mass and Biochemical Markers of Bone Turnover in Postmenopausal Women with Osteoporosis" (Adami et al. 1995). This study was a 24-month trial in postmenopausal women with osteoporosis (low bone density). Patients were randomized into four treatment groups: placebo, alendronate 10 mg, alendronate 20 mg, or calcitonin 100 IU. The upper panel (Figure 2.2a) shows the mean percent changes $\pm$SE in lumbar spine bone-mineral density (L-spine BMD) at 6, 12, 18, and 24 months. Based on this information, consider the following questions: Why was there an increase in L-spine BMD in the placebo group at month 6? What did that placebo effect represent?

One might suspect that the placebo effect was due to the calcium supplements (500 mg daily) provided to all of the participants in the trial. This guess seems reasonable but, if it is true, why was there no similar placebo effect shown on the lower panel for the trochanter BMD at month 6? A more plausible reason for the placebo effect can be found in the participant selection and eligibility section of the paper. The trial required that at baseline each participant have an L-spine BMD >2 SD below the mean for young premenopausal women (<0.99 g/cm^2 for Lunar® densitometers and <0.86 g/cm^2 for Hologic®, Norland®, and Sophos®), while there was no restriction for the trochanter BMD. Thus, regression toward the mean might be what the placebo effect represents in this case. Interestingly, Cummings et al. (2000) published a later article that supports this reasoning.

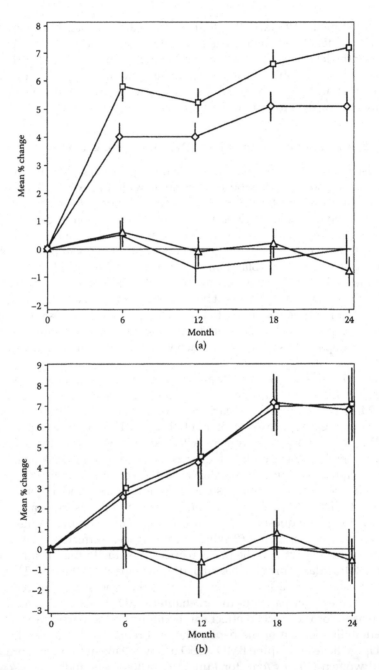

FIGURE 2.2
(a) Lumbar spine bone-mineral density (L-spine BMD). Mean percent changes (SE) in BMD
with placebo, alendronate 10 mg (◊), alendronate 20 mg (□), and intranasal salmon calcitonin
100 IU (Δ), baseline to 24 months; (b) trochanter BMD. Mean percent changes (SE) in BMD with
placebo, alendronate 10 mg (◊), alendronate 20 mg (□), and intranasal salmon calcitonin 100 IU
(Δ), baseline to 24 months. (From Adami S, et al., *Bone*, 17: 383–390, 1995, with permission.)

2.4.2 Effect of Regression toward the Mean as a Form of Bias

Because clinical trials are follow-up studies, there must be at least two observations per subject: the baseline and the follow-up measurements. In this two-dimensional setting, the notion of bivariate distribution is needed. The bivariate normal distribution and the expression of simple linear regression are very helpful when continuous variables are involved. Let the random variable X_1 be the baseline measurement for one treatment group and X_2 be the follow-up measurement for that same group. Assume a bivariate normal distribution for the paired measurements (X_1, X_2), with the mean vector and covariance matrix shown as follows:

$$\begin{pmatrix} X_1 \\ X_2 \end{pmatrix} \sim N\left(\begin{pmatrix} \mu_1 \\ \mu_2 \end{pmatrix}, \begin{pmatrix} \sigma_1^2 & \rho\sigma_1\sigma_2 \\ \rho\sigma_1\sigma_2 & \sigma_2^2 \end{pmatrix} \right)$$

Recall that, in statistical terms, regression is a conditional analysis. This approach addresses the following question: Given what I observe now (at baseline) as X_1, what should I *expect* to see later (at follow-up) as X_2? We can answer this question by using the simple linear regression expression

$$E(X_2 \mid X_1) = \alpha + \beta X_1$$
$$= \mu_2 + \rho\frac{\sigma_2}{\sigma_1}(X_1 - \mu_1) \tag{2.1}$$

where $\alpha = \mu_2 - \beta\mu_1$ and $\beta = \rho\dfrac{\sigma_2}{\sigma_1}$.

Readers may review the notion of bivariate normal distribution and the simple linear regression expression from an introductory biostatistics textbook (e.g., Daniel 2009).

Assuming no treatment effect in this treatment group (i.e., $\mu_1 = \mu_2 = \mu$ and $\sigma_1 = \sigma_2 = \sigma$), the regression equation can be rewritten for a specific value $X_1 = x_1$ as

$$E(X_2 \mid x_1) = \mu + \rho(x_1 - \mu) \tag{2.2}$$

Subtracting μ from both sides and taking the absolute value, it is clear that the following inequality holds:

$$\left| E(X_2 \mid x_1) - \mu \right| = |\rho| |x_1 - \mu| \le |x_1 - \mu| \tag{2.3}$$

This inequality tells us that, even with no treatment effect, if the initial value $X_1 = x_1$ is an extreme case (larger or smaller than the population mean μ), the follow-up value X_2 will be, on average, closer to the population mean than x_1. Also known as the "ceiling effect" or "floor effect," the phenomenon of regression toward the mean is a form of bias; that is, no treatment effect seemingly produces an effect!

Equation 2.2 also implies

$$|E(X_2 | x_1) - x_1| = |(\rho - 1)(x_1 - \mu)| \tag{2.4}$$

This expression says that the magnitude of the effect of regression toward the mean (left-hand side of Equation 2.4) for a specific case $X_1 = x_1$ is usually not zero. It will be zero when $\rho = 1$ (perfect correlation), or if the specific case x_1 is a perfect sample in which it is equal to the population mean μ (Homework 2.1).

In-Class Exercise: Assume that you are conducting a placebo-controlled antihypertensive clinical trial. One of the inclusion criteria says that, in order to be included in the trial, the participant's baseline sitting diastolic blood pressure (SDBP) has to be between 90 and 110 mmHg. Suppose the normal population of the same age group has a mean SDBP of 85 mmHg. If the correlation between the baseline and follow-up SDBP is 0.5, what would you expect the magnitude of the effect of regression toward the mean to be for participants whose baseline SDBP is 95 mmHg?

Answer: Using Equation 2.4, $|E(X_2 | x_1) - x_1| = |(\rho - 1)(x_1 - \mu)| = |0.5 - 1||95 - 85| = 5$ (mmHg).

2.5 Random Samples and Randomization of Samples

We should distinguish the two kinds of randomness that occur in clinical trials. We should also be sensitive to the perception that a phrase with randomness might imply that the situation is chaotic, without purpose, or out of control to a layman (Featherstone and Donovan 1998). Hence, we should be cautious in our communication.

Randomness as Used Herein: As discussed in Section 2.1 ("External Validity"), consideration of subjects who participate in a clinical trial as conceptually random "samples" is key for generalizing the trial results to the target population in medical practice. This is not the survey type of sampling, where samples are drawn from a fixed, finite, cross-sectional population. The random samples in clinical trials are conceptually drawn from the current, as well as future, cohorts of users of the medication under study.

When there are two or more interventions in a comparative trial, that is, in a controlled clinical trial, randomization of subjects to treatment groups is a methodology for reaching a certain degree of *internal validity* for the given trial. Random sampling and randomization of samples (subjects) are two distinct types of randomness.

2.5.1 What Is Randomization?

Randomization is a process by which subjects are assigned to treatments (or treatment sequence in the case of a study with a crossover design) such that each subject has an equal nonzero chance of being allocated to any given treatment (or treatment sequence) in the study. We may say, for example, that the first subject was randomized to Treatment A. If there are two treatments and a patient's chances of being assigned to each treatment are the same, we can randomize a patient using the flip of a fair coin. In such a case, the second subject could potentially also be randomized to Treatment A, but in the case of many entries, we would see a balance in those randomized to A and B. *Clinical equipoise* (Freedman 1987), which means that there is genuine uncertainty in the expert medical community over whether a test treatment will be beneficial compared to the control, provides the ethical basis for equal randomization.

2.5.2 Why Randomization?

First, we need some background. The outcome of a study is the response that is measured (before and) after administration of a treatment; we expect it to be influenced differentially by the alternative treatments in the study. A prognostic factor is defined as a subject characteristic (such as sex) that may contribute to the outcome. Randomization avoids the potential for subjects with specific prognostic profiles to get assigned preferentially to a particular treatment (resulting in an "allocation bias"). Furthermore, and more importantly, the statistical methods that will be used to analyze the data are based on mathematical theories that assume that random allocation has occurred. If subjects were not randomly assigned to treatment, then such analyses would be less valid or invalid. Observational studies do not have randomization involved. Again, random allocation of treatments is ethical in clinical trials in the case of clinical equipoise—when the treating doctor does not know which of the treatments is best for the patients in terms of the ultimate benefits and risks (Doll 1998).

2.5.3 Logistics of Randomization and Blinding

Randomization of patients to treatment (or treatment sequence) avoids or minimizes *allocation bias*. A related but different method that often accompanies randomization is *blinding*. Blinding is a way to mask the treatment assignment and contains several layers. Basic blinding is implemented as subjects are recruited into the study, to avoid *selection bias*. During the randomization and study, we mask the subject, the investigator, or both to prevent them from knowing the (random) treatment assignment and avoid *assessment bias*. *Single-blind* trials are those where only subjects are masked. A *double-blind* trial refers to one where both subjects and investigators are masked. Some pharmaceutical companies also implement the so-called *triple-blinding* in which the project statistician is also masked when analyzing the data. In contrast, *open-label* trials are those where neither patients nor investigators are masked. Schultz et al. (1995) reanalyzed 250 randomized trials from 33 meta-analyses and found that treatment effects were 30%–40% larger in trials without adequate concealment of treatment allocation. Kunz and Oxman (1998) also reported empirical evidence of bias in trials without random allocation or adequate concealment of allocation.

2.5.4 The Process of Randomization

First, a person who is *not* involved in patient recruitment, the consent process, administrating treatment, or assessment of subjects creates a *randomization schedule*. This person is often the trial biostatistician. The randomization schedule is the sequential list of treatment assignments for subjects who will be enrolled in the study.

Randomization must involve an element of unpredictability. After the randomization schedule is created, the treatment allocation is fixed on the schedule. What is actually random (unpredictable) is the order in which subjects arrive for treatment. Therefore, it is important that the next treatment in sequence be kept confidential to avoid the possibility of *selection bias*. This fact should be communicated to the medical research staff and the patients.

Conventionally, the person who generated the randomization schedule also keeps the schedule (in a centralized location in the case of a multicenter trial). This person (or designee) is contacted once a subject is deemed eligible for the study and has provided consent. This person then informs the investigator or pharmacy of the subject's treatment assignment. Alternatively, sealed envelopes, vials, or medication bottles are numbered and kept by the investigator or pharmacy. These are then used successively as each eligible and consenting patient begins on the study. A sealed sequentially numbered envelope, for example, helps assure the confidentiality of the next randomization.

Many trials sponsored by the pharmaceutical industry now commonly use a centralized, automated, interactive voice or web response system (IVRS or IWRS) instead of a contact person. The IVRS or IWRS usually also provides 24-hour code-breaking capability for investigators when an emergency occurs. In a recent paper, Goodale and McEntegart (2013) described various sources of bias and how technology can be used to eliminate or reduce the risk of occurrence of bias. This paper also cited various references covering examples and the effects of bias. For example, Zhao, Hill, and Palesch (2012) used the Captopril Prevention Project trial as an example to describe how selection bias can occur when technology is not used for the implementation of randomization.

In summary, as presented in the study by Armitage (1982), randomization (i) helps to align treatment groups with similar distributions of prognostic factors; (ii) permits the use of probability theory to express quantitatively the extent to which any difference in response between treatment groups is likely to be due to chance; and (iii) allows various devices for masking the identity of treatment, including the possible use of a placebo, which are often essential for an unbiased assessment of efficacy by the subject or the observer, or both.

2.6 Methods for Randomization

We now turn our attention to several randomization methods and their merits, from simple to more sophisticated approaches. More detail on this topic can be found in Rosenberger and Lachin (2002). For any randomization method, we desire not only to achieve a certain fixed ratio of subjects in each treatment group, but also to ensure that subject groups are similar with respect to prognostic factors such as age, stage or severity of disease, and many others.

2.6.1 Completely Randomized Design

For a randomized trial with two treatments with even allocation, the simplest method is to toss a fair (balanced) coin over and over again (for more than two groups, to roll a dice). Although reasonable, these manual methods are rather antiquated. Computer-generated random numbers are now commonly used instead. Completely randomized design, also called simple (unrestricted) randomization, is the design where no blocking or stratification is involved. The advantage of such a simple design is that each treatment assignment is completely unpredictable, hence with a minimal chance of selection bias by investigators. For a large trial, the number of subjects in each treatment group will not be drastically different. However, for a trial with a small size or for an (early) interim analysis, the possibility exists that treatment groups will end up with considerably unequal numbers of subjects. For example, for a trial with 20 patients, the probability of getting 12 or more patients (60% or more) on a single treatment is approximately 50%. For a trial with 40 patients, the probability of getting 24 or more patients (60% or more) on a single treatment is approximately 27%. Additionally, sometimes known prognostic factors can be unevenly distributed in small groups, and a simple randomization may not distribute such factors evenly. In other words, without proper stratification, treatment groups also might be imbalanced with respect to influential prognostic factors. Therefore, blocked randomization and stratified randomization, or both combined, are often implemented in clinical trials (Homework 2.2).

2.6.2 Blocked Randomization

Blocked randomization is used to perform simple randomization within blocks in order to avoid severely imbalanced allocation to treatment groups. Suppose we have J treatments and s replicates. For a block size of s×J, we then produce a different simple randomization for each s×J patients. We should keep the block size confidential and especially not write it in the protocol. The block size should not be too small (e.g., $s = 1$ is not a good idea), nor should it be too large (e.g., $s > 5$ would be considered large). A small s makes the randomization sequence somewhat predictable. A large s, on the other hand, defeats the purpose of using blocks for balanced allocation. We also can vary s from block to block, which will then create a "varying block size randomization" design. Varying block size randomization, together with masking or blinding for double-blind trials, makes prediction of future allocations difficult, thus minimizing selection bias and achieving the desirable ratio of patient numbers between treatment groups (Homework 2.3).

2.6.3 Stratified Randomization

In clinical trials, we prefer to have similar treatment groups with regard to certain baseline characteristics of subjects. For example, in many instances gender and age relate to disease severity and outcome. If we recognize a factor that is known to influence the subject's outcome, it would be problematic if the treatment groups were not comparable in that prognostic factor. Even though there do exist methods of statistical analysis that can be used to address this issue, we would see a loss of statistical efficiency and would need to make additional efforts to convince others that the conclusion is valid. When such factors are chosen, strata are formed. Stratified randomization can be a complete (simple) randomization, or a blocked randomization within each stratum. However, most believe it advisable to limit the number of strata in a feasible manner. This technique also critically relates to the overall number of subjects to be enrolled in the trial. For example, for a cancer trial that considers age (<55 vs. ≥55), gender (male vs. female), performance status (score 1–2 vs. 3–4), and time since diagnosis (<6 months vs. ≥6 months), there will be $2 \times 2 \times 2 \times 2 = 16$ combinations for strata, each requiring a separate randomization. When there are many prognostic factors, we may consider another method for allocation of patients to treatment groups: the *minimization method*.

Aside: Stratified randomization in clinical trials is similar to the so-called "randomized block design" in classical experimental design, such as that used in agriculture, the agricultural "blocks" being analogous to the clinical strata, rather than to the blocks that are permutated for balanced allocation. The agricultural blocks are a fixed size, whereas the strata in clinical trials are initially of unknown size; the balancing therefore should occur in a sequential manner.

2.7 Minimization

When there are many prognostic factors to consider, often the need is to balance the *marginal distributions* rather than the *joint distribution*. That is, we desire to balance each of the factors individually and simultaneously, when the number of combinations of factors is too large to be feasible. The method of minimization works toward this goal.

The minimization method was first described by Taves (1974), and then by Pocock and Simon (1975). It is a dynamic allocation method, which may be viewed as a special form of adaptive design that is non-response dependent. (An example of response-dependent adaptive design is given in Appendix 3.3 in Chapter 3. More about adaptive designs is discussed in later chapters with sequential designs and methods.) Patients are assigned to treatment as they are enrolled in the study, rather than through a preset randomization schedule. Treatment groups are balanced only with respect to the potential main effects of the prognostic factors. There is no need to prespecify the number of patients within each stratum of each variable. We describe the method by a common case as follows.

Suppose we have two treatment groups, A and B, in a trial. Consider three prognostic factors that have I, J, and K levels (e.g., $I = J = K = 2$). At any time during the trial, let n_{ijk}^A represent the number of subjects randomized to Treatment A at levels i, j, and k of the prognostic factors, respectively, and n_{ijk}^B represent those within the same stratum randomized to Treatment B, with $n_{ijk} = n_{ijk}^A + n_{ijk}^B$. Under simple stratification, we have $n_{ijk}^A \approx n_{ijk}^B$.

The notation n_{i++}^A represents the number of individuals at the i-th level of the first prognostic factor that are randomized to Treatment A, summed over the second and third prognostic factors. The same is true for n_{i++}^B. These are the marginal totals for the first prognostic factor at level i in treatment groups A and B, respectively. To balance the marginal distribution of the first prognostic factor in treatment groups A and B is to ensure that $n_{i++}^A \approx n_{i++}^B$ for all i.

Likewise, to balance the second factor, we need to ensure $n_{+j+}^A \approx n_{+j+}^B$ for all j, and for the third factor, we need to reach $n_{++k}^A \approx n_{++k}^B$ for all k.

For each patient enrolled, we note their levels of the prognostic factors, say, i*, j*, and k*, respectively. Calculate the quantity

$$G = \left(n_{i^*++}^A - n_{i^*++}^B\right) + \left(n_{+j^*+}^A - n_{+j^*+}^B\right) + \left(n_{++k^*}^A - n_{++k^*}^B\right) \qquad (2.5)$$

G represents the total amount of imbalance. Treatment assignment depends on whether G is negative, positive, or zero. If G is negative, indicating a deficit of assignment to A, then the new patient is allocated to A (with probability π). If G is positive, meaning a deficit of assignment to B, then the patient is allocated to B (with probability π). If G equals zero, the treatment assignments are at equilibrium and the patient is allocated to A or B (with initialization probability 1/2). Note that for the first patient, the above quantity is zero. The probability $\pi = 0.7$ might be a suitable choice to prevent advanced predictions of the next treatment assignment. The International Conference on Harmonization (ICH) *E9, Statistical Principles for Clinical Trials*, recommends that a random element should be incorporated into deterministic dynamic allocation procedures like minimization (Lewis 1999). Xu, Proschan, and Lee (2016) conducted simulation studies and concluded that when minimization is used, the subsequent test procedure always needs to take into account the specific design scheme to protect the type I error rate and achieve higher power. They recommended to use $\pi = 0.7$ in the minimization process.

The above method can easily accommodate many numbers of prognostic factors as well as different numbers of levels of each prognostic factor. Additionally, if balance is more important among some prognostic factors than others, the quantity above can be modified to be a weighted sum. The minimization method with a random element is commonly and most efficiently implemented by an automated IVRS/IWRS.

We now give an example for illustration (with $\pi = 1$). Suppose a trial with two treatment groups (experimental and control) has already enrolled 18 participants. Table 2.1 summarizes the three characteristics (sex, age range, and disease stage) for the 18 participants that the trial wishes to balance between treatment groups. If the next (19th) subject is male, aged 46, and at a moderate disease stage, the decision to allocate to the experimental or control group can be made by computing the imbalance quantity G (Equation 2.5) as illustrated below the table. In this case, $G = -1$; hence, the 19th participant would be assigned to the experimental group.

As we can see from the illustration, if the weight to disease stage is double or more than that of age and sex as prognostic factors, the allocation could be different. This method can be generalized to more treatments. Other more complicated minimization methods also exist (see Cook and DeMets, 2007). A good review and recommendation can be found in Scott et al. (2002).

Note that minimization with $\pi = 1$ in the above example just for illustration is a deterministic method in that the allocation of the next subject to treatment is determined by the previous allocations of subjects enrolled. Technically, correct statistical analysis following minimization is complicated

TABLE 2.1

Example to Illustrate the Minimization Method

Prognostic Factor	Experimental Group	Control Group
Sex		
Male	4	5
Female	5	4
Age range		
18–40	4	3
41–65	2	3
>65	3	3
Disease stage		
Moderate	5	4
Severe	4	5

Note: If the 19th patient is male, aged 46, and with moderate disease stage, imbalance quantity $= (4-5)+(2-3)+(5-4) = -1$. Therefore, allocate the 19th patient to the experimental group.

and involves simulation of multiple datasets (100,000) under the assumption of no treatment effect and the practiced allocation strategy. Then, observed results are compared to the distribution of simulated possible results in order to obtain a p-value. In practice, however, analyses may be conducted with the minimization factors used as covariates in the model. Simulation studies have shown the power and type I error rate to be similar between these two approaches (e.g., Forsythe and Stitt 1977, Green et al. 2001). Senn (1995) even argued that factors used in the minimization must also be included in the analysis and that using minimization but not including the covariates in the model is not legitimate.

Concerns were raised (e.g., Berger 2006, 2011) that randomization with more restrictions such as blocked randomization and deterministic methods such as minimization without a random element preclude allocation concealment and invite selection bias by a sophisticated person who can figure out future treatment assignment when the trial is not masked. To alleviate such concerns, trials should be adequately designed and executed to mask the treatment assignment. Recent advances in technology, as described by Goodale and McEntegart (2013), should be utilized to achieve this goal. Setting the probability $\pi = 0.7$ in the allocation of treatment is one way to incorporate a random element in the deterministic dynamic allocation procedure (Homework 2.4).

2.8 Table of Patient Demographics and Baseline Characteristics

The first table in the results section of a clinical trial paper often has a heading such as "Patient Demographics and Baseline Characteristics," and the display is often by treatment groups as well as with treatment groups combined. Sometimes the table also provides p-values for these baseline variables (covariates). (The reference given in Homework 4.1 of Chapter 4 is such an example.) In a nonrandomized clinical study, showing p-values for comparability between groups is meaningful and very necessary to investigate possible *confounding factors*. However, if the trial is randomized (at least titled as such), then we should ask whether these p-values are meaningful. What is the intended purpose of such a table? Take a minute to contemplate this question.

Such a table display may serve multiple purposes. The overall column obviously describes the enrolled participants so as to inform the reader about the applicability of the trial result to the medical practice in general (see Section 2.1, "External Validity"). The display by treatment groups, however, can be more interesting, especially when significance tests are performed for each baseline variable. Many authors have discussed this topic (e.g., Altman 1985, Senn 1989, and Begg 1990). One school of thought states that it is not meaningful to calculate p-values there, because we know the trial is randomized, and the characteristics are baseline values (without treatment effect), so the null hypothesis of no difference between groups is true. Therefore, any statistical significance indicated by a low p-value is simply a type I error, and it is thus pointless and should be avoided. Furthermore, if we examine many baseline variables, as this kind of table often does, we expect to find some "significance" by chance alone. For example, in the report of the Coronary Drug Project (1973), 420 drug–placebo comparisons on baseline characteristics were carried out. The authors correctly pointed out that they would "expect to find about 21 of the differences to be significant at the 0.05 level." They actually observed 22, and concluded that "... there is no evidence of lack of comparability of the treatment groups at baseline." Is this a correct conclusion? (The answer is no, as we explain in the next paragraph.)

Others may ask the question: How do we know the randomization process, as described, was actually carried out properly and that it worked as intended? The editor, the reader, and the FDA authority may wish to check on this by such a table display. In other words, the significance tests are meaningful for the hypothesis that the treatments are randomly allocated, or whether the supposedly randomized trial was in actuality a randomized trial. For the Coronary Drug Project mentioned above, the significance tests only indicated that the randomization was fair. Incidentally, more powerful approaches to analyzing these observed p-values for testing the null hypothesis of randomization also exist; for example, Schweder and Spjotvoll (1982) focused on this in greater detail.

However, if the purpose of doing significance tests here is to check randomization, then we can simply ask the patient irrelevant questions and test the distributions of answers to questions such as "What is your favorite color (or sport)?"—which carry no prognostic importance whatsoever to the outcome of the study. Obviously, the intention of the table is to examine the "baseline comparability," not merely for checking the fairness of randomization. What then does a p-value tell us about a treatment group's comparability? Can we judge what factor to adjust in the statistical analysis by looking at the p-values? The answer to both questions is obviously no.

Baseline comparability of treatment groups may be represented by the treatment–covariate association. The p-values in the baseline table of a medical paper could not measure the strength of the treatment–covariate association; each p-value is simply testing the hypothesis of null *treatment assignment* association with a covariate. As significance tests are not appropriate for assessing baseline comparability in RCTs, how should the comparability be done? Altman (1985) recommended it be initially judged "using a combination of clinical knowledge and common sense." Here, previous experience plays a key role. The actual implication of comparability or lack thereof is whether to adjust for a covariate or not in the analysis.

In a (truly) randomized trial, we can choose to analyze the treatment effect without any covariate and the conclusions will be valid, irrespective of the observed treatment–covariate association. In this regard, the p-values in the baseline table of a medical paper are not needed. However, the observed p-value for the treatment–covariate distribution is very informative about the probability, say, that a significant treatment effect is a false positive. For example, suppose that in a trial, the treatment effect is on the borderline of being significant, and that the treatments are not well balanced with respect to some covariate that is strongly prognostic to the outcome. Then conditional on the observed treatment–covariate distribution, the probability of a significant treatment effect under the null hypothesis will be much different than the nominal significance level. The converse is true when the treatments are especially well balanced with respect to the covariate (Begg 1990).

As a common practice, we usually adjust a prognostic factor that is unbalanced between the groups. In Chapter 5, we write an analysis of covariance (ANCOVA) model to demonstrate the appropriateness of the above practice. We show that the degree of adjustment and the variance reduction depend on two factors: the covariate's correlation or association with the outcome variable and the degree of between-group imbalance. The p-values in the baseline table of a medical paper have no bearing on the adjustment of covariates.

HOMEWORK 2.1

Write out the formula in Equation 2.4 for a control group labeled as Y. Discuss how randomization in treatment allocation and blinding in assessing treatment effects can help cancel out the bias of the effect of regression to the mean.

HOMEWORK 2.2

1. Use the SAS® or R software to generate a completely randomized allocation schedule for a trial with total sample size N = 50, two treatment groups, and an even allocation design. Comment on the actual sample size of each group.

   Hint: Use the R software to generate a list of 50 random numbers from the uniform (0, 1) distribution. Assign Patient 1 the first random number, Patient 2 the second random number, etc. If a patient's random number is <0.5, then assign that patient to Treatment A; otherwise, assign the patient to Treatment B. SAS has a procedure called PROC PLAN that you may also use.

2. Use either a mathematical derivation or run your computer program repeatedly 10,000 times to show that in this case (N = 50) the probability is greater than 5% that the design will end up as an uneven treatment allocation in the ratio of 18:32 or more extreme.

HOMEWORK 2.3

Use the SAS or R software to generate a blocked randomization schedule for a trial with total sample size N = 180, three treatment groups (J = 3), and an even allocation design. Vary the block size (s×J) by permuting s = 1, 2, 3. How many blocks will there be? Comment on the actual sample size of each group.

HOMEWORK 2.4[1]

Suppose that 32 patients will be recruited for a clinical trial comparing Treatments A and B. After completing the consent process for these patients, they will be allocated to one of the treatments. Suppose that age (categories 18–25, 26–39, and 40–60) and gender (M and F) are expected to be important prognostic factors for the outcome being studied. Using the minimization approach, create a randomization schedule using an initialization probability of 1/2 and the probability of $\pi = 1$ afterward. When G = 0, use the following uniform random numbers in the allocation procedure (rather than generating your own):

0.26, 0.69, 0.11, 0.51, 0.22, 0.56, 0.23, 0.98, 0.11, 0.43, 0.53, 0.98, 0.29, and 0.23

Note: Setting $\pi = 1$ here is for convenience so that you need not to do any computer programming for this problem.

The following are the ages and genders of the 32 subjects in the order in which they were enrolled in the study:

---

[1] Homework 2.4 was contributed by Pamela Ohman-Strickland.

ID	Age	Gender
1	26	F
2	32	F
3	18	M
4	29	F
5	35	F
6	35	M
7	38	F
8	55	M
9	56	M
10	34	F
11	22	M
12	22	F
13	23	F
14	35	F
15	34	F
16	22	F
17	34	M
18	56	F
19	59	F
20	29	M
21	45	F
22	43	F
23	33	F
24	23	M
25	49	F
26	51	F
27	23	F
28	38	F
29	34	M
30	19	F
31	39	F
32	40	M

According to the randomization schedule you created:

1. How many subjects are allocated to Treatments A and B within each age–gender subcategory?
2. How many subjects are allocated to Treatments A and B within each age group?
3. How many within each gender group?
4. How many overall?

References

Adami S, Passeri M, Ortolani S, Broggini M, Carratelli L, Caruso I, and Gandolini G. (1995). Effects of oral alendronate and intranasal salmon calcitonin on bone mass and biochemical markers of bone turnover in postmenopausal women with osteoporosis. *Bone* 17: 383–390.

Altman DG. (1985). Comparability of randomized groups. *The Statistician* 34: 125–136.

Armitage P. (1982). The role of randomization in clinical trials. *Statistics in Medicine* 1: 345–352.

Begg CB. (1990). Significance tests of covariate imbalance in clinical trials. *Controlled Clinical Trials* 11: 223–225.

Berger VW. (2006). Misguided precedent is not a reason to use permuted blocks. *Headache* 46: 1210–1212.

Berger VW. (2011). Minimization: not all it's cracked up to be. *Clinical Trials* 8: 443.

Bland JM and Altman DG. (1994). Regression towards the mean. *British Medical Journal* 308: 1499.

Cook TD and DeMets DL. (2007). *Introduction to Statistical Methods for Clinical Trials.* New York: Chapman & Hall/CRC.

Cummings SR, Palermo L, Browner W, Marcus R, Wallace R, Pearson J, and Blackwell T. (2000). Monitoring osteoporosis therapy with bone mineral density: misleading changes and regression to the mean. *Journal of the* American Medical Association 283: 1318–1321.

Daniel WW. (2009). *Biostatistics: A Foundation for Analysis in the Health Sciences.* New York: Wiley.

Doll R. (1998). Controlled trials: the 1948 watershed. *British Medical Journal* 317: 1217–1220.

Downs JR, and Clearfield M. (1998). Primary prevention of acute coronary events with lovastatin in men and women with average cholesterol levels: results of AFCAPS/TexCAPS. Air Force/Texas Coronary Atherosclerosis Prevention Study. *Journal of the American Medical Association* 27: 1615–1622.

Evidence-Based Medicine Working Group. (1992). Evidence-based medicine – a new approach to teaching the practice of medicine. *Journal of the American Medical Association* 268: 2420–2425.

FDA (US Food and Drug Administration). (2019). Demonstrating Substantial Evidence of Effectiveness for Human Drug and Biologic Products. https://www.federalregister.gov/documents/2019/12/20/2019-27524/demonstrating-substantial-evidence-of-effectiveness-for-human-drug-and-biological-products-draft (accessed February 14, 2021).

Featherstone K and Donovan JL. (1998). Random allocation or allocation at random? Patients' perspective of participation in randomized controlled trial. British Medical Journal 317: 1177–1180.

Forsythe AB and Stitt FW. (1977). *Randomization or Minimization in the Treatment Assignment of Patient Trials: Validity and Power of Tests. Technical Report No. 28.* Health Sciences Computing Facility, Los Angeles: UCLA.

Freedman, B (1987). Equipoise and the ethics of clinical research. *The New England Journal of Medicine,* 317: 141–145.

Friedman LM, Furberg CD, and DeMets DL. (1996). *Fundamentals of Clinical Trials.* New York: Springer.

Goodale H and McEntegart D. (2013). The role of technology in avoiding bias in the design and execution of clinical trials. Open Access Journal of Clinical Trials 5: 13–21. doi:10.2147/OAJCT.S40760.

Green H, McEntegart DJ, Byrom B, Ghani S, and Shepherd S. (2001). Minimization in crossover trials with non-prognostic strata: theory and practical application. *Journal of Clinical Pharmacy and Therapeutics* 26: 121–128.

Horton R. (2000). Common sense and figures: the rhetoric of validity in medicine (Bradford Hill Memorial Lecture 1999). *Statistics in Medicine* 19: 3149–3164.

Julian DG and Pocock SJ. (1997). Interpreting a trial report. In *Clinical Trials in Cardiology*. Pitt B, Julian D, and Pocock S (eds.). London: WB Saunders.

Kunz R and Oxman AD. (1998). The unpredictability paradox: review of empirical comparisons of randomised and non-randomised clinical trials. *British Medical Journal* 317: 1185–1190.

Lewis JA. (1999). Statistical principles for clinical trials (ICH E9): an introductory note on an international guideline. *Statistics in Medicine* 18: 1903–1942.

Pocock SJ and Simon R. (1975). Sequential treatment assignment with balancing for prognostic factors in the controlled clinical trial. *Biometrics* 31: 103–115.

Rosenberger W and Lachin JM. (2002). *Randomization in Clinical Trials: Theory and Practice*. New York: John Wiley and Sons.

Rothwell PM. (2005). External validity of randomized controlled trials: "To whom do the results of this trial apply?" *Lancet* 365: 82–93.

Schultz KF, Chalmers I, Hayes RJ, and Altman DG. (1995). Empirical evidence of bias. Dimensions of methodological quality associated with estimates of treatment effects in controlled trials. *Journal of the American Medical Association* 273: 408–412.

Schweder T and Spjotvoll E. (1982). Plots of P-values to evaluate many tests simultaneously. *Biometrika* 69: 493–502.

Scott NW, McPherson CG, Ramsay CR, and Campbell MK. (2002). The method of minimization for allocation to clinical trials: a review. *Controlled Clinical Trials* 23: 662–674.

Senn SJ. (1989). Covariate imbalance and random allocation in clinical trials. *Statistics in Medicine* 8: 467–475.

Senn SJ. (1995). A personal view of some controversies in allocating treatment to patients in clinical trials. *Statistics in Medicine* 14: 2661–2674.

Simvastatin Scandinavian Survival Study Group. (1994). Randomised trial of cholesterol lowering in 4444 patients with coronary heart disease: the Scandinavian Simvastatin Survival Study (4S). *Lancet* 19; 344: 1383–1389.

Taves DR. (1974). Minimization: a new method of assigning patients to treatment and control groups. *Clinical Pharmacology and Therapeutics* 15: 443–453.

The Coronary Drug Project Research Group. (1973). The coronary drug project: design, methods and baseline results. *Circulation* 47 & 48 (Suppl. 1): I-1–I-50.

Xu Z, Proschan M, Lee S. (2016) Validity and power considerations on hypothesis testing under minimization. *Statistics in Medicine* 35(14):2315–2327.

Zhao W, Hill MD, and Palesch Y. (2012). Minimal sufficient balance – a new strategy to balance baseline covariates and preserve randomness of treatment allocation. *Statistical Methods in Medical Research* January 26, 2012.

3

Efficiency with Trade-Offs and Crossover Designs

The two primary concerns of statistical design are *bias* and *efficiency*. We have discussed the concept of bias and methods to help avoid or minimize bias in the last chapter. In this chapter, we explore the concept of efficiency. We begin with two simple examples. In each example, we see that sample size and variance of the outcome variable (endpoint) play the main roles in defining statistical efficiency. Efficiency gains also involve trade-offs when considering trial design. We use the crossover design for an illustration of the trade-offs in efficiency. The crossover design is also useful as a way to introduce the analysis of variance (ANOVA) cell-means model. In Appendices 3.1 through 3.3, we also briefly introduce designs that maximize the benefit of treatment, for example, measured by the expected number of responders, as an alternative to efficiency for the purpose of designing trials optimally in terms of ethics.

3.1 Statistical Efficiency of a Design

We first consider two conceptual examples:

Example 3.1

Consider a study to compare two treatments, X and Y. Let the endpoint be a continuous variable so that the mean difference is the parameter of interest. We have two design options: For Design A, we recruit n pairs of identical twins and randomly assign each sibling to a treatment group. (If one sibling gets treatment X randomly, the other will automatically get treatment Y.) For Design B, we randomize 2n unrelated individuals with 1:1 (equal) allocation to the treatment groups, with the same eligibility as in Design A. Assume both designs use the same bias-avoiding procedures. Which design is more efficient?

Given that Design A uses twins, each member of the pair serves as the control for the other member of the pair, whereas in Design B the 2n individuals are unrelated. Design A will use a paired t-test, and Design B will use a two-sample t-test to compare the means. The paired t-test statistic is expected to be larger than its two-sample t-test statistic counterpart

DOI: 10.1201/9781003176527-3

because, although the two statistics have the same numerator (sample mean difference), the paired t-test has a smaller denominator (standard error). Design A is thus more efficient (Homework 3.1).

However, the smaller standard error (higher efficiency) resulting from non-negative correlation between the twins comes with a trade-off: Paired twins are more difficult to recruit than unrelated individuals.

Example 3.2

Consider a randomized study to compare two treatment groups, again with a continuous outcome variable. Let the total sample size be fixed and, for simplicity, be large enough that we can comfortably use the standardized normal distribution z-test (rather than a t-test). We have two design options. Design A uses 1:1 allocation, and Design B uses 1:2 (unequal) allocation. Assume the outcome variable has the same variance in both treatment groups. Which design is more efficient?

Design A is more efficient because a statistical test with a balanced design has a smaller variance. The proof is shown in Appendix 3.1.

Discussion: Sometimes we would like to place more patients in the group receiving the investigational medicine than in the control (e.g., placebo) to gain more knowledge about the new compound. In that case, we may use a less efficient unequal allocation. Also note that an unequal allocation design is more efficient when the variances are not the same in the treatment groups. In this case, more patients are needed for the treatment group with greater variance. See Appendix 3.2 for details.

Let the treatment effect be estimated by the observed $\hat{\delta}$ and its *standard error* (se) be expressed as $se(\hat{\delta})$. From the above examples involving t-tests and the z-test, and in general, the form of a Wald test or a score test is

$$T = \frac{\hat{\delta}}{se(\hat{\delta})}$$

We see that T increases as $se(\hat{\delta})$ decreases, implying a more significant result. This would then imply a higher power. The above $se(\hat{\delta})$ usually involves sample size n and an estimate of the population standard deviation (SD). Aiming for a target statistical power, a more efficient design means fewer patients are needed. Alternatively, with a fixed sample size, a more efficient design provides the study with a greater power. In Chapter 4, we discuss the topic of sample size and power. Before we proceed, we look at the cross-over design. This design provides good illustrations for (i) another kind of randomization—randomizing the treatment sequence, (ii) the commonly used concept of the ANOVA cell-means model, and (iii) some trade-offs to be considered in a trial design to gain efficiency.

3.2 Crossover Designs

Crossover designs are commonly used in Phase I *bioavailability* (BA) and *bioequivalence* (BE) pharmacology trials to study the pharmacokinetics (PK)—absorption, distribution, metabolism, and elimination (ADME)—of a new compound in the human body. PK variables of interest include the measurements of peak concentration in blood or urine, time to peak concentration, half-life, and exposure (area under the curve, or AUC) within a certain period of time, usually 24 or 48 hours. A characteristic of a crossover design is that each patient receives the test compound as well as the control agent. In this way, each patient serves as the control for himself or herself. There are many varieties; we study the simplest 2×2 crossover for the purpose of highlighting the trade-offs with efficiency (Table 3.1).

For example, if $n_1 = n_2 = n = 10$, then a total of 20 subjects are in the trial, where all 20 receive A and also B. (In contrast, for a parallel-group design with 20 subjects per treatment group, there would be 40 subjects in total.) Subjects are randomized into the two sequences (AB or BA). The major advantage is an increase in efficiency (i.e., a decrease in the number of subjects). This is due to *pairing*, as we saw in Section 3.1 when we compared the paired identical twins to the unrelated individuals. A trade-off here is the increase in study duration—two periods, plus a *washout period* in between. In addition, a major concern of a crossover design is that, if the washout period is not sufficiently long, based on the half-life of the compounds under study, there may be a *residual effect* from the treatment in the first period added to the (direct) treatment effect of the second period. (For a 3×3 crossover, there would be first-order and second-order residual effects to be concerned about.) Moreover, the residual treatment effects, if they exist, may not be equal in magnitude for the two treatment sequences. Even if there is no residual effect, the experimenter should also check whether a confounding *period effect* is a possibility (e.g., temporal or seasonal effects if the periods occur over different times). Statistically, one can test whether

TABLE 3.1

A 2×2 Crossover Layout

Sequence	Patient	Period 1	Washout Period	Period 2
1	1	A		B
1	2	A		B
1	n_1	A		B
2	1	B		A
2	2	B		A
2	n_2	B		A

Note: Usually, $n_1 = n_2 = n$ (balanced allocation is usually most efficient).

the period effect is (statistically) significant or not. But we should be aware that this test may not have adequate power to test the issue. The statistical nonsignificance does not prove the nonexistence of an effect.

Note that in the literature *residual effect* and *carryover effect* are used interchangeably, and treatment *sequence* and *group* are also used interchangeably in this context.

After the washout period, and before receiving the second-period treatment, subjects' condition should return to the same baseline as in the first period. This is the main reason why the crossover design is suitable for BA/BE studies with healthy volunteers, where returning to the baseline condition after a period of time is achievable. However, this may be greatly influenced by the pharmacokinetics (how long the agent lasts) and the pharmacodynamics (how long the biological effects of the agent last). For example, a cytotoxic agent may clear quickly, whereas the biological effect may last weeks. It is obvious that the crossover design is never used in survival studies. Drugs that elicit an immune response are also not ideal for crossover designs. More discussion on this topic, including drawbacks and limitations of crossover designs, can be found in Louis et al. (1984).

3.3 Analysis of 2 × 2 Crossover Designs

First, consider a model for a general crossover design. Let y_{ijk} be the continuous outcome of the subject k in treatment sequence/group i and period j. A linear model for a general crossover design is expressed in the following:

$$y_{ijk} = E\left(y_{ijk}\right) + e_{ijk}$$

where

$$E\left(y_{ijk}\right) = \mu + \pi_j + \tau_{d[i,j]} + \lambda_{d[i,j-1]} \tag{3.1}$$

and e_{ijk} is the random error with normal distribution $N(0, \sigma^2)$, μ is the grand mean, π_j is the j-th *period effect*, $\tau_{d[i,j]}$ is the *(direct) treatment effect* from sequence i and period j, and $\lambda_{d[i,j-1]}$ is the *residual effect* from the previous period on the same subject. Note that, if there is no residual effect $\left(\lambda_{d[i,j-1]} = 0\right)$ and no period effect $\left(\pi_j = 0\right)$, then the above model reduces to a one-way ANOVA with a paired-data design.

For a 2 × 2 crossover design, i = j = 1, 2. The analysis can be conveniently carried out by a series of t-tests (or rank tests when the distribution is skewed), with the expansion of the above expression to the following cell-means model. That is, in each (Sequence, Period) cell, we write down the mean of the observations as follows:

Sequence	Period 1	Period 2	
1(AB)	$\mu + \pi_1 + \tau_1$	$\mu + \pi_2 + \tau_2 + \lambda_1$	(3.2)
2(BA)	$\mu + \pi_1 + \tau_2$	$\mu + \pi_2 + \tau_1 + \lambda_2$	

The first step is to test for the equality of residual (carryover) effects: $\lambda_1 = \lambda_2$. (Note that this is a weaker condition than no residual effects, $\lambda_1 = \lambda_2 = 0$.) This test can be done as follows. We sum the measurements over the two periods for each subject of the two treatment sequences:

$$t_{1k} = y_{11k} + y_{12k}$$
$$t_{2k} = y_{21k} + y_{22k} \qquad (3.3)$$

Note that

$$E(t_{1k}) = 2\mu + \pi_1 + \pi_2 + \tau_1 + \tau_2 + \lambda_1$$
$$E(t_{2k}) = 2\mu + \pi_1 + \pi_2 + \tau_1 + \tau_2 + \lambda_2$$

Hence, $E(t_{1k} - t_{2k}) = \lambda_1 - \lambda_2$. We can compare the sums t_{1k} and t_{2k} by an independent t-test and obtain T_λ with $n_1 + n_2 - 2$ degrees of freedom (df). Grizzle (1965) suggested to perform this preliminary test at the two-sided $\alpha = 0.10$ level.

The second step is to test for the equality of treatment effects: $\tau_1 = \tau_2$, assuming *equal* residual effects $\lambda_1 = \lambda_2$ (tested by the previous step).

We subtract the measurements between the two periods for each subject of the two treatment sequences:

$$d_{1k} = y_{11k} - y_{12k}$$
$$d_{2k} = y_{21k} - y_{22k} \qquad (3.4)$$

We find:

$$E(d_{1k}) = \pi_1 - \pi_2 + \tau_1 - \tau_2 - \lambda_1$$
$$E(d_{2k}) = \pi_1 - \pi_2 - \tau_1 + \tau_2 - \lambda_2$$

Therefore, $E(d_{1k} - d_{2k}) = 2(\tau_1 - \tau_2)$, since $\lambda_1 = \lambda_2$. We can compare the differences d_{1k} and d_{2k} by an independent t-test and obtain T_τ with df $= n_1 + n_2 - 2$. If the residual effects are not equal, then $E(d_{1k} - d_{2k}) = 2(\tau_1 - \tau_2) - (\lambda_1 - \lambda_2) = (2\tau_1 + \lambda_2) - (2\tau_2 + \lambda_1)$. In this case, the residual effects are *confounded* with the direct treatment effects; hence, we cannot separate τ_1 and λ_2, τ_2 and λ_1.

We can further test the equality of the period effect $\pi_1 = \pi_2$, assuming *no* residual effects $\lambda_1 = \lambda_2 = 0$. To do this, we only need to reverse the second difference in (3.4). Let

$$c_{1k} = d_{1k} = y_{11k} - y_{12k}$$
$$c_{2k} = -d_{2k} = y_{22k} - y_{21k} \qquad (3.5)$$

We find $E(c_{1k} - c_{2k}) = 2(\pi_1 - \pi_2)$. Therefore, we can compare the differences c_{1k} and c_{2k} by an independent t-test and obtain T_π with df $= n_1 + n_2 - 2$. (If the residual effects exist, then they are *confounded* with the period effect.)

Example 3.3

In this example, we examine the data in Table 3.2. For this dataset, $T_\lambda = -1.623$ with $n_1 + n_2 - 2 = 15$ df (p-value>0.10). Thus, we proceed to test for equal direct treatment effects by $T_\tau = -2.162$ with 15 df (p<0.05). Furthermore, we test the equality of the period effect $\pi_1 = \pi_2$, assuming *no* residual effects $\lambda_1 = \lambda_2 = 0$, by $T_\pi = 1.172$ with 15 df (p>0.20) (In-Class Exercise).

TABLE 3.2

A 2×2 Crossover Trial of Acute Bronchial Asthma

Sequence 1 (AB)				Sequence 2 (BA)				
Subject	Period 1	Period 2	Total	Difference	Subject	Period 1	Period 2	Total	Difference
1	1.28	1.33	2.61	−0.05	9	3.06	1.38	4.44	1.68
2	1.6	2.21	3.81	−0.61	10	2.68	2.1	4.78	0.58
3	2.46	2.43	4.89	0.03	11	2.6	2.32	4.92	0.28
4	1.41	1.81	3.22	−0.4	12	1.48	1.3	2.78	0.18
5	1.4	0.85	2.25	0.55	13	2.08	2.34	4.42	−0.26
6	1.12	1.2	2.32	−0.08	14	2.72	2.48	5.2	0.24
7	0.9	0.9	1.8	0	15	1.94	1.11	3.05	0.83
8	2.41	2.79	5.2	−0.38	16	3.35	3.23	6.58	0.12
					17	1.16	1.25	2.41	−0.09

Source: Jones, B$_v$ and Kenward, M. G., *Design and Analysis of Cross-Over Trials*, Chapman and Hall, New York, 1989.

Note: The outcome variable is the forced expired volume (liters) in one second (or FEV_1).

Appendix 3.1: Efficiency of the 1:1 Allocation Assuming Equal Variance

Compare the means of the primary endpoint of two independent treatment groups with a common variance. Show that a balanced design is more efficient than an imbalanced design. In particular, show that a 1:1 allocation is more efficient than a 1:2 allocation.

Proof:

Let $x_1, x_2, \ldots, x_{n_1}$ be the n_1 samples from the treatment group X and $y_1, y_2, \ldots, y_{n_2}$ be the n_2 samples from the treatment group Y. $N = n_1 + n_2$. Assume X and Y are independent and normally distributed with means μ_X and μ_Y, respectively, with common known variance σ^2. To test the hypothesis of $\mu_X = \mu_Y$, the z-test statistic is

$$Z = \frac{\bar{X} - \bar{Y}}{\sqrt{\dfrac{\sigma^2}{n_1} + \dfrac{\sigma^2}{n_2}}} = \sqrt{\frac{n_1 n_2}{n_1 + n_2}} \frac{\bar{X} - \bar{Y}}{\sigma} \tag{3A.1}$$

If $n_1 = n_2 = N/2$, then $\sqrt{\dfrac{n_1 n_2}{n_1 + n_2}} = \sqrt{\dfrac{N}{4}}$.

If $n_1 = N/3, n_2 = 2N/3$, then $\sqrt{\dfrac{n_1 n_2}{n_1 + n_2}} = \sqrt{\dfrac{2N}{9}}$.

Since $1/4 > 2/9$, then the 1:1 allocation results in a larger expected Z-statistic.

In general, let $n_1 = g \times N$, then $\dfrac{n_1 n_2}{n_1 + n_2} = \dfrac{g(1-g)N^2}{N} = g(1-g)N$.

Find the maximum of $g(1-g)$ by solving $\dfrac{dg(1-g)}{dg} = 0$, yielding $g = 1/2$. The second derivative is $-2 < 0$. Therefore, $g = 1/2$ maximizes the expected Z.

Appendix 3.2: Optimal Allocation under Unequal Variance

Using the above setting, let σ_X^2 and σ_Y^2 be the variances of the treatment groups X and Y, respectively. Suppose $\sigma_X^2 \neq \sigma_Y^2$ are known. The z-test statistic for the hypothesis of $\mu_X = \mu_Y$ is

$$Z = \frac{\bar{X} - \bar{Y}}{\sqrt{\dfrac{\sigma_X^2}{n_1} + \dfrac{\sigma_Y^2}{n_2}}} \tag{3A.2}$$

To achieve the maximum power, we would minimize $\dfrac{\sigma_X^2}{n_1} + \dfrac{\sigma_Y^2}{n_2}$ by choosing appropriate n_1 and n_2 subject to $n_1 + n_2 = N$, a prefixed constant. Show that the optimal allocation to treatment group X is $n_1 = g \times N$, where $g = \dfrac{\sigma_X}{\sigma_X + \sigma_Y}$. Equation 3A.1 is a special case where $\sigma_X = \sigma_Y$.

The proof is a homework assignment (Homework 3.3).

Appendix 3.3: Optimizing the Number of Responders

The above discussion on optimal efficiency was designed to maximize the power of testing the hypothesis of equal means of the primary endpoint of two treatment groups by optimally allocating the sample sizes n_1 and n_2 to the two treatment groups, subject to $n_1 + n_2 = N$, a prefixed total N subjects. It boils down to minimizing the denominator of the Z-statistic in Equation 3A.2. There is also another kind of strategy that focuses on maximizing, not the power, but the expected number of "responders" for the trial, subject to a prefixed total N and fixed denominator of Z in Equation 3A.2. The rationale for this kind of strategy is based on optimizing ethics rather than optimizing efficiency. Below is an example similar to Biswas and Mandal (2004).

Suppose that a larger value is more desirable to patients and that there is a threshold constant c such that the subject is a responder if the endpoint value is larger than c. The probability of a non-response in group X is

$P(X < c) = \Phi\left(\dfrac{c - \mu_X}{\sigma_X}\right)$, where $\Phi(\cdot)$ is the cumulative density function

(cdf) of the standard normal distribution. The same is true for group Y. We then minimize the total expected number of non-responders by choosing n_1 and n_2

$$\min\left\{n_1\Phi\left(\frac{c - \sigma_X}{\sigma_X}\right) + n_2\Phi\left(\frac{c - \mu_X}{\sigma_Y}\right)\right\} \tag{3A.3}$$

subject to $n_1 + n_2 = N$, as well as $\dfrac{\sigma_X^2}{n_1} + \dfrac{\sigma_Y^2}{n_2} = K$. Both N and K are prefixed

constants. The restriction on $\dfrac{\sigma_X^2}{n_1} + \dfrac{\sigma_Y^2}{n_2}$ will preserve a specified level of power

for the test of equal means. The solution of Equation 3A.3 with the restrictions yields g, the optimal allocation proportion of subjects to treatment group X, as

$$g = \frac{\sigma_X\sqrt{\Phi\left(\dfrac{c - \mu_Y}{\sigma_Y}\right)}}{\sigma_X\sqrt{\Phi\left(\dfrac{c - \mu_Y}{\sigma_Y}\right)} + \sigma_Y\sqrt{\Phi\left(\dfrac{c - \mu_X}{\sigma_X}\right)}} \tag{3A.4}$$

Proof:
Homework 3.4.
In practice, the design is implemented by assuming some initial values, then estimating the parameters using the available data up to the first cohort of patients, and finally plugging them into Equation 3A.4 to find the optimal allocation proportion to treatment X for the next cohort of patients. Relating this procedure to the minimization method for sequential allocation of the

next patient based on balancing the distribution of baseline covariates of previous enrollments (see Chapter 2), this procedure is a response-adaptive design for continuous endpoints. Other designs of this kind include Zelen's (1969) "play the winner rule."

HOMEWORK 3.1

Review the independent t-test and the paired t-test statistics and show the answer statement for Example 3.1.

HOMEWORK 3.2[1]

Table 3.3 (Weight Loss Data) displays outcome data and calculations of Equations 3.3 and 3.4 from a clinical trial on weight loss (kg) with the test drug mCPP versus placebo using a 2×2 crossover design. The test drug mCPP is denoted by D (drug) and the placebo by P.

1. First, we simply assume that there are no carryover and no period effects. Because this is a small dataset, we prefer to carry out the basic nonparametric sign test for equal treatment effects. The readers should review the sign test from an introductory-level statistics textbook (Daniel 2009; see also Chapter 2) and apply it to these data.

2. Second, use the cell-means model to test the hypothesis regarding the assumption of equal carryover effect, whether there is a treatment effect, and whether there is a period effect (with necessary assumptions) by (a) independent t-tests (available in SAS PROC ttest) and by (b) Wilcoxon rank-sum test (available in SAS PROC npar1way) due to the small sample size.

TABLE 3.3

Weight Loss Data (kg)

	Sequence 1 (DP)				Sequence 2 (PD)			
Subject (k)	Period 1 (y_{11k})	Period 2 (y_{12k})	Total (t_{1k})	Difference (d_{1k})	Subject (k)	Period 1 (y_{21k})	Period 2 (y_{22k})	Total (t_{2k})	Difference (d_{2k})
1	1.1	0.0	1.1	1.1	6	−0.2	0.1	−0.1	−0.3
2	1.3	−0.3	1.0	1.6	7	0.6	0.5	1.1	0.1
3	1.0	0.6	1.6	0.4	8	0.9	1.6	2.5	−0.7
4	1.7	0.3	2.0	1.4	9	−2.0	−0.5	−2.5	−1.5
5	1.4	−0.7	0.7	2.1					

---

[1] Homework problem 3.2 was contributed by Dirk F. Moore.

HOMEWORK 3.3

Prove the assertion of Appendix 3.2.

HOMEWORK 3.4

Prove the assertion of Appendix 3.3.

References

Biswas A and Mandal S. (2004). Optimal adaptive designs in Phase III clinical trials for continuous responses with covariates. In *m0Da 7—Advances in Model-Oriented Design and Analysis*, Di Bucchianico A, Lauter H, and Wynn HP (Eds.), Heidelberg, Germany: Physica-Verlag; 51–58.

Daniel WW. (2009). *Biostatistics: A Foundation for Analysis in the Health Sciences*. New York: Wiley.

Grizzle JE. (1965). The two-period change-over design and its use in clinical trials. *Biometrics* 21: 467–480.

Jones B and Kenward MG. (1989). *Design and Analysis of Cross-Over Trials*. New York: Chapman and Hall.

Louis TA, Lavori PW, Bailar JC, and Polansky M. (1984). Crossover and self-controlled designs in clinical research. *New England Journal of Medicine* 310: 24–31.

Zelen M. (1969). Play the winner rule and the controlled clinical trial. *Journal of the American Statistical Association* 64:131–146.

4

Sample Size and Power Calculations

Some authors choose to refer to the topic of sample size calculation as sample size *estimation*. This word choice is understandable because the calculation of the sample size for a clinical trial is based on design parameters whose values are *estimated* from previous data, or some other form of external information or assumptions. On the other hand, some authors prefer to use the term *calculation* for sample size to distinguish from the estimation of a model parameter in the context of making statistical inferences; these estimated values are usually assumed as fixed in the calculation, and seldom considered for their uncertainty. We use calculation and estimation interchangeably in this book.

In previous chapters, we discussed how clinical trials should be designed to minimize potential bias and to balance efficiency and generalizability (homogeneous versus heterogeneous samples). We should also check feasibility and ensure enough resources are available to conduct the study, in order to detect a clinically meaningful treatment effect that impacts medical practice, which is the ultimate goal of a clinical trial. The aspects of feasibility and resources are also relevant to sample size and study power.

In Chapter 3, we briefly discussed the concept of efficiency of a trial in terms of sample size and power. If one design, say Design A, can achieve the same power to detect the same effect size as another design, say Design B, but with a smaller sample size, then Design A is more efficient. Equivalently, if Design A, with the same sample size, can achieve a higher power than Design B can, then Design A is more efficient.

When the sample size is inadequate, the study is underpowered. An underpowered study will render inconclusive results; that is, the study may not be able to detect an existing important treatment effect. On the other hand, when the sample size is too large, the study is overpowered. An overpowered study wastes resources and affects its feasibility. That is, it may be unaffordable or not fundable or it may detect a small, nonmeaningful treatment effect. The question is: how can we design a trial with an appropriate sample size that is "just right?"

4.1 Fundamentals and General Formula

The readers are expected to have understood the basics of hypothesis testing, including the notion of a null hypothesis (H_0) versus an alternative hypothesis (H_A), and the associated type I error (false-positive) rate (often denoted as α) and type II error (false-negative) rate (often denoted as β), and power (which equals $1 - \beta$). A two-sided test at an α level, or a one-sided test at an $\alpha/2$ level, is commonly used in industrial and regulatory practice, but not necessarily followed by academic studies that are more exploratory in nature. Conventionally, α is set to be 1% or 5%, and β may be 10%, 15%, or 20%.

Although there are many software available such as PROC POWER in SAS, R package pwr (Champely 2018), a menu-driven Stata program for the calculation of sample size or power for complex clinical trial designs under a survival time or binary outcome (Barthel, Royston and Babiker 2005), and http://powerandsamplesize.com/Calculators/ on the web, the readers need to understand the basic concept and the assumptions of the formulas of sample size and power calculations. The general formula is presented here first and then applied to the specific outcomes in the following sections. We also discuss the Monte Carlo simulation method in the final section.

Follow the notation in Chapter 3. Denote the true (unknown) treatment effect by δ, which is estimated by the observed $\hat{\delta}$. Let its associated *standard error* (se) be expressed as $\text{se}(\hat{\delta})$. The null hypothesis of equal treatment effect between two treatment groups is denoted by

$$H_0 : \delta = 0$$

It is convenient to think that we are interested in the one-side alternative hypothesis:

$$H_A : \delta > 0.$$

The form of a Wald test statistic or a score test statistic is expressed as

$$T = \frac{\hat{\delta}}{\text{se}(\hat{\delta})}$$

We shall see that $\text{se}(\hat{\delta})$ involves the sample size. For a score test, $\text{se}(\hat{\delta})$ is always derived under the null hypothesis. For a Wald test, $\text{se}(\hat{\delta})$ may be different under the null from that under the alternative hypothesis. To be explicit, we write $\text{se}(\hat{\delta})_0$ and $\text{se}(\hat{\delta})_A$, respectively, for the two situations T_0 and T_A. In general, $\hat{\delta}$ should be an unbiased estimate of δ. We also assume that the sample

TABLE 4.1

Commonly Used Upper Quantiles of the Standard
Normal Distribution

$z_{0.01}$	=	2.326	=	$-z_{0.99}$
$z_{0.025}$	=	1.96	=	$-z_{0.975}$
$z_{0.05}$	=	1.645	=	$-z_{0.95}$
$z_{0.10}$	=	1.28	=	$-z_{0.90}$
$z_{0.15}$	=	1.04	=	$-z_{0.85}$
$z_{0.20}$	=	0.84	=	$-z_{0.80}$

size is large enough to justify that $\hat{\delta}$ is normally distributed by the Central Limit Theorem.

As seen in Appendix in Chapter 3, the *cumulative distribution function* (cdf) of the standard normal distribution is denoted by $\Phi(z) = \Pr(Z < z)$. The upper $100 \times \alpha$ percentile of Φ is denoted by $z_\alpha = \Phi^{-1}(1 - \alpha) = -\Phi^{-1}(\alpha) = -z_{1-\alpha}$. Table 4.1 gives examples of z_α that are useful for common practice of statistics in clinical trials.

Under the null hypothesis, $T_0 = \dfrac{\hat{\delta}}{se(\hat{\delta})_0}$ has a standard normal distribution.

To satisfy the type I error rate requirement, under the null hypothesis, the critical value c for the test is $\alpha/2 = \Pr(T_0 > c \mid H_0)$, which implies that the critical value $c = z_{\alpha/2} = -z_{1-\alpha/2}$. The desired power, by definition, is, under the alternative hypothesis,

$$1 - \beta = \Pr\left(T_0 > c \mid H_A\right) = \Pr\left(T_0 > z_{\alpha/2} \mid H_A\right)$$

$$= \Pr\left(\frac{\hat{\delta}}{se(\hat{\delta})_0} > z_{\alpha/2} \mid H_A\right)$$

$$= \Pr\left(\frac{\hat{\delta}}{se(\hat{\delta})_0} \times \frac{se(\hat{\delta})_0}{se(\hat{\delta})_A} - \frac{\delta}{se(\hat{\delta})_A} > z_{\alpha/2} \times \frac{se(\hat{\delta})_0}{se(\hat{\delta})_A} - \frac{\delta}{se(\hat{\delta})_A} \mid H_A\right)$$

$$= \Pr\left(\frac{\hat{\delta} - \delta}{se(\hat{\delta})_A} > b \mid H_A\right)$$

$$= 1 - \Phi(b)$$

$$\text{where } b = z_{\alpha/2} \times \frac{\text{se}\left(\hat{\delta}\right)_0}{\text{se}\left(\hat{\delta}\right)_A} - \frac{\delta}{\text{se}\left(\hat{\delta}\right)_A} = \Phi^{-1}(\beta) = -z_\beta$$

Therefore, a general formula is:

$$\left(z_{\alpha/2}\right)\text{se}\left(\hat{\delta}\right)_0 - \delta = \left(-z_\beta\right)\text{se}\left(\hat{\delta}\right)_A \quad\quad\quad (4.1)$$

Or, $\left(z_{\alpha/2}\right)\text{se}\left(\hat{\delta}\right)_0 + \left(z_\beta\right)\text{se}\left(\hat{\delta}\right)_A = \delta = \text{E}\left(\hat{\delta}\right)$

In the following sections, we apply this general formula to different situations of comparisons of two treatment groups with different kinds of outcome variables (endpoints).

4.2 Comparing Means for Continuous Outcomes

For a randomized design with an equal allocation, which compares two parallel (independent) treatment groups with a continuous outcome, let $Y_{11}, \ldots, Y_{n1}$ be the n independent observations from Treatment 1 and $Y_{12}, \ldots, Y_{n2}$ be the other n independent observations from Treatment 2, so that the total sample size is $N = 2n$. Y could also be a change or percent change from baseline for each patient's laboratory or clinical measurements. We would like to test the null hypothesis of equal means as denoted by

$$H_0 : \delta = \mu_1 - \mu_2 = 0$$

The difference of the sample means $\hat{\delta} = \bar{Y}_1 - \bar{Y}_2$ is the estimated treatment effect. We apply *large sample theory* to the sample means so that there is no need to assume the parent distribution is normal, but an equal variance for the distribution of the two groups ($= \sigma^2$) is a convenient assumption. Recall that this equal variance leads to the optimal balanced allocation $n_1 = n_2 = n$ (see Chapter 3). Let s^2 be the sample variance estimator pooled from both groups. The squared standard error (se) of $\hat{\delta} = \bar{Y}_1 - \bar{Y}_2$ is equal to $2s^2/n$ either under the null or under the alternative hypothesis, and the Wald test statistic is

$$T = \frac{\hat{\delta}}{\text{se}\left(\hat{\delta}\right)}$$

$$= \sqrt{\frac{n}{2}} \frac{(\bar{Y}_1 - \bar{Y}_2)}{s} \qquad (4.2)$$

T follows the t distribution with $2(n-1)$ degrees of freedom. With a large sample size, the t distribution approaches the normal distribution. When designing a study, we assume a known value for σ^2. Then $T = Z$ (replacing s^2 in T with σ^2), whose distribution is the standard normal, $N(0,1)$, under the null hypothesis. Under the alternative hypothesis, T is normally distributed with mean $\delta\sqrt{\frac{n}{2\sigma^2}}$ and variance 1. The required sample size can be obtained from Equation (4.1), where we plug in $se(\hat{\delta})_0 = se(\hat{\delta})_A = \sqrt{\frac{2\sigma^2}{n}}$.

Hence, we obtain

$$n = \frac{2\sigma^2 \left(z_{\alpha/2} + z_\beta\right)^2}{\delta^2} \qquad (4.3)$$

That is, we require a sample size of n in each treatment group to detect a mean difference of δ with a power of $1 - \beta$ by a one-sided test with type I error rate of $\alpha/2$. The total $N = 2n$. If there are three treatment groups of equal size, then $N = 3n$, etc. The same formula (Equation 4.3) applies to an evenly split α-level two-sided test $|T| > z_{\alpha/2}$ as well. This is because

$$\Pr(|T| > z_{\alpha/2}) = \Pr(T < -z_{\alpha/2}) + \Pr(T > z_{\alpha/2}) \approx \Pr(T > z_{\alpha/2})$$

where the first term is almost 0 under H_A. Formula (4.3) is for even $(1:1) = (\frac{1}{2} : \frac{1}{2})$ allocation. For $r:(1-r)$ allocation, $n_1 = rN$, $n_2 = (1-r)N$, then we express the total sample size N:

$$N = \frac{1}{r(1-r)} \frac{\sigma^2 \left(z_{\alpha/2} + z_\beta\right)^2}{\delta^2} \qquad (4.4)$$

Note that Equation (4.4) is minimum when $r = 1/2$ (equal allocation). The form of Equation (4.3) or (4.4) will also be useful for other sample size calculations in the next few sections for different endpoints.

The power and alpha level are set more or less by convention (Table 4.1). The factors that are not preset and matter the most for estimating the required sample size are σ and δ. The ratio of δ/σ is the *standardized treatment difference*, which is also referred to as *(treatment) effect size*. Its reciprocal is the *coefficient of variation* σ/δ. The power curve is a function of the sample size and the treatment effect size for a given trial. As shown in Equation 4.4, a smaller effect size δ/σ (or, equivalently, a larger coefficient of variation) requires a larger sample size. A general idea for the magnitude of sample size is listed below for $\alpha/2 = 0.025$ and $1 - \beta = 0.80$:

$$\delta/\sigma \quad \approx 0.2\,(\text{small effect size}) \text{ requires } n \approx 400$$
$$\approx 0.5\,(\text{medium effect size}) \text{ requires } n \approx 70$$
$$\approx 0.8\,(\text{large effect size}) \text{ requires } n \approx 25$$

In practice, one should review the literature or prior studies to obtain an idea of the control group's μ_2 and σ. If the control is a placebo, then the disease's natural history provides valuable background information. The project statistician should consult with the clinical investigator regarding a meaningful or expected treatment difference δ. Note that clinical investigators often express expected treatment effect in terms of the relative change, $r = (\mu_1 - \mu_2)/\mu_2$, instead of the absolute change $\delta = \mu_1 - \mu_2$. With the information on μ_2 and r, it is just a simple step to convert r to $\delta = r\mu_2$.

Information regarding the within-group σ is more difficult to obtain. A homogeneous patient cohort will have a smaller σ, and from Equation 4.3, we can see that a smaller σ results in a smaller n (i.e., a more efficient design). However, a homogeneous cohort comes at the expense of limited generalizability to a wider, more heterogeneous population. A method to include a heterogeneous population while maintaining study efficiency is the stratified randomization design. With a stratified randomization, using a prognostic factor as a covariate in the analysis reduces the variance σ^2. (That is, it reduces the variance from marginal to conditional variance.) This fact also reminds us that, when using data from another study as a reference, we need to be sure to use the right *mean squared error* (MSE) from the ANOVA or ANCOVA (analysis of covariance) for an appropriate estimate of σ^2. Unfortunately, the medical literature usually publishes little information about variance. Sometimes we need to go several steps into a paper's summary table to find a useful estimate of the variance. For example, it sometimes is hidden in the confidence intervals. A recent medical paper by Puntoni et al. (2013) provides a good exercise (Homework 4.1).

Specifically, for a linear regression model (which includes ANOVA/ANCOVA) with several covariates expressed as

$$Y = \beta_0 + \beta_1 X_1 + \beta_2 X_2 + \ldots + \beta_k X_K + e \qquad (4.5)$$

the marginal variance of Y, $\text{Var}(Y) = \sigma_Y^2$, could be very large. (This would induce a large, conservative sample size.) The conditional variance (adjusted for covariates), $\text{Var}(Y \mid X) = \text{Var}(e) = \sigma_e^2$, is more suitable for the sample size estimation formula (Equation 4.3), if the same covariates are used in the new trial as in the literature. In fact, the derivation setting we considered was just for treatment group being the only covariate in Equation (4.5). Note that, in general, $\sigma_e^2 = (1 - R^2)\sigma_Y^2$, where R is the multiple correlation of the covariates with the outcome Y. The reduction in the variance depends on the prognostic importance of the covariates to the outcome Y. More discussion of ANCOVA is given in Chapter 5. The readers may want to review linear regression analysis (e.g., Weisberg 1985) as homework (Homework 4.2).

In practice, because investigators are often not certain about the effect size, it is useful to present a table or a power function graph for a range of (per group) sample sizes and possible effect sizes via Equation 4.6 when preparing a study proposal or trial protocol. From (4.3), the power is:

$$1 - \beta = \Phi\left(\sqrt{\frac{n}{2}}\frac{\delta}{\sigma} - z_{\alpha/2}\right) \tag{4.6}$$

where, as noted before, $\sqrt{\frac{n}{2}}\frac{\delta}{\sigma} = E(Z \mid H_A)$. Equation (4.6) also indicates $E(Z \mid H_A) = z_{\alpha/2} + z_\beta$.

Example 4.1

A randomized trial was conducted to assess the effectiveness of Relenza, a new treatment for influenza, compared with placebo. The primary variable of interest was the number of days to alleviation of symptoms. A previous study suggested that a sensible value for σ was 2.75 days. The minimally clinically relevant difference, δ, that the trial should have a good power to detect, was taken to be 1 day. The investigators used a significance level of $\alpha = 0.05$ (two-sided) and aimed for 90% power ($\beta = 0.1$). We calculate the sample size per group to meet these design parameters as follows:

$$n = \frac{2(z_{\alpha/2} + z_\beta)^2}{(\delta/\sigma)^2} = \frac{2(1.96 + 1.28)^2}{(1/2.75)^2} = 158.8 \approx 160$$

Rounding the sample size up to a convenient integer is a common-sense practice for conservativeness. Sample size estimation is not exact mathematics because the design factors we assume (such as $\sigma = 2.75$) are approximations. Figure 4.1 presents a power curve for a range of alternative values $\delta = \mu_1 - \mu_2$ for $n = 160$ per group. It is also informative to depict the power functions for different scenarios of sample size, as shown in Figure 4.2. When showing a power curve as a function of δ, values of δ are interpreted as detectable differences, for which the minimally clinically relevant difference is one of them with the targeted power.

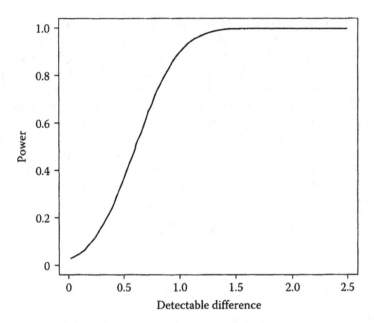

FIGURE 4.1
Power curve versus detectable $\delta = \mu_1 - \mu_2$ for n = 160 per group.

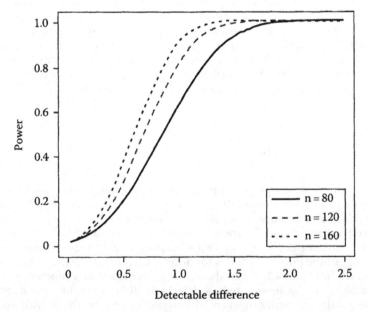

FIGURE 4.2
Power plot: Power versus detectable difference in means for different n.

4.3 Comparing Proportions for Binary Outcomes

For a randomized design with an equal allocation that compares two parallel treatment groups with a binary outcome, let $Y_i = 0$ or 1 ($= 1$ with probability π_i) for group $i = 1$ or 2. Without loss of generality, we let $Y = 1$ when observing an outcome event. The mean and variance parameters are

$$E(Y_i) = \pi_i$$

$$Var(Y_i) = \pi_i(1 - \pi_i)$$

The treatment effect of interest may be the difference in the probability of an event in the two treatment groups: $\delta = \pi_1 - \pi_2$. Other measures such as rate ratio π_1/π_2 or odds ratio $\pi_1(1 - \pi_2)/\pi_2(1 - \pi_1)$ are not considered in this section. The rate ratio can be transformed by taking the (natural) logarithm, and the variance for the difference in the log scale can be derived using the delta method (Homework 4.4). See Appendix 4.3 for the delta method. A method for odds ratio is included as a special case in Section 4.7. The null hypothesis of equal probability of the event occurring in both treatment groups is H_0: $\delta = 0$.

Sample estimates of the event probability π_1 and π_2 are proportions p_1 and p_2, respectively. Under H_0 ($\pi_1 = \pi_2$), the variance of $p_1 - p_2$ is

$$V_0 = \frac{2\bar{\pi}(1 - \bar{\pi})}{n}$$

where $\bar{\pi} = (\pi_1 + \pi_2)/2$ is the average probability of event over the treatment groups. That is, $se(\hat{\delta})_0 = \sqrt{V_0}$.

Under H_A, the variance of $p_1 - p_2$ is

$$V_1 = \frac{\pi_1(1 - \pi_1) + \pi_2(1 - \pi_2)}{n}$$

That is, $se(\hat{\delta})_A = \sqrt{V_1}$.

There are two kinds of formulas given for tests of proportions in many introductory biostatistics books. One is

$$n = \frac{2\bar{\pi}(1 - \bar{\pi})(z_{\alpha/2} + z_\beta)^2}{\delta^2} \tag{4.7}$$

which is based on the *score test*. The derivation follows the same procedure as Equation 4.3 using the variance of $(p_1 - p_2)$ under H_0. (For the score test, the se in the denominator of the test is derived under the null hypothesis.)

The other formula is based on the *Wald test*, also derived from the general formula (4.1), where we plug in $se\left(\hat{\delta}\right)_0 = \sqrt{V_0}$ and $se\left(\hat{\delta}\right)_A = \sqrt{V_1}$ to obtain:

$$n = \frac{\left(z_{\alpha/2}\sqrt{2\bar{\pi}(1-\bar{\pi})} + z_{\beta}\sqrt{\pi_1(1-\pi_1) + \pi_2(1-\pi_2)}\right)^2}{\delta^2} \qquad (4.8)$$

Again, n is the number of subjects required for each treatment group in order to detect a difference of at least δ with power $(1-\beta) \times 100\%$ using a two-sided α-level or one-sided $\alpha/2$-level test. The Wald test and the score test are asymptotically equivalent; hence, the n calculated from these two formulas should not be too different. The formula based on the score test is certainly simpler; thus, it is also used in many other places, such as the group sequential design, as we see in Chapter 9.

4.4 Comparing Time-to-Event (Survival) Endpoints

4.4.1 Outcome Event

For a trial with time-to-event data, it is important to define the *outcome event*. Often, the primary and the secondary endpoints refer to different sets of events. The event for the *overall survival* (OS) endpoint is death from any cause; that is, the event is all-cause mortality. For the endpoint of *progression-free survival* (PFS), both death and disease progression are counted as the outcome event, whichever occurs first. For the endpoint of *time to progression* (TTP), however, only disease progression is counted as the outcome event, whereas death prior to progression is considered a *censoring event*. TTP is used mostly in tumor recurrence studies. A good reference that discusses the merits of OS, PFS, and TTP in cancer trials is the FDA guidance document *Guidance for Industry: Clinical Trial Endpoints for the Approval of Cancer Drugs and Biologics* (CDER and CBER 2005). In cancer trials, determining disease progression in solid tumors involves measuring the tumor size physically or by radiologic images/scans and the radiologist's subjective assessment. How to standardize and maintain the quality of the progression assessment is an important issue of design and conduct for clinical trials with this type of data. Without ambiguity, we use the general term "survival" for all types of time-to-event variables in the following discussion.

4.4.2 Exponential Distribution Model with and without Censoring

Commonly used tests for comparing two time-to-event (survival) curves can be derived in several different ways: nonparametrically by combining a sequence of hypergeometric 2×2 tables, semi-parametrically by using the partial likelihood function, or parametrically by assuming a distribution such as the exponential or the Weibull distribution model (see, e.g., Collett 1994). Some basic points of survival data analysis are given in Appendices 4.2–4.5 of this chapter. More on survival data analysis methods are given in Chapter 6. For a simple sample size calculation, the parametric approach is the easiest. In this section, we derive a formula for sample size under the exponential distribution without and with censoring.

Assume equal allocation of two treatment groups in a randomized trial. Let $y_{11}, ..., y_{1n}$ be the times to event in the test group; they are identically, independently distributed (iid) from the exponential distribution with the probability density function (pdf)

$$f_1(y) = \lambda_1 e^{-\lambda_1 y}$$

And let $y_{21}, ..., y_{2n}$ be the times to event in the control group, iid with pdf

$$f_2(y) = \lambda_2 e^{-\lambda_2 y}$$

The parameter $\lambda > 0$ in the exponential model is called the *hazard rate*. With the exponential model, we explicitly assume that the hazard rate is a constant over time. First, let us assume no censoring; that is, everyone has an event, so that the event number $d = n$ per treatment group, and the total event number is $D = 2n = 2d$. This is similar to assuming no missing data in the continuous or the binary case; actually, without censoring, this endpoint is also a continuous variable: time. The adjustment of randomly missing data in a continuous case or randomly censored data in this case is explained in Section 4.8.3.

We are interested in comparing the hazard rates between the two treatment groups. This is typically done by testing the (natural) log of the hazard ratios, log(HR). The null hypothesis of equal hazard rates is

$$H_0 : \log(\lambda_1/\lambda_2) = 0$$

Let $\bar{Y}_1 = \sum_1^n y_{1i}/n$. The *maximum likelihood estimate* (MLE) of the hazard rate λ_1 and its asymptotic distribution are

$$\hat{\lambda}_1 = \frac{1}{\bar{Y}_1} \sim AN\left(\lambda_1, \frac{\lambda_1^2}{n}\right)$$

(See Appendix 4.3. The notation *AN* above stands for *asymptotic normal distribution*.) However, $\log(\hat{\lambda}_1)$ has a better normal approximation than $\hat{\lambda}_1$. Using the delta method, we can find the distribution of $\log(\hat{\lambda}_1)$:

$$\log\left(\hat{\lambda}_1\right) \sim N\left(\log \lambda_1, \frac{1}{n}\right) \qquad (4.9)$$

The same is true for the hazard rate λ_2. (See Appendix 4.3 for the delta method.)

We then apply the same formula as in the continuous case (Equation 4.3), where Equation 4.9 corresponds to the form of $\overline{X} \sim N\left(\mu, \frac{\sigma^2}{n}\right)$. By switching parameters: $\delta = \log(\lambda_1/\lambda_2)$ and $\sigma = 1$ (since n = d without censoring), we have

$$d = \frac{2\left(Z_{\alpha/2} + Z_\beta\right)^2}{\delta^2}$$

Or, as commonly used for a survival study, the total number of events:

$$D = \frac{4\left(Z_{\alpha/2} + Z_\beta\right)^2}{\delta^2} \qquad (4.10)$$

In Equation 4.10, we need to determine the value of $\delta = \log(\lambda_1/\lambda_2)$. This is often accomplished by finding out the reference hazard rate, λ_2, from the literature and proposing a percent decrease for the test agent for λ_1. Medical literature often reports a landmark survival time (e.g., 5-year survival probability) or a median survival time (if reached). Because the cumulative survival function $S(y) = 1 - F(y)$, and then for the exponential model,

$$S(y) = \exp(-\lambda y) \qquad (4.11)$$

we can convert the landmark survival probability or the median survival time to the hazard rate (Homework 4.5). Table 4.2 lists survival summaries for three different exponential distribution models.

Equation 4.10 is simple in the sense that it unrealistically assumes no censoring and that all patients reach the endpoint (i.e., there is no definite study end time). Now, let us consider censoring in the following scenario:

Suppose that the random censoring time C (perhaps as a result of a competing risk such as adverse events in a time-to-pain-relief study or death

TABLE 4.2

Survival Summaries with Exponential Distribution Models

Hazard Rate (λ)	Mean Survival Time ($1/\lambda$)	Standard Deviation of Survival Time ($1/\lambda$)	Median Survival Time (($\log 2)/\lambda$)
1.5	0.67	0.67	0.46
1.0	1.00	1.00	0.69
0.5	2.00	2.00	1.39

in a TTP cancer study) is independent of the (outcome) event time and is also exponentially distributed with the same parameter η for both treatment groups. Then the probability of observing an outcome event in the test group during the study (of length L) is

$$P_1 = \Pr(Y_1 < L, Y_1 < C) = \int_0^L \left[\int_u^\infty \eta e^{-\eta c} dc \right] \lambda_1 e^{-\lambda_1 u} du$$

(4.12)

$$= \frac{\lambda_1}{\lambda_1 + \eta} \left(1 - e^{-(\lambda_1 + \eta)L} \right)$$

Likewise,

$$P_2 = \frac{\lambda_2}{\lambda_2 + \eta} \left(1 - e^{-(\lambda_2 + \eta)L} \right)$$

With an equal allocation of patients, n, per group, the total expected number of events is

$$D = d_1 + d_2 = n(P_1 + P_2)$$

Hence, to adjust for censoring, we can first calculate D from Equation 4.10, and then the number of patients needed per group is

$$n = D/(P_1 + P_2)$$

(4.13)

The hazard rate of the censoring due to withdrawal, $\eta > 0$, has to be assumed as well for Equation 4.12. Like the hazard rate for the outcome event, one can assume a cumulative censoring rate and convert it to η. The case $\eta = 0$ reduces to the case where the censoring of outcome event is only due to the finite study end time L. That is, $P_i = \Pr(Y_i < L) = 1 - e^{-\lambda_i L}$ for $i = 1, 2$ (Homework 4.6).

Alternatively, one can use the assumed cumulative censoring rate directly to make an adjustment. Section 4.8.1 uses this simple approach. Note that Equation 4.13 assumes that all patients are enrolled at time 0, which is not realistic in practice. However, the same formula applies to the more realistic case of random (right) censoring due to staggered entry of patients with the same study duration for each patient. When patients have different follow-up durations (e.g., early entries have longer follow-up than later entries for the same study end time), the entry pattern will determine the differential follow-up times; hence, a more complicated formula involving entry distribution within recruitment time is needed. Further information about this topic is discussed in Chapter 10.

In addition, clinical trials with a time-to-event endpoint, especially when the event is fatal or life-threatening (myocardial infarction, stroke, cancer progression, etc.), usually involve group sequential designs with interim analyses. In Chapter 9, we cover the maximum sample size and expected sample size for group sequential trials. In Chapter 10, we discuss the monitoring of the maximum sample size.

4.4.3 Log-Rank Test under Weibull Distribution

The hazard rate under the exponential model is constant over time. Sometimes, the hazard rate may not be constant, but increasing or decreasing over time. In that case, it is a function of time, which can be denoted as $h(t)$, and a Weibull distribution is a better choice of model. If a random variable $X \sim \exp(\lambda)$, then $Y = X^{1/k} \sim \text{Weibull}(\lambda, k)$. The parameter k (>0) controls how the hazard function $h(t)$ varies with time (i.e., the shape of the hazard function). If $k > 1$, then the hazard is increasing with time; otherwise, if $0 < k < 1$, it is decreasing with time. For sample size calculation, one needs to first assume a value for this shape parameter (a common k value for both treatment groups). To be specific, the hazard function of a Weibull(λ, k) is

$$h(t) = k\lambda^k t^{k-1} \tag{4.14}$$

and the survival distribution is

$$S(t) = e^{-(\lambda t)^k} \tag{4.15}$$

The null hypothesis can be expressed in terms of the median survival time:

$$m = [\log(2)]^{(1/k)} / \lambda \tag{4.16}$$

or, equivalently, in terms of transformed λ as

$$\theta = \lambda^k = \log(2) / m^k \tag{4.17}$$

That is, the null hypothesis is that the two treatment groups have equal median survival times or equal θ. Note that Y^k (= X) is $\exp(\theta)$. Comparing Equation 4.15 to Equation 4.11, we find that for a specific k, if we regard $\theta = \lambda^k$ as the parameter of interest, with the transformed time t^k, then the model simplifies to the exponential model and we can utilize the result found there. From Equation 4.10, we obtain the needed total number of events:

$$D = \frac{4(Z_{\alpha/2} + Z_\beta)^2}{\delta^2}$$

$$= \frac{4(Z_{\alpha/2} + Z_\beta)^2}{\left[\log\left(\frac{\theta_1}{\theta_2}\right)\right]^2} \tag{4.18}$$

where θ_1 and θ_2 are the median survival times m_1 and m_2, respectively, from Equation 4.17 for the two treatment groups under the alternative hypothesis.

4.4.4 Log-Rank Test under Proportional Hazards Model

The formulas in Equations 4.10 and 4.18 are based on parametric model assumptions. Semi-parametrically, we can also work out a sample size formula for a general proportional hazards model as argued in the following, without going through mathematical details.

First, we note whether the hazard rate is a constant (as in the exponential model) or a function of time (as in the Weibull model); the null hypothesis uses the log of median survival times. The median survival time is a function of the parameter(s) that is (are) not a function of time. The proportional hazards model is a general setting, which says that the ratio of the hazards is a constant, although the hazards may change over time. Specifically, the general model is expressed as

$$h_1(t) = \varphi h_2(t) \qquad (4.19)$$

where $h_i(t)$ is the hazard function of the outcome event for the treatment group i, $i = 1, 2$. In terms of the survival function, it is

$$S_1(t) = \left[S_2(t)\right]^\varphi \qquad (4.20)$$

without specifying a parametric distribution.

The null hypothesis of interest is $\varphi = 1$, or $\log(\varphi) = 0$. The parameter φ is the *hazard ratio* (HR), where $\varphi = \lambda_1/\lambda_2$ for the exponential model, and $\varphi = \theta_1/\theta_2 = (\lambda_1/\lambda_2)^k$ for the Weibull model.

Using the large sample theory of the score statistic, one can derive the nonparametric version of the log-rank test. The general formula for the total number of events needed is the same as before:

$$D = \frac{4\left(Z_{\alpha/2} + Z_\beta\right)^2}{\delta^2}$$

where δ is the treatment effect expressed in the alternative hypothesis, which is the log of the hazard ratio, or $\log(\text{HR}) = \log(\varphi)$.

4.5 Clustered (or Correlated) Observations

In some clinical trials, *subunits* are clustered within the *main unit* (*cluster*). The treatment is randomized and administered to the main unit, but measurements are taken on the subunit. Hence, the subunits nested within a main unit are correlated observations. Examples include the following:

- Dental studies, in which a tooth is the subunit, nested in a patient (main unit or cluster).
- A repeated measures design, where an observation at each time point is a subunit, nested in the subject.
- Community trials, such as trials on teaching methods, in which students are taught in classes. The class is the main unit, and the students are the subunits nested in each class.

In a randomized trial that compares Group X versus Group Y with equal allocation, let the observations in Group Y be denoted as

$$Y_{ij}; \ i = 1, \ldots, n \ (\text{main unit}); j = 1, \ldots, m_i \ (\text{subunit})$$

By design, we often set $m_i = m$ for all i so that all main units contain the same number of subunits. In this setting, the treatment group is a "fixed" effect, and the main unit (cluster) is a "random" effect. Together, we have a "mixed" effect model. To simplify the notation, we can write down a simple random effect model separately for each treatment group, just like we did previously for the two independent treatment groups before we combine them in a linear model setting with a covariate designated for the fixed treatment group. The random effect model is useful to induce the correlation among the subunits as follows: Let

$$Y_{ij} = \mu_i + e_{ij}; \ \mu_i \text{ and } e_{ij} \text{ are independent} \qquad (4.21)$$

with

$$E(\mu_i) = \mu_Y, \ \text{Var}(\mu_i) = \sigma_b^2 \ (\text{between-cluster variability})$$
$$E(e_{ij}) = 0, \ \text{Var}(e_{ij}) = \sigma_w^2 \ (\text{within-cluster, between-subunit variability})$$

Therefore, the total variance of an observation Y_{ij} and the covariance between observations Y_{ij} and Y_{ik} within the i-th cluster are

$$\text{Var}(Y_{ij}) = \sigma^2 = \sigma_b^2 + \sigma_w^2$$
$$\text{Cov}(Y_{ij}, Y_{ik}) = \text{Var}(\mu_i) = \sigma_b^2$$

The correlation (corr) among subunits within a cluster equals

$$\rho = \frac{\sigma_b^2}{\sigma^2} \qquad (4.22)$$

This correlation is the same across all subunits and is called the *compound symmetry* model in the repeated measures context.

We model the data from Group X the same way, except that $E(\mu_i) = \mu_X$ for clusters of X.

We now take advantage of the form of Equation 4.3 again. We first average over the subunits within each cluster i in the group Y to obtain $\bar{Y}_{i\cdot}$ and note that

$$E(\bar{Y}_{i\cdot}) = E(Y_{ij}) = \mu_Y$$

$$Var(\bar{Y}_{i\cdot}) = \frac{1}{m^2} Var\left(\sum_j Y_{ij}\right)$$

$$= \frac{1}{m^2}\left[Var(Y_{i1}) + \ldots + Var(Y_{im}) + Cov(Y_{i1}, Y_{i2}) + \ldots + Cov(Y_{i(m-1)}, Y_{im})\right]$$

$$= \frac{1}{m^2}\left[m\sigma^2 + m(m-1)\sigma_b^2\right]$$

$$= \frac{1}{m}\left[\sigma^2 + (m-1)\rho\sigma^2\right]$$

$$= \frac{1}{m}\left[1 + (m-1)\rho\right]\sigma^2 \tag{4.23}$$

The same is true for Group X.

We can see that the cluster average remains to be an unbiased estimate of the population mean. However, as shown by Equation 4.23, the variance is modified by an extra multiplier, $1 + (m-1)\rho$, in comparison with the average of m independent samples. If $m > 1$ and $\rho > 0$, then there is an inflation of the variance due to the positive correlation among the subunits.

We next calculate the number of clusters needed per group (n) for testing H_0: $\delta = \mu_X - \mu_Y = 0$, using the cluster averages as the observations. Plug the appropriate variance in Equation 4.23 into Equation 4.3 to obtain the following:

$$n = \frac{2\sigma^2\left[1 + (m-1)\rho\right]\left(z_{\alpha/2} + z_\beta\right)^2}{m\delta^2} \tag{4.24}$$

The total number of main units (clusters) equals $N = 2n$, and the total number of subunits (observations) equals $N \times m$.

In the above setting, the treatment group is a "fixed" effect, and the main unit (cluster) is a "random" effect. Together, we have a "mixed" effect model. If a pilot study is conducted for only the control group to collect information for a future study with this kind of design, we would need to fit an ANOVA model to obtain the right variance components. Caution is required to identify the right MSE for the right variances for Equation 4.24. The following in-class exercise and Homework 4.7 illustrate this point.

In-Class Exercise: Mental 2-Inch Experiment Students should first put away their rulers. (Note that rulers will be needed at a later point.) Student will each be given a piece of paper and asked to draw a 2-inch segment on it without a ruler, write their initials on it, and hand in the piece of paper. After all papers have been collected, more blank sheets of paper will be distributed, and the students will be asked to again draw a 2-inch segment and mark their initials. All papers will again be collected, shuffled, and redistributed to the class, in such a way that no one receives their own papers or papers with the same initials. Students will then be asked to take out a ruler, measure the length of each segment, and record the length next to the segment. The length should be recorded in a standard fashion: (integer: a)+(integer: b)/16. Analyzing the collected data and comparing it with data from a previous class will be a homework assignment for the class (Homework 4.7).

This exercise has multiple purposes: (i) to illustrate the thought process of a statistical model to describe the data from an experiment; (ii) to let the readers practice some of the procedures in SAS for data analysis; (iii) to introduce the concept of a mixed-effect model, and to find the estimates of variance components for sample size estimation for clustered (correlated) data; and (iv) to construct a confidence interval to estimate the true mean, which is known (2 inches).

4.6 Sample Size for Testing a Noninferiority or Equivalence Hypothesis

The Helsinki Declaration (1976) published by the World Medical Association (WMA) has a mandate that all clinical research should avoid unnecessary suffering and injury and that, for a clinical trial, the investigator should make sure that there is no reasonable alternative to conducting the experiment. With the advancement of medicine in the last few decades, these ethical principles have now been updated by the WMA to include the consideration of avoiding the use of placebo as the control in a clinical trial whenever there is a standard medical practice available to treat the disease with an approved active medicine. Many clinical trials use an add-on design that includes having the placebo and the test drug added to the standard care. There are also trials that compare the test compound head-to-head with an active control that has been approved and used in practice. In the latter scenario, the hypothesis of superiority may require an unaffordable sample size to detect a miniscule improvement. In this case, a common approach is to test the null hypothesis of inferiority versus the alternative hypothesis of noninferiority within a designated margin of acceptance for the test compound compared to the active control. In the meantime, the trial also has the purpose of showing that the new compound has other advantages such as lower cost, more convenient administration, and better safety profile.

For a noninferiority trial, the first step is to establish a margin, $\Delta > 0$, to define the boundary between inferiority and noninferiority. For the case of continuous endpoints where a greater value implies a better outcome and the mean difference is $\delta = \mu_X - \mu_Y$, the setup of hypotheses is

$H_0 : \delta < -\Delta$ (implying X is inferior to Y by more than $-\Delta$ for the mean)

$H_A : \delta \geq -\Delta$ (implying X is NOT inferior to Y by more than $-\Delta$ for the mean)

This is a one-sided test. It is convenient to carry out an α-level test by constructing a one-sided $(1-\alpha) \times 100\%$ confidence interval (CI) for $\delta = \mu_X - \mu_Y$. We reject H_0 when the lower bound of the $(1-\alpha) \times 100\%$ CI is greater than $-\Delta$, as shown in Figure 4.3. For pharmaceutical industry, one-sided alpha is usually $\alpha = 0.025$, that is, one-sided 97.5% CI.

The power of this test is equal to

$$\Pr\left(\hat{\delta} - z_\alpha se\left(\hat{\delta}\right) \geq -\Delta \mid -\Delta \leq \delta\right) = 1 - \beta \qquad (4.25)$$

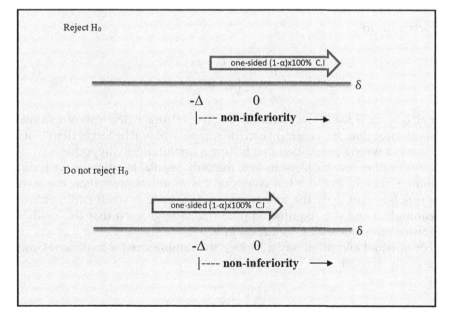

FIGURE 4.3
Graphical representation of a noninferiority test.

Usually, we pick a specific value for δ in the H_A space, say $\delta = \delta^* > -\Delta$, to achieve a desired power. Then,

$$\hat{\delta} - \delta^* = \bar{X} - \bar{Y} - \delta^* \sim N\left(0,\ \frac{2\sigma^2}{n}\right)$$

and

$$\left(\hat{\delta} - \delta^*\right) - z_\alpha se\left(\hat{\delta}\right) \geq -\Delta - \delta^*$$

if and only if

$$\frac{\left(\bar{X} - \bar{Y}\right) - \delta^*}{\sqrt{\frac{2\sigma^2}{n}}} \geq z_\alpha - \frac{\left(\Delta + \delta^*\right)}{\sqrt{\frac{2\sigma^2}{n}}}$$

From Equation 4.25 and the assumption of $\delta = \delta^*$, we have

$$-z_\beta = z_\alpha - \frac{\left(\Delta + \delta^*\right)}{\sqrt{\frac{2\sigma^2}{n}}}$$

which leads to

$$n = \frac{2\sigma^2 \left(z_\alpha + z_\beta\right)^2}{\left(\Delta + \delta^*\right)^2} \tag{4.26}$$

for all $\delta^* > -\Delta$. If $\Delta = 0$, we return to (4.3). If $\delta^* < 0$ (that is, the test compound is less effective than the control), then the sample size will be larger than that in (4.3). It is a wrong perception that testing a noninferiority hypothesis would always require less subjects. In fact, the only justifiable rationale for testing noninferiority is that the test compound is more effective than the active control; however, only the magnitude of difference is small (still clinically meaningful) and the required sample size is large such that the available resource prohibits testing for superiority.

For unequal allocation, say $n_X = k n_Y$, the sample size for treatment Group Y is easily derived:

$$n_Y = \frac{\frac{(k+1)}{k}\sigma^2 \left(z_\alpha + z_\beta\right)^2}{\left(\Delta + \delta^*\right)^2}$$

The corresponding formula for a binary endpoint with $\delta = \pi_X - \pi_Y$ is

$$n_Y = \frac{\left[\dfrac{\pi_X(1-\pi_X)}{k} + \pi_Y(1-\pi_Y)\right](z_\alpha + z_\beta)^2}{\left(\Delta + \delta^*\right)^2}$$

For testing the equivalence hypotheses, H_0: $|\delta| \geq \Delta$ (nonequivalence) versus H_A: $|\delta| < \Delta$ (equivalence), we would construct a two-sided $(1 - 2\alpha) \times 100\%$ confidence interval for δ to see if the CI falls entirely within $(-\Delta, \Delta)$. For the sample size and power calculation, we may set $\delta = \delta^* = 0$ for the alternative hypothesis (as being "truly" equivalent). Comparing this hypothesis to the two-sided hypothesis situation in Section 4.2, the only difference is that the null and the alternative hypotheses are switched. Therefore, we only need to switch the type I and type II errors in Equation 4.3 to obtain the sample size per group for a power of $1 - \beta$ in this situation:

$$n = \frac{2\sigma^2\left(z_{\beta/2} + z_\alpha\right)^2}{\Delta^2} \tag{4.27}$$

The above heuristic argument can be formally derived as shown in the following text. The resemblance of Equations 4.26 and 4.27 to Equation 4.3 highlights the role of the (non)inferiority margin Δ.

$$\alpha = \Pr\left(\text{Reject } |\delta| \geq \Delta \mid |\delta| \geq \Delta\right)$$

$$= \Pr\left(|T| < c \mid |\delta| \geq \Delta\right) \text{ where } T \sim N\left(\delta\sqrt{\frac{n}{2\sigma^2}}, 1\right)$$

$$\leq \Pr\left(|T| < c \mid |\delta| = \Delta\right) \qquad \text{(for a positive } c\text{)}$$

If $\delta = \Delta$, $\alpha \leq \Pr(T < c \mid \delta = \Delta) - \Pr(T < -c \mid \delta = \Delta)$

$$= \Pr\left(T - \Delta\sqrt{\frac{n}{2\sigma^2}} < c - \Delta\sqrt{\frac{n}{2\sigma^2}} \mid \delta = \Delta\right) - \Pr\left(T - \Delta\sqrt{\frac{n}{2\sigma^2}} < -c - \Delta\sqrt{\frac{n}{2\sigma^2}} \mid \delta = \Delta\right)$$

$$\leq \Pr\left(T - \Delta\sqrt{\frac{n}{2\sigma^2}} < c - \Delta\sqrt{\frac{n}{2\sigma^2}} \mid \delta = \Delta\right) \qquad \text{(the second positive term} \approx 0\text{)}$$

$$= \Pr\left(Z < c - \Delta\sqrt{\frac{n}{2\sigma^2}}\right)$$

Hence, $z_{1-\alpha} = c - \Delta\sqrt{\dfrac{n}{2\sigma^2}}$, $c = -z_\alpha + \Delta\sqrt{\dfrac{n}{2\sigma^2}}$.

That is, we reject H_0 when $T < -z_\alpha + \Delta\sqrt{\dfrac{n}{2\sigma^2}}$.

If $\delta = -\Delta$, $\alpha \le \Pr\left(T < c \mid \delta = -\Delta\right) - \Pr\left(T < -c \mid \delta = -\Delta\right)$

$= \Pr\left(T + \Delta\sqrt{\dfrac{n}{2\sigma^2}} < c + \Delta\sqrt{\dfrac{n}{2\sigma^2}} \mid \delta = -\Delta\right)$

$\quad - \Pr\left(T + \Delta\sqrt{\dfrac{n}{2\sigma^2}} < -c + \Delta\sqrt{\dfrac{n}{2\sigma^2}} \mid \delta = -\Delta\right)$

$= \Pr\left(Z < c + \Delta\sqrt{\dfrac{n}{2\sigma^2}}\right) - \Pr\left(Z < -c + \Delta\sqrt{\dfrac{n}{2\sigma^2}}\right)$

$\le 1 - \Pr\left(Z < -c + \Delta\sqrt{\dfrac{n}{2\sigma^2}}\right) \qquad$ (the first term is ≈ 1)

$= \Pr\left(Z \ge c - \Delta\sqrt{\dfrac{n}{2\sigma^2}} \mid \delta = -\Delta\right)$

Hence, $z_\alpha = c - \Delta\sqrt{\dfrac{n}{2\sigma^2}}$, $c = z_\alpha - \Delta\sqrt{\dfrac{n}{2\sigma^2}}$.

That is, we reject H_0 when $T \ge z_\alpha - \Delta\sqrt{\dfrac{n}{2\sigma^2}}$.

Note that the above shows that the two-sided $(1 - 2\alpha) \times 100\%$ CI approach is equivalent to rejecting H_0 (nonequivalence) when $|T| < -z_\alpha + \Delta\sqrt{\dfrac{n}{2\sigma^2}}$. (Note that when n is large enough, $-z_\alpha + \Delta\sqrt{\dfrac{n}{2\sigma^2}}$ is always positive.)

The power function is

$$g(\delta) = \Pr\left(T < -z_\alpha + \Delta\sqrt{\dfrac{n}{2\sigma^2}} \text{ and } T \ge z_\alpha - \Delta\sqrt{\dfrac{n}{2\sigma^2}} \mid |\delta| < \Delta\right).$$

Set power $= 1 - \beta$ at $\delta = 0$,

$$1 - \beta = \Pr\left(T < -z_\alpha + \Delta\sqrt{\dfrac{n}{2\sigma^2}} \text{ and } T \ge z_\alpha - \Delta\sqrt{\dfrac{n}{2\sigma^2}} \mid \delta = 0\right) \text{ implies}$$

$$\Pr\left(T \ge -z_\alpha + \Delta\sqrt{\dfrac{n}{2\sigma^2}}\right) = \beta/2$$

Hence, $-z_\alpha + \Delta\sqrt{\dfrac{n}{2\sigma^2}} = z_{\beta/2}$. This leads to Equation 4.27.

For binary outcomes with $\delta = \pi_X - \pi_Y$, we simply replace $2\sigma^2$ by $\pi_X(1 - \pi_X) + \pi_Y(1 - \pi_Y)$ in both formulas of sample size for noninferiority (Equation 4.26) and equivalence (Equation 4.27).

Example 4.2[1]

Two inhalers, A and B, used for the relief of asthma attacks, are to be assessed for equivalence. They will be considered equivalent if the two-sided 90% CI for the treatment difference measured by the morning peak expiratory flow rate (liters/min) falls entirely within the range of ±15 liters/min. That is, $\Delta = 15$. From a previous trial, the prior estimate of σ^2, the between-subject variance, is 1600 (L/min)^2. We would like to claim equivalence, if they in fact are identical, with 80% power. From Table 4.1, we use $z_\alpha = z_{0.05} = 1.645$, $z_{\beta/2} = z_{0.10} = 1.28$ in Equation 4.26 to obtain:

$$n = \frac{2 \times 1600 \times (1.645 + 1.28)^2}{15^2} \approx 122$$

Each group should include 122 patients. If we construct a 95% CI for the equivalence test, then $z_\alpha = z_{0.025} = 1.96$ and $n \approx 150$.

4.7 Comparing Ordinal Endpoints by the Wilcoxon–Mann–Whitney Test

Ordinal endpoints in clinical trials are usually used for quality-of-life questionnaires such as the Short Form 36 (SF-36) (Fayers and Machin 2000). When there are many (say, five or more) categories, one can assign a score to each category and treat the change from the baseline of the score as a continuous variable, and then apply Equation 4.3 for the sample size calculation. Otherwise, using methods for ordered categorical data would be more appropriate. The Wilcoxon–Mann–Whitney (WMW) test, also known as the two-sample Wilcoxon rank-sum test (Wilcoxon 1945; Mann and Whitney 1947), is a popular method to compare two distributions $F(x)$ and $G(y)$ for two independent treatment groups. Because there is no specification of the shape and form of these distributions, it is a nonparametric test. The general null hypothesis is that the two distributions are the same. In the case of a continuous endpoint, any difference between distributions implies that $Pr(X < Y)$ no longer equals 1/2. Therefore, the WMW test is often also used to test the null hypothesis of $Pr(X < Y) = 1/2$. When ties exist (which is the case for ordinal data), $Pr(X = Y) \neq 0$, so we split the ties between $Pr(X < Y)$ and $Pr(X > Y)$. The null hypothesis would then be

$$Pr(X < Y) + 0.5Pr(X = Y) = 1/2$$

---
[1] From Jones, B., et al., *British Medical Journal*, 313, 36–39, 1996.

If one wants to test a specific aspect of the distributions such as $E(X) = E(Y)$, which is true if $F(x) = G(y)$, against $E(X) \neq E(Y)$, assuming means exist, then we need to add the following assumption: If there is a difference between the two distributions, then it is in the location shift. That is, $F(x) = G(y+c)$, where c is some nonzero constant. However, when the outcome is bounded, as in the case of ordinal data presented in a contingency table, this shift hypothesis is not applicable. Thus, McCullagh (1980) suggested using the odds ratio (OR) as the effect size with the assumption of a proportional odds model. (In Section 4.4.4, we discussed the use of the semi-parametric log-rank test under the proportional hazards model for comparing two survival distributions.) With fewer ordered categories (typically, no more than five), the proportional odds assumption is more likely to hold.

Specifically, suppose the outcome measure of interest has J ordered categories, $j = 1, ..., J$. Let π_{jX} be the probability of being in category j for a subject in treatment Group X and $S_{jX} = \sum_{i=1}^{j} \pi_{iX}$ be the (cumulative) probability of being in category j or less in Group X. (Note that $S_{JX} = 1$.) Likewise, assume π_{jY} and S_{jY} for the control group Y. π_{j+} is the marginal probability of category j. The proportional odds assumption states that

$$OR_j = \frac{S_{jX}(1-S_{jY})}{S_{jY}(1-S_{jX})} \text{ is the same } (OR_j = OR) \quad \text{for all } j = 1, \ ..., J-1$$

The null hypothesis in terms of OR is

$$H_0: OR = 1 \text{ or } \log(OR) = 0$$

By specifying a particular OR value for the alternative hypothesis and assuming values for π_{jX}, $j = 1, ..., J$ (if X is the control group), we have

$$S_{jY} = \frac{S_{jX}}{OR(1-S_{jX})+S_{jX}}, \quad j = 1, ..., J-1$$

Then, π_{jY} for each category $j = 1, ..., J$ can be calculated. Finally, the marginal probability π_{j+} of category j is obtained for each $j = 1$ to J. Whitehead (1993) provided a formula of sample size per group:

$$n = \frac{6(Z_{\alpha/2}+Z_{\beta})^2}{OR^2\left(1-\sum_{j=1}^{J} \pi_{j+}^3\right)} \tag{4.28}$$

Equation 4.28 is given here without derivation. There is a homework assignment to compare Equation 4.28 with the result based on the simulation of the WMW test (Homework 4.8).

4.8 Sample Size Adjustments

Note for teachers and readers: Since this chapter is long and homework may be assigned before finishing the whole chapter, this section may be taught right after Section 4.2 prior to Section 4.3 in order for Homework 4.1 to be done correctly.

4.8.1 Adjustment for Loss to Follow-Up

In almost all clinical trials, some subjects are *lost to follow-up*; that is, they fail to complete the study and cannot be traced for their outcomes. The data lost will affect the study power. A possible problem that is more serious is that the missing data will also bias the result. We discuss this possibility in more detail in Chapter 15. Here we make an important assumption that the missing data from loss to follow-up are *missing at random* (MAR). MAR will be precisely defined in Chapter 15, but this essentially assumes that the missing data only affect the power and do not result in bias for the result.

Suppose f is the *projected* proportion of subjects that are lost to follow-up in the trial, and N is the total number of subjects necessary to be recruited, taking into account loss to follow-up. With loss to follow-up, N* is the number of patients available for analysis at the completion of the trial, based upon which we would like to detect a significant treatment effect with a desirable power.

We first use the formulas in the above sections to obtain the appropriate unadjusted sample size N*. Then the sample size adjusted for the possible loss to follow-up is simply

$$N = N^* / (1 - f) \tag{4.29}$$

The same applies to random right-censoring for the survival time case.

4.8.2 Adjustment for Nonadherence/Noncompliance

In almost all clinical trials, subjects sometimes fail to adhere to their assigned treatment regimen. This is also called a noncompliance issue. For example, in an open-label active control study, because the active control agent is already approved and available on the market, it is possible for a patient to stop the experimental treatment and take the active control treatment if the patient feels the test treatment is not working well for him or her. Another possible scenario is that in a placebo-controlled trial, patients receiving the test treatment may discontinue the assigned treatment and leave untreated because of some intolerable side effect. Although medical principles mandate that subjects in a clinical trial may withdraw from the study treatment at will at any time and the investigator has the obligation to withdraw the subject for any foreseeable risk, the study protocol should be designed in such a way that these patients' condition can still be followed up on, so that their outcome and other useful data can still be collected. The *intention-to-treat* (ITT) principle states that patients' data should be analyzed according to the original treatment group to which they were randomized and that all patients should be accounted for in an ITT analysis (for internal validity).

To understand the impact of noncompliance, we use the continuous outcome in a randomized trial of two treatment groups for illustration. This method is similar to other types of outcomes. Assume the true treatment means are μ_1 and μ_2. Let p be the proportion of subjects who are assigned to treatment group A but take Treatment B, and let q be the proportion of subjects who are assigned to treatment group B but take Treatment A. Under nonadherence, the resulting treatment means become

$$\mu_1^* = (1-p)\mu_1 + p\mu_2$$
$$\mu_2^* = q\mu_1 + (1-q)\mu_2 \tag{4.30}$$
$$\text{Then, } \mu_1^* - \mu_2^* = (1-p-q)(\mu_1 - \mu_2)$$

This treatment difference in Equation 4.30 should be used as the detectable treatment effect in the sample size calculation. We can see that $\mu_1^* - \mu_2^* \leq \mu_1 - \mu_2$. Hence, the required sample size will need to be larger to take into account the possible noncompliance.

4.8.3 Adjustment for Loss to Follow-Up and Nonadherence/Noncompliance

The combined impact of loss to follow-up and noncompliance on the required sample size can be calculated for a range of possible loss-to-follow-up proportion f and noncompliance proportions p and q. This impact is calculated by first making the adjustment described in Section 4.8.2, followed by the adjustment described in Section 4.8.1 (Equation 4.29).

4.8.4 Adjustment for Multiple Testing

The issue of multiple hypothesis testing can have different appearances, such as multiple endpoints or objectives, multiple treatment groups, multiple time points, and multiple (interim) analyses. For a clinical trial, especially a Phase III confirmatory trial, the FDA, EMA (European Medicines Agency), and health authorities in other regions require that the overall (familywise) type I error rate be maintained, at most, at the 5% level for a two-sided test. Although there are more efficient ways to deal with the issue in the data analysis, for sample size calculation, the *Bonferroni correction* is considered the simplest and most conservative method to control the familywise error rate. That is, we simply replace the type I error rate α in the above formulas with α/k, where k is the number of statistical tests that contribute to the claims on the label of the medication. This correction will dramatically increase the sample size if k is large. Therefore, it is advisable for a Phase III trial to have a limited number of objectives, endpoints, and treatment group comparisons. In Chapter 10, we will discuss in more detail the methods for addressing multiplicity issues.

4.9 Sample Size by Simulation and Bootstrap

In some situations when it is not straightforward to derive a sample size or power function formula in closed forms by conventional methods, we can use computer simulations to estimate the sample size or plot the power function. An illustration is given in Homework 4.7 with the Wilcoxon rank-sum test, which is the most popular nonparametric test when the outcome is ordinal with a limited number of categories. This test is also popular in cases where the outcome is continuous with a highly skewed distribution, while data transformation is undesirable for interpretation and the trial size is not large enough for applying the Central Limit Theorem to the mean. In a simulation study for sample size and power estimation, data are generated and test statistics are calculated from the given models under the null as well the alternative hypotheses. If a reliable pilot dataset is available, one can try anticipating the outcome of the trial by bootstrapping (repeated sampling with replacement) based on the available pilot data. Simulation and bootstrapping are very useful tools for design, development of methods, and analyses in clinical trials. See Tsodikove, Hasenclever, and Loeffler (1998) for an example in a chronic myelogenous leukemia trial, and Walters and Campbell (2005) for trials with health-related quality-of-life outcomes.

There are also packages in statistical software programs, such as the *simglm* R package for power by simulation (LeBeau 2019). The *simglm* package offers users the ability to simulate data from general(-ized) linear (mixed) models and contains wrappers that aids users in replicating the analysis. Once the data have been simulated, the package contains functionality to fit models to the generated data for power estimation. The *simglm* R package can simulate continuous, binary, and count outcome data from the general linear model with and without random effects. The user may add heterogeneity of variance and various missing data mechanisms for longitudinal data, and specify different distributional assumptions for fixed and random model attributes.

Appendix 4.1: Sample Size for 2 by 2 Crossover Design

In Chapter 3, we studied the 2 by 2 crossover design. Using the same notation in Section 3.3, after passing equal residual effects, we test the hypothesis of treatment effect: $H_0 : \delta = \tau_1 - \tau_2 = 0$. Equation 3.4 indicated that $E(d_{1k} - d_{2k}) = 2(\tau_1 - \tau_2)$, where $d_{1k} = y_{11k} - y_{12k}$ and $d_{2k} = y_{21k} - y_{22k}$. Hence, $\hat{\delta} = (\bar{d}_1 - \bar{d}_2)/2 = [(\bar{y}_{11} - \bar{y}_{12}) - (\bar{y}_{21} - \bar{y}_{22})]/2$ is an unbiased estimator of δ. The sample averages are taken over n = the number of subjects in a treatment sequence (AB or BA). Hence, $\mathrm{Var}(\bar{y}_{11}) = \mathrm{Var}(\bar{y}_{12}) = \mathrm{Var}(\bar{y}_{21}) = \mathrm{Var}(\bar{y}_{22}) = \dfrac{\sigma^2}{n}$. Furthermore, Cov $(\bar{y}_{11}, \bar{y}_{12}) = \mathrm{Cov}(\bar{y}_{21}, \bar{y}_{22}) = \rho \dfrac{\sigma}{\sqrt{n}} \dfrac{\sigma}{\sqrt{n}}$. We obtain the variance of $\hat{\delta}$ as

$$\mathrm{var}(\hat{\delta}) = \frac{1}{4}\left[\frac{4\sigma^2}{n} - 4\rho\frac{\sigma^2}{n}\right] = (1-\rho)\frac{\sigma^2}{n}$$

Usually, the correlation of the paired observations from the same individual $\rho > 0$. Just like other parameters, at the design stage we do not have its value unless we obtain it from a pilot study. We may conservatively set $\rho = 0$ so that the $\mathrm{Var}(\hat{\delta}) = \dfrac{\sigma^2}{n}$ is the largest possible value for sample size estimation. Compared to the parallel-group design, it is half of the corresponding variance of the estimated effect of treatment mean difference. Hence,

$$n = \frac{\sigma^2\left(z_{\alpha/2} + z_\beta\right)^2}{\delta^2}$$

As n is the number of subjects in a treatment sequence, for two sequences (AB and BA) of the same size, the total sample size is

$$N = \frac{2\sigma^2\left(z_{\alpha/2} + z_\beta\right)^2}{\delta^2}$$

Assuming $\rho = 0.5$ so that the $\mathrm{Var}(\hat{\delta}) = \dfrac{\sigma^2}{2n}$, the total sample size is

$$N = \frac{\sigma^2\left(z_{\alpha/2} + z_\beta\right)^2}{\delta^2}$$

Appendix 4.2: Fundamentals of Survival Data Analysis

Survival distribution is the probability that an individual is event-free, "survives," to a certain time, t:

$$S(t) = \Pr(T > t) = 1 - \Pr(T \le t) = 1 - F(t)$$

If the time-to-event random variable T has an exponential distribution with the parameter $\lambda > 0$, then (Figure 4.4)

$$S(t) = \int_{T=t}^{\infty} f(T)dT = \int_{t}^{\infty} \lambda e^{-\lambda T} dT = e^{-\lambda t}$$

Hazard function is the instantaneous event rate that the given individual has survived to that point in time:

$$h(t) = \lim_{\delta \to 0} \frac{\Pr(t < T < t + \delta \mid T > t)}{\delta} = \frac{f(t)}{S(t)}$$

Hazard rate is also called *failure rate* or *instantaneous risk*, which are often interchangeably used in the literature. It relates to the same type of information as that implied by the question: "What is the probability of surviving two years after therapy if a patient has already survived one year?"

For exponential T, $h(t) = \lambda$, and the expected failure time for an individual is

$$E(T) = \int_{t=0}^{\infty} tf(t)dt = \int_{0}^{\infty} t\lambda e^{-\lambda t} dt = \frac{1}{\lambda}$$

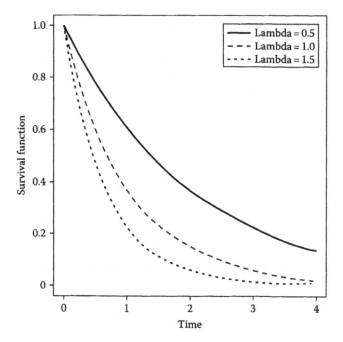

FIGURE 4.4
Survival function with exponential distribution models.

Appendix 4.3: Exponential Distribution Model

In the following, we continue to use the simple exponential distribution for summaries of basic concepts.

Likelihood:

$$L(\lambda; t_1, \ldots t_n) = \prod_{i=1}^{n} f(t_i) = \prod_{i=1}^{n} \lambda e^{-\lambda t_i} = \lambda^n \prod_{i=1}^{n} e^{-\lambda t_i}$$

Log-likelihood:

$$l(\lambda) = n \log \lambda - \lambda \sum_{i=1}^{n} t_i$$

MLE maximizes the (log-)likelihood. It is derived by taking the derivative of the log-likelihood with respect to λ, setting the resulting score function equal to 0 and solving for λ.

The derivative of the log-likelihood is called *score function:* $\dfrac{n}{\lambda} - \sum_{i=1}^{n} t_i$

MLE: The solution of the score function is MLE, $\hat{\lambda} = \dfrac{n}{\sum_{i=1}^{n} t_i} = \dfrac{1}{\bar{t}}$

The variance of the MLE is estimated as the inverse of the *Fisher information:*

$$I(\lambda) = -E_\lambda \left[\frac{\partial^2}{\partial \lambda^2} l(\lambda) \right]$$

Fisher information:

$$I(\lambda) = -E_\lambda \left[\frac{\partial^2}{\partial \lambda^2} l(\lambda) \right] = E_\lambda \left[\frac{n}{\lambda^2} \right] = \frac{n}{\lambda^2}$$

Therefore, $\mathrm{Var}\left[\hat{\lambda} \right] = \dfrac{\lambda^2}{n}$.

Statistical theory shows that for all practical purposes, with a suitably large sample size, the MLE is normally distributed and unbiased. Thus,

$$\hat{\lambda} = \frac{1}{\bar{t}} \sim AN\left(\lambda, \frac{\lambda^2}{n} \right)$$

The notation *AN* stands for *asymptotic normal distribution.*

Example 4.3

Suppose that in a study of chemoradiotherapy for patients with pancreatic cancer, the average survival time among 20 patients was found to be 15.1 months. We can calculate the 95% CI for the hazard around the point estimate of $1/15.1$ ($= 0.066$) deaths per month.

$$\left(\hat{\lambda} - z_{1-\alpha/2} \times \frac{\hat{\lambda}}{\sqrt{n}}, \ \hat{\lambda} + z_{1-\alpha/2} \times \frac{\hat{\lambda}}{\sqrt{n}} \right)$$

$$= \left(\frac{1}{15.1} - 1.96 \times \frac{1}{15.1\sqrt{20}}, \ \frac{1}{15.1} + 1.96 \times \frac{1}{15.1\sqrt{20}} \right)$$

$$= (0.037, \ 0.095)$$

Delta method: If $X \sim AN(\mu, V(X))$, then $g(X) \sim AN(g(\mu), g'(\mu)^2 V(X))$ for continuous and differentiable function g.

$$\text{For } \hat{\lambda} - AN\left(\lambda, \frac{\lambda^2}{n} \right), \text{ then } \frac{1}{n}\sum_{i=1}^{n} t_i = \frac{1}{\hat{\lambda}} \sim AN\left(\frac{1}{\lambda}, (-\lambda^{-2})^2 \frac{\lambda^2}{n} \right) = AN\left(\frac{1}{\lambda}, \frac{1}{n\lambda^2} \right)$$

$$\text{and } \log\left(\hat{\lambda} \right) \sim AN\left(\log(\lambda), \left(\frac{1}{\lambda} \right)^2 \frac{\lambda^2}{n} \right) = AN\left(\log(\lambda), \frac{1}{n} \right).$$

Appendix 4.4: Survival with Independent Censoring

A censoring event should be distinguished from an outcome event. The outcome event is the primary interest. The censoring event might be a competing risk, which truncates the time to the outcome event when occurring before the outcome event. Without a competing risk, the fixed finite study duration could also censor the outcome event. Because the timescale starts at the origin (time zero) and extends to the right, this censoring due to a fixed study end time is usually called "right-censoring."

Right-censoring may happen in two possible ways: (i) All patients enter the study simultaneously and complete the study at the same calendar time, or more likely (ii) patients enter and end the study at different calendar times but are followed up with the same duration of time. The study ends completely after the last patient completes the study. If an event has not occurred for a subject by his/her study end time, all we can say is that his/her time to event is greater than the observed follow-up time.

Notation

Y_i = time of event for subject i
C_i = time of censoring for subject i
$T_i = \min(Y_i, C_i)$

$\delta_i = 1$ if event was observed (i.e., $C_i > Y_i$)

$\quad = 0$ if censored at time C_i before event was observed (i.e., if $C_i < Y_i$)

The observed data: T_i and δ_i.

Appendix 4.5: MLE with Censoring under the Exponential Model

Likelihood:

$$L(\lambda; t_1, \ldots t_n) = \prod_{i:\delta_i=1} f(t_i) \prod_{i:\delta_i=0} S(t_i)$$

$$= \prod_{i=1}^{n} \left[\lambda e^{-\lambda t_i} \right]^{\delta_i} \left[e^{-\lambda t_i} \right]^{1-\delta_i}$$

$$= \prod_{i=1}^{n} \lambda^{\delta_i} e^{-\lambda t_i}$$

Log-likelihood:

$$l(\lambda) = \left(\sum_{i=1}^{n} \delta_i \right) \log \lambda - \lambda \sum_{i=1}^{n} t_i = D \log \lambda - \lambda \sum_{i=1}^{n} t_i$$

Score equation:

$$\frac{D}{\lambda} - \sum_{i=1}^{n} t_i = 0$$

where D is total outcome events and $\sum_{i=1}^{n} t_i$ is the total follow-up time.

MLE: $\hat{\lambda} = \dfrac{D}{\sum_{i=1}^{n} t_i}$

Fisher information:

$$I(\lambda) = -E\left[\frac{\partial^2}{\partial \lambda^2} l(\lambda) \right] = E\left[\frac{D}{\lambda^2} \right] = \frac{n\left(1 - e^{-\lambda C}\right)}{\lambda^2}$$

since $E(D) = n\Pr(\delta_i = 1) = n\Pr(Y_i < C_i) = n(1 - e^{-\lambda C})$ when all $C_i = C$ (i.e., all patients are subject to the same study duration C).

Therefore,

$$\mathrm{Var}\left(\hat{\lambda}\right) = \frac{\lambda^2}{n\left(1 - e^{-\lambda C}\right)} = \frac{\lambda^2}{E(D)}$$

Appendix 4.6: Use the POWER Procedure of SAS for Log-Rank Test

The following is an example of using the TWOSAMPLESURVIVAL statement with the TEST=LOGRANK option to compute the required sample size for the log-rank test.

```
proc power;
   twosamplesurvival test=logrank
      curve("Standard") = 5 : 0.5
      curve("Proposed") = (1 to 5 by 1):(0.95 0.9 0.75 0.7
0.6)
      groupsurvival = "Standard" | "Proposed"
      accrualtime = 2
      followuptime = 3
      groupmedlosstimes = 10 | 20 5
      power = 0.8
      npergroup = .;
run;
```

NOTE: The CURVE= option defines the two survival curves. The "Standard" curve has only one point, specifying an exponential form with a survival probability of 0.5 at year 5. The "Proposed" curve is a piecewise linear curve defined by the five points. The GROUPSURVIVAL= option assigns the survival curves to the two groups, and the ACCRUALTIME= and FOLLOWUPTIME= options specify the accrual and follow-up times. The GROUPMEDLOSSTIMES= option specifies the years at which 50% loss is expected to occur. The POWER= option specifies the target power, and the NPERGROUP= option identifies sample size per group as the parameter to compute. Default values for the SIDES= and ALPHA= options specify a two-sided test with = 0.05. Other features of PROC POWER are detailed in the SAS manual.

HOMEWORK 4.1

Study the paper "A Randomized, Placebo-Controlled, Preoperative Trial of Allopurinol in Subjects with Colorectal Adenoma" (Puntoni, M., et al., *Cancer Prevention Research*, 2013, 6: 74–81) and do the following:

1. Find the primary endpoint. Comment on Table 1 in light of our discussion in Chapter 2.
2. Do your own sample size calculation for this study: Set up the null and alternative hypotheses; define your notation, alpha,

and power; and list all the necessary parameters, just as if you were the statistician of that project and were writing the study design in the protocol. Compare your results with their calculation. Discuss your reading of the "Study power and statistical analysis" section of the paper.

3. Assume that the rate of loss to follow-up is 15% and the nonadherence rate is 5% for one group and 3% for the other group. How many total patients do you then need to recruit for the study?

4. Write an SAS or R program for the above sample size calculation, make a "power curve plot" (i.e., power versus detectable delta/treatment effect) for three different sample sizes of your own choice to show the sensitivity of power versus n, just like Figure 4.2.

5. Note that this exercise is like "playing detective" to guess "what happened when that study was planned" from the manuscript. Also note that this study was not a positive study. Suppose that later, researchers want to conduct another study of this kind and ask you to use the results in this study as a reference to plan a new study. What would you recommend for the (revised) sample size for this new study? The paper might not have all the necessary information explicitly written. You should derive information as needed. (Hint: Find information regarding σ from the 95% CIs in their Table 2.)

HOMEWORK 4.2

1. Review the multiple linear regression formula $\sigma_e^2 = (1-R^2)\sigma_Y^2$ from a linear regression textbook. Interpret the R^2.

2. Formulate the two independent samples of continuous outcome setting in Section 4.2 by using the linear model structure given by Equation (4.5) with the treatment group as the only covariate to see that the within-group variance σ^2 is $Var(e) = \sigma_e^2$ of the linear model.

HOMEWORK 4.3

1. Read the article "Effect of Continuous Glucose Monitoring on Glycemic Control in Adults With Type 1 Diabetes Using Insulin Injections -- The DIAMOND Randomized Clinical Trial" (Beck et al. JAMA. 2017;317(4):371–378). For readers who are not mathematics oriented, apply formula (4.4) to verify the sample size calculation of the paper. For statistical readers, derive formula (4.4) for unequal treatment allocations.

2. Read the article "Continuous Glucose Monitoring vs Conventional Therapy for Glycemic Control in Adults With Type 1 Diabetes Treated With Multiple Daily Insulin Injections – The GOLD Randomized Clinical Trial" (Lind et al. JAMA. 2017;317(4):379–387). For readers who are not mathematics oriented, apply the sample size formula in Appendix 4.1 and verify the sample size calculation of the paper. For statistical readers, derive the $\text{Var}\left(\hat{\delta}\right) = (1-\rho)\dfrac{\sigma^2}{n}$ in more detailed steps in Appendix 4.1 for the 2 by 2 crossover trial design with equal allocation to the treatment sequence.

HOMEWORK 4.4

The relative treatment effect for a binary outcome may also be measured by the ratio of event probabilities in the two treatment groups: $\delta = \pi_1/\pi_2$. Form the hypothesis test, and obtain the sample size per group using the log transformation and delta method.

HOMEWORK 4.5

With an exponential model, $S(t) = \exp(-\lambda t)$. Show that the median survival time $m = \log(2)/\lambda$. With a Weibull(λ, k) model, show that the median survival time is $m = [\log(2)]^{1/k}/\lambda$.

HOMEWORK 4.6

A randomized clinical trial was planned to examine whether the glucocorticoid prednisone could prolong life relative to an inactive placebo treatment for patients with histologically verified liver cirrhosis. Historical data suggest that, when untreated, 50% of patients with liver cirrhosis die within 4.2 years. Estimate how many patients are needed to attain 90% power to test the null hypothesis of no effect of hormone at the 0.05 significance level when the treatment can increase median survival time by 0.5, 1, 1.5, 2, or 2.5 years (five scenarios).

1. Assume the exponential model with no censoring in the problem above and use the log(HR) as the effect size of interest. Organize all the results in a single table of required sample sizes and comment on these results.
2. Consider terminating the observation of each individual after they have been followed up for 4, 6, and 10 years (three different scenarios). Use the log(HR) as the effect size/estimate of interest. Organize all of these results as well as the results under no censoring in a single table of required sample sizes, and provide an interpretation of and comment on these results. How much will the sample sizes be inflated to account for this censoring?

HOMEWORK 4.7

Referring to the "Mental 2-Inch Experiment" (Section 4.5) conducted in class:

1. Discuss briefly how the data of the experiment can be modeled by Equation 4.21. What are the model parameters and what process when generating the data ensures the assumptions?
2. Input the data collected from n = 15 students (of a previous class) into SAS. This is our "control" group. Obtain estimates of the within-subject variance, the between-subject variance, and the population true value we are trying to estimate (here, we know the true value = 2 inches); and calculate the correlation between the first and second within-subject repeated measures. Practice that this task can be accomplished by the following different ways available in SAS:
   a. Use a variance component model in PROC VARCOMP
   b. Use a model in PROC ANOVA
   c. Use a model in PROC GLM
   d. Use a random effect model in PROC MIXED

(Hint: You may need to read the "expect mean square", EMS, column of the ANOVA table in these SAS procedures to find the right variance components. PROC VARCOMP and PROC GLM with "random" statement can output EMS.)

Data

Student	Sequence	Measurement (inch)	Student	Sequence	Measurement (inch)
1	1	1.375	9	1	2.125
	2	1.375		2	2.0625
2	1	1.5625	10	1	1.625
	2	1.5		2	1.25
3	1	1.1875	11	1	2.28125
	2	1.175		2	2.4375
4	1	1.375	12	1	2
	2	1.25		2	2.375
5	1	2.46875	13	1	1.875
	2	2.34375		2	1.875
6	1	2.46875	14	1	1.5625
	2	2.3125		2	1.625
7	1	1.625	15	1	1.8125
	2	1.625		2	1.8125
8	1	2.0625			
	2	1.9375			

3. Verify that the within-class correlation obtained from Equation 4.22 matches the *Pearson correlation* from PROC CORR in SAS for paired data. For students of biostatistics, prove the theoretical equivalence of these two representations of correlation.

4. Using the above information of the control group for designing a comparative study, find the right estimate for the variance components and calculate the sample size needed for the main trial with the same clustered/correlated measures. (Specify your own delta, alpha, and power.)

5. (Only for class teaching) Now we have two datasets, one from the previous class of 15 students as shown in the above data table and another one from the current class (collected after performing the in-class experiment). We may suppose these two classes as two randomized groups and perform a comparison between them. The null hypothesis of interest would be an "equivalence" hypothesis. Let the equivalence margin be $(-0.45, 0.45)$ inches. Construct a 90% CI to test this hypothesis.

HOMEWORK 4.8

Carry out simulations to calculate power and sample size for the WMW test for testing the general null hypothesis of identical distributions, and compare the result with that from Equation 4.28 with the proportional odds alternative hypothesis.

Data: Let x_i ($i = 1, ..., n$) be random samples from population $F(x)$ and y_j ($j = 1, ..., m$) be random samples from population $G(y)$. Assign the ranks 1 to $N = n+m$ to them together. Let $R(x_i)$ denote the rank assigned to x_i and $R(y_j)$ be the rank assigned to y_j.

The WMW test statistic and critical value: If there are no ties, or just a few ties, the sum of the ranks assigned to treatment Group X can be used as a test statistic:

$$T = \sum_i^n R(x_i)$$

For n or m greater than 20, the p-th quantile w_p of T is approximated by

$$w_P = n(N+1)/2 + z_p\sqrt{nm(N+1)/12}$$

Thus, we reject the null hypothesis of identical distributions at alpha level, α, if $|T| > w_{1-\alpha}$ for a two-sided alternative hypothesis. If there are many ties, then we use:

$$T_1 = \frac{\sum_i^n R(x_i) - n(N+1)/2}{\sqrt{\dfrac{nm}{N(N-1)}\sum_i^N R_i^2 - \dfrac{nm(N+1)^2}{4(N-1)}}}$$

where $\sum_{i=1}^N R_i^2$ refers to the sum of the squares of all N of the ranks or average ranks actually used in both samples. T_1 is approximately $N(0,1)$ under the null hypothesis of identical distributions for n or m greater than 20. You can use SAS PROC npar1way to find the test statistic T_1 to perform the Wilcoxon–Mann–Whitney test.

Simulate the power for the WMW test as follows:

1. We should first verify the test gives the correct type I error level. Generate $n = m = 50$ observations from two identical ordinal distributions (with four categories c1, c2, c4, and c6):

$Pr(X = c1) = Pr(Y = c1) = 0.05, \quad Pr(X = c2) = Pr(Y = c2) = 0.30,$
$Pr(X = c4) = Pr(Y = c4) = 0.25,$ and $Pr(X = c6) = Pr(Y = c6) = 0.40$

Calculate the test T_1, and compare it to $z = -1.96$ for one-sided test (see below). If $T_1 < -1.96$, then we reject the null hypothesis; otherwise, we do not reject it. Do this 100,000 times. Count the number of times that the null hypothesis is rejected. Check if the proportion of rejection is close to 0.025. Construct a 95% CI based on this proportion. Does this CI include 0.025?

2. Then we test a specific alternative hypothesis: Generate $n = m = 50$ observations from the following two different ordinal distributions:

   $F(x)$ is still the same as above. But for $G(y)$, it is now:
   $Pr(Y = c1) = 0.01, \quad Pr(Y = c2) = 0.25, \quad Pr(Y = c4) = 0.30,$ and $Pr(Y = c6) = 0.44.$

   Notice that Group Y has more subjects in higher categories c4 and c6 than Group X.

   Again, do the WMW test T_1 as above.

   Do this 10,000 times. Find the proportion of times the null hypothesis is rejected. This is the estimated power for the WMW test for this specific alternative.

3. If the above power is much lower than 80%, the usual target for a reasonable Phase II or Phase III study, then do the simulation again, using a larger sample size for n and m. If the power is much higher than 80%, then do the simulation again, using a smaller sample size for n and m. Record these results, and make a table (n, m) versus power.

4. Does the alternative hypothesis in (2) above meet the assumption of proportional odds? Suppose we now specify an alternative hypothesis in terms of proportional odds ratios. Construct $G(y)$ accordingly first. Then carry out a simulation to find the sample size ($n = m$) for detecting $OR = 2$ with power = 80% at one-sided $\alpha = 0.025$. Compare the result with that from Equation 4.28.

References

Barthel FMS, Royston P, and Babiker A. (2005). A menu-driven facility for complex sample size calculation in randomized controlled trials with a survival or a binary outcome: update. *Stata Journal* 13: 123–129.

CDER and CBER (US Department of Health and Human Services Food and Drug Administration Center for Drug Evaluation and Research and Center for Biologics Evaluation and Research). (2005). *Guidance for Industry: Clinical Trial Endpoints for the Approval of Cancer Drugs and Biologics*. Rockville, MD.

Champely S. (2018). Pwr: Basic Functions for Power Analysis. https://CRAN.R-project.org/package=pwr.

Collett D. (1994). *Modelling Survival Data in Medical Research*. New York: Chapman & Hall.

Fayers PM and Machin D. (2000). *Quality of Life Assessment, Analysis and Interpretation*. Chichester, UK: Wiley.

Jones B, Jarvis P, Lewis JA, and Ebbutt AF. (1996). Trials to assess equivalence: the importance of rigorous methods. *British Medical Journal* 313: 36–39.

LeBeau B. (2019). Simglm: Simulate Models Based on the Generalized Linear Model. https://CRAN.R-project.org/package=simglm.

Mann HB and Whitney DR. (1947). On a test of whether one of two random variables is stochastically larger than the other. *Annals of Mathematical Statistics* 18: 50–60.

McCullagh P. (1980). Regression models for ordinal data (with discussion). *Journal of the Royal Statistical Society, Series B* 42: 109–142.

Puntoni M, Branchi D, and Argusti A, et al. (2013). A randomized, placebo-controlled, preoperative trial of allopurinol in subjects with colorectal adenoma. *Cancer Prevention Research* 6: 74–81.

Tsodikove A, Hasenclever D, and Loeffler M. (1998). Regression with bounded outcome score: evaluation of power by bootstrap and simulation in a chronic myelogenous leukaemia clinical trial. *Statistics in Medicine* 17: 1909–1922.

Walters SJ and Campbell MJ. (2005). The use of bootstrap methods for estimating sample size and analyzing health-related quality of life outcomes. *Statistics in Medicine* 24: 1075–1102.

Weisberg S. (1985). *Applied Linear Regression*. New York: Wiley.

Whitehead J. (1993). Sample size calculation for ordered categorical data. *Statistics in Medicine* 12: 2257–2271.

Wilcoxon R. (1945). Individual comparisons by ranking methods. *Biometrics* 1: 80–83.

5

Analysis of Covariance and Stratified Analysis

Having discussed some key concepts of statistical design in previous chapters, we turn to the topic of methods for analyzing data from clinical studies including clinical trials. We begin with the principles of data analysis and stress the importance of purpose-driven analysis. Often we read data analyses that involve regression models, where the outcome measure of each subject is regressed on treatment plus other covariates. We should first distinguish the purpose of such regression analyses. There could be two kinds of purposes. One is to study the treatment and covariate association with respect to outcome. The purpose can be to study how some covariates may influence the treatment effect so that, when planning a clinical trial, we can properly choose a population based on the information gathered from the data. Here the attention is on the covariates. Another kind of purpose is for assessing the treatment effect "adjusted for" covariates. The focus is on the treatment effect. Our interest in this and next chapter is placed on the latter.

As we have alluded to in Section 2.8, in a randomized trial, we can choose to analyze the treatment effect without any covariate and the conclusions will be valid, irrespective of the observed treatment–covariate association. As a common practice, we usually adjust a covariate—prognostic factor— that is unbalanced between the groups. In this chapter, we study the method of analysis of covariance (ANCOVA), where the endpoint is a continuous outcome, to discuss the appropriateness of this common practice. We show that the degree of adjustment and the variance reduction depend on two factors: the covariate's correlation or association with the outcome variable and the degree of between-group imbalance. We also extend the discussion on stratified analysis and logistic regression for categorical data. We continue the topic of covariate adjustment in survival data analysis in the next chapter.

5.1 Principles of Data Analysis

Data analysis should be tied to the study design, especially the study objective, and consequently provide appropriate interpretation of the results. For a formal data analysis, two common types of inferences are *hypothesis testing* and *estimation with confidence interval*. (Other possibilities include prediction and posterior probability; some basic Bayesian methods are introduced

DOI: 10.1201/9781003176527-5

in Chapter 7.) The framework of hypothesis testing was used for sample size calculation in Chapter 4. Testing and estimation are both used for two aspects of the data analysis: within-group and between-group comparisons. We examine these comparisons in this chapter.

A key concept of interpretation of the results is *statistical significance* versus *clinical significance*. The former asks the question, "To what extent is the observed difference attributable to random variation?" The latter asks, "Is the observed difference clinically meaningful in magnitude?" Statistical significance is assessed by probability theory. Clinical significance is judgmental and based on consensus or expert opinion by the clinical community.

For statistical significance, the phrase "to what extent..." is often measured by the tail probability under the null hypothesis of "no difference." This tail probability is termed *p-value*. The proper use of p-values is very important; we already discussed the misuse of p-values found in baseline characteristics tables in the medical literature (see Section 2.8). We will further discuss the limitations of p-values in Chapter 14. For assisting a proper interpretation of the result versus clinical significance, we should always provide a 90% or 95% confidence interval with the point estimate of the treatment effect in addition to the p-value.

As we have mentioned when discussing sample size calculation, the methods of data analysis depend on the type of the outcome variable (i.e., *"endpoint"*); in a regression context, the outcome variable is also called the response or dependent variable:

- Continuous response—for example, blood pressure, serum cholesterol level, bone-mineral density, and weight. Analyses are often performed using analysis of variance (ANOVA) or analysis of covariance (ANCOVA) on change from baseline, percent change from baseline, or the posttreatment outcomes adjusted by the baseline.

- Categorical—binary and ordered categorical response. For a binary response, analyses are often performed using *logistic regression* with covariates. The same is true for an ordinal categorical response using cumulative logit models. When treatment group is the only covariate and sample size is not large, Fisher's exact test is often used for a 2×2 table. When other prognostic covariates are involved and are also categorical, stratified analyses are performed. The Cochran–Mantel–Haenszel (CMH) test (Cochran 1954, 1957; Mantel and Haenszel 1959; Mantel 1963) is a popular stratified method to combine summary statistics from each stratum formed by the categorical prognostic variable.

- Survival response (time to event) with censoring—this endpoint is in between binary and continuous. Cox regression assuming proportional hazard rates and the stratified log-rank test are often used. We will cover survival data analysis with covariate adjustment in Chapter 6, including proportional and non-proportional hazards.

We have seen some ANOVA and ANCOVA models and their roles in previous chapters when discussing the crossover design, baseline comparability, and sample size calculations. In this chapter, we further study ANCOVA and stratified analysis as commonly used tools for data analysis in clinical trials to adjust for prognostic factors (covariates). We also use a simple form of ANCOVA (a continuous response and a continuous covariate along with treatment group) and stratified analysis (a binary response and a binary covariate besides treatment group) to tie analysis together with some of the key design methods such as stratification and randomization covered in previous chapters.

In clinical trials, there could be many covariates collected, many possibly correlated with each other. To avoid ambiguity caused by having many possibilities of different covariates and their interactions in the data analysis, which could lead to the problem of multiplicity and/or multicollinearity for inference, it is good practice to prespecify a set of prognostic covariates in the statistical analysis plan before the study is unmasked for treatment comparisons.

5.2 Continuous Response—ANOVA and ANCOVA

An ANCOVA model contains the continuous outcome as the response variable, and the covariates often include the baseline value of the outcome variable and other continuous or categorical variables in addition to the treatment group. The subject's age at baseline is often a meaningful covariate to consider, because in many situations it is correlated with the subject's disease status. It can be treated as a continuous variable or be grouped on certain ranges and become a categorical variable. Therefore, ANCOVA is a method that combines ANOVA and linear regression analysis, and all of these methods are in the larger class called the general linear model (GLM). (Note: Another even larger class called "generalized linear model", abbreviated as GLM as well, includes categorical and survival response variables; see Section 6.7.3.) The basic idea of ANCOVA can be illustrated as shown in Figure 5.1.

Figure 5.1a shows that the observed difference in response between treatment groups can be a result of an imbalance of a prognostic factor (covariate) or combination of factors. In this case, the treatment effect is said to be confounded with the prognostic factor(s). Hence, randomization is very important to minimize this possibility. However, imbalance can still occur by chance with randomization, especially for trials with a small sample size.

Figure 5.1b shows that even when balance is reached in the prognostic factor, the two treatment groups may still have different relationships, expressed by the slopes, between the response and the prognostic factor. Treatment differences vary at different levels of the prognostic factor. Treatment effect is shown by the difference in the slopes/correlations.

Figure 5.1c shows that there is a little imbalance (which can and often does occur even with randomization) and a little heterogeneity in slopes. We could use a common slope model to ease the analysis and interpretation. When using a common slope derived from the pooled data, the treatment

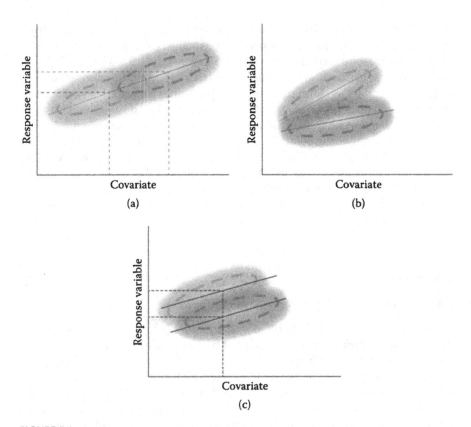

FIGURE 5.1
(a) The two treatment groups are not comparable because of the differences in the covariate. (b) The two treatment groups have different correlations between response and covariate. (c) The two treatment groups are approximately comparable and have similar correlations between response and covariate.

difference is then considered to be constant within the range of the prognostic factor, and it simplifies the interpretation of the treatment comparison. This is the essence of ANCOVA.

In Sections 5.2.1–5.2.3, we use SAS procedures to conduct an ANCOVA step by step.

5.2.1 Test for Equal Slopes

Denote the treatment group by T, the baseline prognostic factor by X, and the outcome variable by Y. The SAS procedure for assessing equality of slopes is

```
PROC GLM;
    Class T;
    Model Y = T X T*X;
Run;
```

The ANCOVA test for the treatment group by covariate interaction, T*X, indicates whether the slopes are the same across treatment groups or not. If the interaction is significant (say at 5% level), we need to interpret the ANCOVA with caution, because this means that the treatment effects vary at different levels of the prognostic factor. In this case, we can say that the treatment effect is shown to affect the relationship, expressed by the slope, between the outcome Y and the prognostic factor X.

When the interaction is not significant, we then omit it from the model statement:

```
PROC GLM;
   Class T;
   Model Y = T X;
Run;
```

In SAS, the order of the effect in the model statement is important for the type I SS (sum of squares), where the latter effect will sequentially be adjusted for the preceding effect, whereas for the type III SS, the order is irrelevant; that is, all the effects will be adjusted for each other. In this case, it is more sensible that the treatment effect, T, is adjusted for the covariate, X. Hence, in writing T before X as seen in the model statement above, the type III SS should be used instead of the type I SS.

When the slope is the same, the treatment comparison is adjusted for the baseline prognostic factor at any level, because the comparison will be the same regardless of the prognostic level. A meaningful choice for comparison would be at the mean level of the pooled baseline prognostic factor across the treatment groups.

When the interaction term is on the borderline of significance, we may still force a common slope (equivalent to combining the groups and fitting one regression line) to ease the interpretation of ANCOVA.

In summary, for ANCOVA, the following steps should be followed:

1. For a single factor, always make a scatter plot with a linear regression fitted for each treatment group.
2. Test the hypothesis of equal slopes.
3. If the hypothesis of equal slopes is not rejected, use a common slope ANCOVA model (i.e., a model without the interaction term) to compare the treatment difference.
4. If the slopes are shown to be significantly unequal, stop the ANCOVA. The slopes themselves express the treatment effects.

Note that the baseline measurement of the outcome variable is always considered an important prognostic factor to control by stratification and randomization methods in the study design and by the regression method in ANCOVA. We should also pay attention to the interpretation of the SAS outputs, as discussed in Section 5.2.2.

5.2.2 ANCOVA Model with a Common Slope

Let y_{ij} be the posttreatment outcome, x_{ij} be the baseline measure, and $d_{ij} = y_{ij} - x_{ij}$ be the change, for the j-th patient in the i-th treatment group; $i = 1$, 2, and $j = 1, \ldots, n_i$. The ANCOVA mean model is expressed by

$$E\left(y_{ij} \mid x_{ij}\right) = \mu + \tau_i + \beta\left(x_{ij} - \bar{x}_{..}\right)$$
$$= \alpha_i + \beta\left(x_{ij} - \bar{x}_{..}\right) \qquad (5.1)$$
$$= \beta_0 + \tau_i + \beta x_{ij}$$

The term μ (or $\beta_0 = \mu - \beta\bar{x}_{..}$) is the grand mean, τ_i (or $\alpha_i = \mu + \tau_i$) represents the effect due to treatment i, and β reflects the common linear relationship between Y and X, which is independent of the treatment group. The above expressions are equivalent, and both are presented here to make some interpretation easier in different occasions. For example, as we previously mentioned, even though the between-treatment comparison in this ANCOVA model with a common slope is the same regardless of the level of X, the first or second line of Equation 5.1 makes it clear that the comparison at the pooled average value of X ($= \bar{x}_{..}$) is often more meaningful than at X = 0.

By the method of least squares (LS), we obtain the LS estimates of the parameters:

$$\hat{\mu} = \bar{y}_{..}$$

$$\hat{\alpha}_i = \bar{y}_{i.} - \hat{\beta}(\bar{x}_{i.} - \bar{x}_{..})$$

$$\hat{\beta} = \frac{\sum_{i=1}^{2} \sum_{j=1}^{n_i} (y_{ij} - \bar{y}_{..})(x_{ij} - \bar{x}_{..})}{\sum_{i=1}^{2} \sum_{j=1}^{n_i} (x_{ij} - \bar{x}_{..})^2}$$

$$= \frac{\sum_{i=1}^{2} \sum_{j=1}^{n_i} y_{ij} x_{ij} - \sum_{i=1}^{2} n_i \bar{y}_{i.} \bar{x}_{i.}}{\sum_{i=1}^{2} \sum_{j=1}^{n_i} x_{ij}^2 - \sum_{i=1}^{2} n_i \bar{x}_{i.}^2} \qquad (5.2)$$

(At this point, if you feel that your memory of linear regression analysis is rusty, you should review this topic immediately; see Weisberg 1985.) The numerator of $\hat{\beta}$ is sometimes denoted as SS_{YX}, and the denominator as SS_{XX}. Hence, in brief, $\hat{\beta} = SS_{YX} / SS_{XX}$.

In Equation 5.2, $\bar{y}_{i.}$ is the raw (unadjusted) mean of treatment group i, and $\hat{\alpha}_i$ is the adjusted mean (LS mean) of the treatment group i, adjusted for the baseline covariate X. The amount of adjustment, $\hat{\beta}(\bar{x}_{i\cdot} - \bar{x}_{\cdot\cdot})$, depends on the product of two factors: correlation of X with Y (expressed by $\hat{\beta}$), and how far the group mean is away from the overall mean (i.e., degree of baseline imbalance). This is enlightening. In Chapter 2, Section 2.8, we discussed the concept of *baseline comparability*. First, using the p-value to indicate baseline comparability, as is sometimes seen in medical publications, is not as meaningful as this amount of LS mean adjustment. If we are sure that the randomization has been carried out properly, then the p-value just reflects the type I error rate. A small and statistically insignificant baseline difference (which is a type I error) of a highly correlated prognostic factor may still induce a greater adjustment than a large difference of a baseline characteristic that has very weak correlation with the outcome endpoint. Second, the design methods of stratification (for categorical covariates) and randomization can enhance the chance of baseline balance, and the method of blinding can protect the assessment bias so that the correlation between the outcome and baseline covariate would be independent of the treatment group (thus implying a common slope).

5.2.3 ANCOVA Using SAS

In addition to the mean model in Equation 5.1, the ANCOVA model also has an additive error term. When the error term is normally distributed, the LS estimators (Equation 5.2) are also the maximum likelihood estimators (MLEs). We can then perform statistical tests and confidence interval estimations. Note that testing the adjusted mean within an individual group i, $\alpha_i = 0$, by itself is not meaningful. Testing between groups, $\alpha_1 = \alpha_2$, is meaningful, by examining

$$\hat{\alpha}_1 = \bar{y}_{1\cdot} - \hat{\beta}(\bar{x}_{1\cdot} - \bar{x}_{\cdot\cdot}); \hat{\alpha}_2 = \bar{y}_{2\cdot} - \hat{\beta}(\bar{x}_{2\cdot} - \bar{x}_{\cdot\cdot});$$

$$\hat{\alpha}_1 - \hat{\alpha}_2 = (\bar{y}_{1\cdot} - \bar{y}_{2\cdot}) - \hat{\beta}(\bar{x}_{1\cdot} - \bar{x}_{2\cdot}) \tag{5.3}$$

The adjustment for the baseline mean difference is clearly shown in the second term of Equation 5.3 here. If the randomization is fair, then $\bar{x}_{1\cdot} - \bar{x}_{2\cdot} \approx 0$, and the adjustment is nearly negligible. Hence, in the context of a properly randomized trial, especially for a randomized trial with a large sample size, one of the purposes of ANCOVA is studying covariates, not adjusting for bias. The study of covariates is a way to understand the disease and treatment mechanisms and to discover relationships that may help the investigator plan future research. Including covariates could also reduce the variance when comparing treatment effects, as another purpose. We discuss this point in Section 5.3.

Instead of y_{ij}, if we use d_{ij} (which is a change from baseline, i.e., $d_{ij} = y_{ij} - x_{ij}$) in the ANCOVA model, what would be the slope (in relation to the above β)? Is it still meaningful to test this new slope = 0? Will the treatment comparison be the same as using y_{ij}? The following examines these questions.

The regression slope of the change, d, on baseline, X, is denoted by $\tilde{\beta}$. Then,

$$\tilde{\beta} = \rho_{dX}\frac{\sigma_d}{\sigma_X} = \frac{\sigma_{dX}}{\sigma_d\sigma_X}\frac{\sigma_d}{\sigma_X} = \frac{cov(Y-X,\,X)}{\sqrt{var(X)\,var(X)}} = \frac{cov(Y,\,X) - var(X)}{var(X)} = \beta - 1$$

Therefore, testing $\tilde{\beta} = 0$ is equivalent to testing $\beta = 1$, which is generally not meaningful, unless $\sigma_Y = \sigma_X$. When $\sigma_Y = \sigma_X$, $\beta = \rho$. Then, testing $\tilde{\beta} = 0$ is equivalent to testing a perfect correlation $\rho = 1$.

Now, let us look at the treatment group comparison. With obvious notation of the estimates, the LS mean of the group i is

$$\tilde{\alpha}_i = \bar{d}_i - \hat{\tilde{\beta}}(\bar{x}_{i\cdot} - \bar{x}_{\cdot\cdot})$$

$$= \bar{d}_i - \left(\hat{\beta} - 1\right)(\bar{x}_{i\cdot} - \bar{x}_{\cdot\cdot})$$

$$= \left(\bar{y}_{i\cdot} - \bar{x}_{i\cdot}\right) - \hat{\beta}(\bar{x}_{i\cdot} - \bar{x}_{\cdot\cdot}) + (\bar{x}_{i\cdot} - \bar{x}_{\cdot\cdot})$$

$$= \bar{y}_{i\cdot} - \hat{\beta}(\bar{x}_{i\cdot} - \bar{x}_{\cdot\cdot}) - \bar{x}_{\cdot\cdot}$$

$$= \hat{\alpha}_i - \bar{x}_{\cdot\cdot}$$

Therefore, the LS mean based on y and that based on d only differ by a constant, that is, the overall average of x. The between-group comparison is the same whether using y or d. It is also interesting to see from the equation

$$\tilde{\alpha}_i = \bar{d}_i - \hat{\tilde{\beta}}(\bar{x}_{i\cdot} - \bar{x}_{\cdot\cdot}) \tag{5.4}$$

that testing the individual $\alpha_i = 0$ using difference, d_{ij}, is now meaningful because in this case it is the *within-group* change from baseline, adjusted for the *regression toward the mean effect* (the second term of Equation 5.4). Note that, in contrast, the pre–post paired t-test only uses the first term of Equation 5.4, $\bar{d}_i$, without accounting for any change attributable to regression to the mean. When the regression to the mean effect is large, we prefer Equation 5.4 for within-group change over the pre–post paired t-test.

5.3 Variance Reduction by Covariates

Following the mean model (Equation 5.1) with the error term being normally distributed with mean 0 and conditional variance $Var(Y|X) = \sigma_{Y|X}^2$, we can compare the unadjusted estimator of the treatment effect with the adjusted estimator in Equation 5.3. Denote the marginal variance of Y as $\text{Var}(Y) = \sigma_Y^2$, and assume a sample size n per group.

If the model in Equation 5.1 is correct, the unadjusted estimator of the treatment effect is $(\bar{y}_1. - \bar{y}_2.)$.

$$E(\bar{y}_1. - \bar{y}_2.) = (\tau_1 - \tau_2) + \beta(\bar{x}_1. - \bar{x}_2.)$$

This then gives a bias of $\beta(\bar{x}_1. - \bar{x}_2.)$ in estimating $\tau_1 - \tau_2$. The variance of $(\bar{y}_1. - \bar{y}_2.) = 2\sigma_Y^2 / n$. The mean squared error of the unadjusted estimator is therefore

$$\beta^2 (\bar{x}_1. - \bar{x}_2.)^2 + 2\sigma_Y^2 / n \tag{5.5}$$

The adjusted estimator of the treatment effect is $\hat{\alpha}_1 - \hat{\alpha}_2 = (\bar{y}_1. - \bar{y}_2.) - \hat{\beta}(\bar{x}_1. - \bar{x}_2.)$. Because $\hat{\beta}$ is an unbiased estimator of β, $E(\hat{\alpha}_1 - \hat{\alpha}_2) = \tau_1 - \tau_2$. The variance of $\hat{\alpha}_1 - \hat{\alpha}_2$ involves the variance of $\hat{\beta}$, or more precisely, the conditional variance of $\hat{\beta}$, given X:

$$\text{Var}(\hat{\beta} \mid X) = \sigma_{Y|X}^2 / SS_{XX}.$$

Hence,

$$\text{Var}(\hat{\alpha}_1 - \hat{\alpha}_2 \mid X) = \sigma_{Y|X}^2 \left[\frac{2}{n} + \frac{(\bar{x}_1. - \bar{x}_2.)^2}{SS_{XX}} \right] \tag{5.6}$$

Because $\hat{\alpha}_1 - \hat{\alpha}_2$ is unbiased, Equation 5.6 is also the mean squared error.

When we compare Equations 5.5 and 5.6, the desirability of adjusting the covariate for the given data relies on the unknown factors of $\sigma_{Y|X}^2$, σ_Y^2, and β. In practice, we can replace them with the corresponding estimates from the data. If the mean squared error (Equation 5.5) is smaller, then we use the unadjusted estimator; otherwise, we use the adjusted estimator. Some simulation studies carried out by Abeyasekera (1984) show that this strategy is better than the "always adjust" or the "always do not adjust" rules in most situations when the correlation between the response variable and the covariate is at least modest (above 0.15). This procedure is easy to do when there are only two treatment groups and only one covariate to consider. For more than one covariate and more than two treatment groups, it is more difficult to carry out.

5.4 Stratified Analysis

For a binary or ordered categorical response and some continuous and categorical covariates, logistic and cumulative logistic regression models are often used to analyze treatment effects adjusted for the covariates; see the next section. Because logistic regression involves an iterative method to obtain the maximum likelihood estimate of the regression coefficient (e.g., McCullagh and Nelder 1989), it is not so obvious to perceive the impact of the distribution of the covariate as in the continuous response case by ANCOVA. However, we can make the point by studying a simple case of comparing two treatment groups (T = A, B) with respect to a binary response (R = 1, 0), stratified by a binary covariate (X = "+", "−"). This stratified analysis is shown in Table 5.1.

In Table 5.1(A), the patient allocation distribution panel indicates that $Pr(T = A) = Pr(T = B) = 1/2$, meaning an even allocation between treatment groups. $Pr(T = A, X = "+") = \pi_A$ and $Pr(T = B, X = "+") = \pi_B$ implies that $Pr(X = "+") = \pi_A + \pi_B$ and $Pr(X = "−") = 1 - \pi_A - \pi_B$. For a stratified randomization, $Pr(T = A \mid X = "+") = \pi_A/(\pi_A + \pi_B) = Pr(T = B \mid X = "+") = \pi_B/(\pi_A + \pi_B)$ if and only if $\pi_A = \pi_B$.

The "Response Rate" panel in Table 5.1(B) indicates that

$$Pr(R = 1 \mid T = A, \ X = "−") = \alpha, \ Pr(R = 1 \mid T = A, \ X = "+") = \varphi\alpha,$$

$$Pr(R = 1 \mid T = B, \ X = "−") = \beta, \ Pr(R = 1 \mid T = B, \ X = "+") = \varphi\beta.$$

Hence,

$$Pr(R = 1 \mid T = A, X = "+") / Pr(R = 1 \mid T = A, X = "−")$$
$$= Pr(R = 1 \mid T = B, X = "+") / Pr(R = 1 \mid T = B, X = "−") = \varphi$$

TABLE 5.1

Stratified Analysis

		Treatment Group (T)	
		A	**B**
(A) *Allocation Distribution*			
Factor (X)	"+"	π_A	π_B
	"−"	$\frac{1}{2} - \pi_A$	$\frac{1}{2} - \pi_B$
Total		$\frac{1}{2}$	$\frac{1}{2}$
(B) *Response Rate*			
Factor (X)	"+"	$\varphi\alpha$	$\varphi\beta$
	"−"	α	β
Ratio		φ	φ

The positive factor X, that is, X = "+", influences the response rate by a multiplier of φ versus the negative factor X, that is, X = "−", independent of the treatment group. This is similar to the parallel slopes in the ANCOVA model.

From Table 5.1, we can calculate the expected response rate for each treatment group combining the strata of X = "+" and X = "−" as follows:

$$P_A = \Pr\left(R=1 \mid T=A\right) = \frac{\Pr\left(R=1,\ T=A\right)}{P\left(T=A\right)}$$

$$= 2\left[\Pr\left(R=1, T=A,\ X="+"\right) + \Pr\left(R=1, T=A,\ X="-"\right)\right]$$

$$= 2\left[\Pr\left(R=1 \mid T=A,\ X="+"\right)\Pr\left(T=A,\ X="+"\right)\right.$$
$$\left. + \Pr\left(R=1 \mid T=A,\ X="-"\right)\Pr\left(T=A,\ X="-"\right)\right]$$

$$= 2\left[\left(\varphi\alpha\right)\pi_A + \alpha\left(1/2 - \pi_A\right)\right]$$
$$= \alpha\left[1 + 2\pi_A\left(\varphi-1\right)\right] \tag{5.7}$$

Similarly,

$$P_B = \Pr\left(R=1 \mid T=B\right) = \frac{\Pr\left(R=1, T=B\right)}{\Pr\left(T=B\right)}$$

$$= 2\left[\left(\varphi\beta\right)\pi_B + \beta\left(1/2 - \pi_B\right)\right]$$
$$= \beta\left[1 + 2\pi_B\left(\varphi-1\right)\right] \tag{5.8}$$

To see how the treatment comparison with balanced factor X, when $\pi_A = \pi_B = \pi$, relates to that with imbalanced case, we let $\pi_A = \pi_B = \pi$ in Equations 5.7 and 5.8 and correspondingly obtain

$$P_A^* = \alpha\left[1 + 2\pi\left(\varphi-1\right)\right]$$

$$= P_A \frac{\left[1 + 2\pi\left(\varphi-1\right)\right]}{\left[1 + 2\pi_A\left(\varphi-1\right)\right]} \tag{5.9}$$

$$P_B^* = \beta\left[1 + 2\pi\left(\varphi-1\right)\right]$$

$$= P_B \frac{\left[1 + 2\pi\left(\varphi-1\right)\right]}{\left[1 + 2\pi_B\left(\varphi-1\right)\right]} \tag{5.10}$$

Because the effect of X on R is expressed in terms of the multiplier φ, we also examine the impact of the distribution of X in terms of ratio of response rates as follows:

$$\frac{P_A}{P_B} = \frac{\alpha}{\beta} \frac{\left[1 + 2\pi_A(\varphi - 1)\right]}{\left[1 + 2\pi_B(\varphi - 1)\right]} = \frac{P_A^*}{P_B^*} \frac{\left[1 + 2\pi_A(\varphi - 1)\right]}{\left[1 + 2\pi_B(\varphi - 1)\right]} \tag{5.11}$$

The imbalance in factor X changed the ratio of response rates by a factor of $\dfrac{\left[1 + 2\pi_A(\varphi - 1)\right]}{\left[1 + 2\pi_B(\varphi - 1)\right]}$, which involves not only the distribution of X in treatment groups (π_A and π_B), but also φ, which is the effect of factor X on the response. This is an adjustment that corresponds to the additive adjustment $\beta(x_{ij} - \bar{x}_{..})$ in Equation 5.1 for ANCOVA.

Rank-based analyses of stratified design such as the Wilcoxon–Mann–Whitney test are often used for ordered categorical endpoints (see Homework 4.7). A good discussion with simulations is given in Mehrotra, Lu, and Li (2010). An application of stratified WMW test in the remdesivir trial for the treatment of severe COVID-19 patients is provided in Shih, Chen, and Xie (2020).

5.5 Logistic Regression Analysis

In Sections 4.3 and 4.7, when we studied power and sample size estimation, we had briefly discussed the comparison of treatment groups for binary and ordinal endpoints without explicitly adjusting for covariates. With covariates, if response categories are few and only categorical covariates are involved, we may carry out (covariate-) stratified analyses, as discussed in Section 5.4. One of the commonly used methods is the CMH (or Mantel–Haenszel) test. CMH (Cochran-Mantel-Haenszel) test is also known as stratified log-rank test in the context of analysis of survival data; we will discuss more in Chapter 6. In Section 5.4, we have seen an illustration of a stratified analysis with the case of a simple binary covariate. For data with a binary or ordered categorical endpoint and continuous and/or categorical covariates, logistic and cumulative logistic regression models are often used to analyze treatment effects adjusted for covariates.

5.5.1 Binary Endpoint and Logistic Regression

Denote the binary outcome variable by Y, with Y = 1 being response and Y = 0 being non-response. Let X_i be a column vector of covariates including the treatment group and other baseline prognostic factors for the individual

i. $\mathbf{X}_i$ is usually augmented with constant 1 in its first row for the intercept of the model, as we have seen in (5.1) for the linear regression ANCOVA model. The conditional mean of Y_i given $\mathbf{X}_i$ (i.e., regression of Y on X) is $\Pr(Y_i = 1 \mid \mathbf{X}_i)$, and it is no longer linear but follows a logistic form:

$$E(Y_i \mid \mathbf{X}_i) = \pi(\mathbf{X}_i) = \frac{e^{\mathbf{X}_i'\beta}}{1 + e^{\mathbf{X}_i'\beta}} \tag{5.12}$$

where $\mathbf{X}_i'$ is the transpose of $\mathbf{X}_i$ and $\beta = \{\beta_0, \ldots, \beta_K\}$ is the column vector of unknown regression coefficients. This is because $\pi(\mathbf{X}_i)$, as probability of response given $\mathbf{X}_i$, is limited in the range of 0 to 1 interval, but $\mathbf{X}_i'\beta$ is not. Expression (5.12) is equivalent to applying the logit transformation on $\pi(\mathbf{X}_i)$ and mapping it to the real line scale:

$$\text{logit}\left[\pi(\mathbf{X}_i)\right] \equiv \log\left[\frac{\pi(\mathbf{X}_i)}{1 - \pi(\mathbf{X}_i)}\right] = \beta_0 + \beta_1 X_{i1} + \ldots + \beta_K X_{iK}$$

This is a log-linear regression model. The coefficient β_j is the log odds ratio of response when the corresponding covariate X_{ij} is to change by one unit, adjusted for other covariates. Log-linear model is a member of the so-called "generalized linear model" as we mentioned it in Section 5.2.

To obtain estimates of the coefficients, we maximize the log-likelihood as follows (as we have seen previously in Appendix 4.3 and Appendix 4.5 for the exponential distribution for survival data). The likelihood function of β based on n observations $(y_i, \mathbf{x}_i)$ is

$$L(\beta; (y_i, \mathbf{x}_i), i = 1, \ldots, n) = \prod_{i=1}^{n} \pi(\mathbf{x}_i)^{y_i} \left[1 - \pi(\mathbf{x}_i)\right]^{1 - y_i}$$

The log-likelihood function is

$$l(\beta; (y_i, \mathbf{x}_i), i = 1, \ldots, n) = \log L(\beta; (y_i, \mathbf{x}_i), i = 1, \ldots, n)$$

$$= \sum_{i=1}^{n} \left\{ y_i \log(\pi(\mathbf{x}_i)) + (1 - y_i)\log\left[1 - \pi(\mathbf{x}_i)\right] \right\}$$

$$= \sum_{i=1}^{n} \left\{ y_i \log\left(\frac{\pi(\mathbf{x}_i)}{1 - \pi(\mathbf{x}_i)}\right) + \log\left[1 - \pi(\mathbf{x}_i)\right] \right\}$$

$$= \sum_{i=1}^{n} \left\{ y_i \left(\mathbf{X}_i'\beta\right) - \log\left(1 + e^{\mathbf{X}_i'\beta}\right) \right\}$$

The so-called score functions are the partial derivatives of the log-likelihood function with respect to each component of β. The score equations are to set the score functions to zero. That is, for $j = 0, \ldots, K$

$$\sum_{i=1}^{n}\left(y_i - \frac{e^{X_i'\beta}}{1+e^{X_i'\beta}}\right)x_{ij} = 0 \qquad (5.13)$$

The MLE of β is obtained by solving all the score equations in (5.13) using the iterative Newton–Raphson numeric method. The standard error of the MLE $\hat{\beta}$ is obtained through the second derivatives of the log-likelihood functions. Note that the estimates of the coefficients are correlated.

5.5.2 Ordinal Endpoint and Cumulative Logistic Regression

When there are $J>2$ ordered response categories, $\pi_j(X) = \Pr(Y = j \mid X)$ is the conditional probability of being in category j given X. We can form cumulative probabilities $F_j(X)$, as we did in Section 4.7, by

$$F_j(X) = \Pr(Y \le j \mid X) = \pi_1(X) + \cdots + \pi_j(X), \qquad j = 1, \ldots, J-1$$

and $F_J(X) = 1$. The cumulative logits are defined as, for $j = 1, \ldots, J-1$,

$$\text{logit } [F_j(X)] = \log\left[\frac{F_j(X)}{1 - F_j(X)}\right] = \log\left[\frac{\pi_1(X) + \cdots + \pi_j(X)}{\pi_{j+1}(X) + \cdots + \pi_J(X)}\right] = \log\left[\frac{\Pr(Y \le j \mid X)}{\Pr(Y > j \mid X)}\right]$$

It is the log odds of being in the categories 1 to j versus being in the categories $j + 1$ to J. So, the cumulative logit model is to view categories 1 to j as a single category and the rest of the categories $j + 1$ to J as another. The proportional odds model comparing two treatment groups with no other covariates was introduced in Section 4.7. Now, with other covariates, the proportional odds model is expressed as

$$\text{logit } [F_j(X)] = \alpha_j + X'\beta, \qquad j = 1, \ldots, J. \qquad (5.14)$$

This model indicates that, for two individuals with covariates X_1 and X_2, respectively,

$$\text{logit } [F_j(X_1)] - \text{logit}\left[F_j(X_2)\right] = X_1'\beta - X_2'\beta = (X_1' - X_2')\beta$$

Or,

$$\log\left\{\left[\frac{\Pr(Y \le j \mid X_1)}{\Pr(Y > j \mid X_1)}\right] \Big/ \left[\frac{\Pr(Y \le j \mid X_2)}{\Pr(Y > j \mid X_2)}\right]\right\} = (X_1' - X_2')\beta$$

That is, the log odds ratio of the cumulative probability of being in categories up to j is proportional to the difference between the values of the covariates and is the same for all categories $j = 1, \ldots, J-1$. The odds of being in the response category $\leq j$ are $e^{(X_1 - X_2)\beta}$ times higher at $X = X_1$ than at $X = X_2$ for all $j = 1, \ldots, J-1$.

For ordered categorical response, the above assumption of proportional odds is often assumed. This proportional odds model is easy to interpret and verify with few (e.g., less than 5) ordered categories.

Example 5.1 Remdesivir for Severe COVID-19 Pandemic

In the first remdesivir trial for treating severe COVID-19 patients, the following WHO (World Health Organization) scoring system for the evaluation of virus infection was used: score = (category): 1 = (live discharge), 2 = (mildly severe), 3 = (moderately severe), 4 = (critically severe), 5 = (very critically severe), and 6 = (death) (Table 5.2). For score ≥ 3, patients require supplemental oxygen in the hospital. Define the "response" criterion as reaching the clinical status of score = 2 or 1 in the 6-category scale (Wang et al. 2020 and Shih et al. 2020). As expressed by clinical experts, sparing severely ill patients from requiring supplemental oxygen amid the pandemic crisis is clinically meaningful to the patients as well as to the healthcare providers, since the supplemental oxygen equipment

TABLE 5.2

Summary of Score Distribution on 6-Category Scale

Scale (Category)		1 (Live discharge)	2 (Mildly severe)	3 (Moderately severe)	4 (Critically severe)	5 (Very Critically severe)	6 (Death)
Baseline	Remdesivir n=153*	0	0	124	27	1	1
	(%)	(0)	(0)	(81.0)	(17.6)	(0.7)	(0.7)
	Placebo						
	n=78	0	3	65	9	1	0
	(%)	(0)	(3.8)	(83.3)	(11.5)	(1.3)	(0)
Day 14	Remdesivir n=151	45	18	59	12	4	13
	(%)	(29.8)	(11.9)	(39.1)	(7.9)	(2.6)	(8.6)
	Placebo n=78	18	11	27	8	7	7
	(%)	(23.1)	(14.1)	(34.6)	(10.3)	(9.0)	(9.0)
Day 28	Remdesivir n=149	99	11	15	2	2	20
	(%)	(66.4)	(7.4)	(10.1)	(1.3)	(1.3)	(13.4)
	Placebo n=76	46	3	12	2	3	10
	(%)	(60.5)	(3.9)	(15.8)	(2.6)	(3.9)	(13.2)

* One death that occurred prior to receiving treatment was excluded from the analysis.
Data Source: Shih et al. (2020), with permission.

may then be cleared to other patients who are in need. We therefore clas-
sify each outcome in the trial a "response" or "non-response" at each
assessment day by examining the 6-point scale status: point = 2 or 1
being a response; otherwise, a non-response. The duration of the trial
was 28 days. We analyze the binary response data using logistic regression. The logistic regression model includes the baseline disease status,
treatment group, assessment day, treatment by day interaction, and treatment by baseline status interaction. Notice that this model will obtain
the treatment effect adjusted for the baseline status and assessment day
in the study. Our main aim is to assess the treatment effect at Day 28
while controlling for baseline status. We also test the treatment effect at
Day 14 to see if there is an early treatment effect 4 days after the 10-day
intravenous regimen of remdesivir. We express the treatment effect of
remdesivir in terms of odds ratio (OR) of response (with 95% confidence
interval) relative to the placebo. The SAS code for the regression analysis
is in Appendix 5.3.

The dataset included 231 patients (153 remdesivir; 78 placebo) for
the 6-point ordinal scale at baseline and 225 patients (149 remdesivir;
76 placebo) on Day 28. The baseline score distribution (%) is: (0, 0, 81.0,
17.6, 0.7, 0.7) for the remdesivir group and (0, 3.8, 83.3, 11.5, 1.3, 0) for the
placebo group, for point=1 (discharged or met discharge criteria) to 6
(death). As seen, majority (81–83%) were point = 3 patients, who were
hospitalized and required supplemental oxygen—the moderately severe
category. About 12–18% were point=4 patients, who were hospitalized
and required non-invasive ventilation (NIV) and/or high-flow oxygen
therapy (HFNC). Very few in the category 5 required extracorporeal
membrane oxygenation (ECMO) and/or invasive mechanical ventilation
(IMV). The proportions of responders (defined as score≤2), uncontrolled

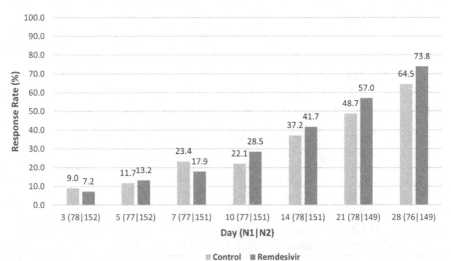

FIGURE 5.2
Response rate (%) by day: Remdesivir versus Control.

TABLE 5.3

Regression Analysis of the Remdesivir Trial for Severe COVID-19 Patients

Baseline Scale	Day	Treatment Group	Model-adjusted response rate*	Odds Ratio	95% Confidence Limits		P-value
3	14	Placebo	0.33		0.28	0.38	
		Remdesivir	0.43		0.39	0.46	
		Remdesivir vs Placebo		1.53	1.17	2.01	0.0022
	28	Placebo	0.70		0.61	0.78	
		Remdesivir	0.85		0.80	0.89	
		Remdesivir vs Placebo		2.38	1.41	4.01	0.0012
4	14	Placebo	0.14		0.07	0.25	
		Remdesivir	0.07		0.04	0.12	
		Remdesivir vs Placebo		0.48	0.19	1.18	0.1082
	28	Placebo	0.44		0.27	0.63	
		Remdesivir	0.37		0.25	0.50	
		Remdesivir vs Placebo		0.74	0.29	1.89	0.5296

Data Source: Shih et al. (2020), with permission. *Logistic regression model includes treatment group, baseline score, day of assessment, treatment by day interaction, and treatment by baseline interaction.

for baseline status, are displayed in Figure 5.2 by treatment groups at each study assessment day. The increasing trend of response is obvious for both treatment groups. Table 5.3 shows the main results from the logistic regression analysis adjusting for covariates. The response rate was 85% for remdesivir-treated patients with baseline status point=3 (moderately severe category) versus 70% response rate for likewise placebo-treated patients on Day 28 (OR = 2.38, p-value = 0.0012). On Day 14, the response rate for these patients was 43% for remdesivir versus 33% for placebo (OR = 1.53, p-value = 0.0022). For patients with baseline status point=4 (critically severe category), which was a much smaller cohort in the study, no similar comparisons were statistically significant, although the placebo group had higher response rate numerically.

Appendix 5.1: Weekly Average Pain Score (WAPS) Data

Obs	WK_0	WK_7	Age	Sex	SubjID	TRT
1	6.8571	4.5714	62	M	30007	Control
2	4.8571	2.8571	64	M	30009	Control
3	5.8571	7.0000	48	M	40003	Control
4	7.7143	5.5714	58	M	60002	Control
5	6.6000	2.0000	59	F	60007	Control
6	5.7143	6.5714	65	F	70004	Control
7	7.5714	2.2857	58	M	70012	Control
8	2.8333	0.5714	67	F	70023	Control

(Continued)

Obs	WK_0	WK_7	Age	Sex	SubjID	TRT
9	8.8571	8.7143	68	M	70037	Control
10	6.0000	1.4000	40	M	90015	Control
11	6.2857	6.0000	56	M	90025	Control
12	8.7143	7.0000	67	M	90031	Control
13	6.1429	6.1429	50	F	110001	Control
14	8.2857	8.5714	67	F	110004	Control
15	9.8000	7.8571	63	F	140014	Control
16	7.1429	5.1429	62	M	170008	Control
17	7.2857	3.8571	69	M	190004	Control
18	4.8571	2.0000	73	M	190010	Control
19	7.0000	7.0000	71	F	190015	Control
20	6.0000	1.0000	65	F	190025	Control
21	7.5714	4.8571	70	F	190036	Control
22	4.4286	2.2857	73	F	190042	Control
23	9.7143	10.0000	44	F	190046	Control
24	5.0000	3.0000	52	M	190055	Control
25	7.2857	3.8333	36	F	200002	Control
26	5.2857	2.0000	51	F	210002	Control
27	9.7143	9.0000	50	M	210009	Control
28	5.4286	3.2857	55	F	210013	Control
29	9.7143	9.3333	48	F	210014	Control
30	9.7143	10.0000	55	F	230011	Control
31	7.7143	5.0000	58	M	240001	Control
32	5.8571	5.5714	60	F	240004	Control
33	8.5714	7.7143	50	F	240012	Control
34	7.7143	8.0000	75	M	240017	Control
35	7.5714	6.0000	60	F	240023	Control
36	9.5714	9.4286	73	F	280003	Control
37	6.7143	5.1429	77	M	280010	Control
38	8.0000	5.2857	75	F	280012	Control
39	8.8571	7.2857	62	F	280015	Control
40	10.0000	0.0000	55	F	280016	Control
41	6.2500	5.1429	52	M	60011	Active
42	8.0000	4.4286	68	M	70010	Active
43	8.4286	9.0000	67	F	70038	Active
44	7.3333	6.8571	54	M	90004	Active
45	6.2857	4.1667	60	F	90026	Active
46	8.7500	3.2857	53	F	130001	Active
47	10.0000	1.5714	57	M	140011	Active
48	7.2857	6.3333	55	F	190054	Active
49	7.0000	5.7143	65	F	190056	Active
50	4.1429	1.1429	28	F	210008	Active
51	7.83333	4.28571	52	F	220001	Active
52	4.14286	3.42857	55	F	230001	Active

(Continued)

Obs	WK_0	WK_7	Age	Sex	SubjID	TRT
53	6.85714	4.80000	63	M	230009	Active
54	7.85714	2.57143	62	F	240005	Active
55	5.28571	5.00000	64	F	290011	Active
56	8.71429	6.00000	63	F	290046	Active
57	5.85714	3.00000	58	F	310005	Active
58	7.00000	6.57143	51	M	310033	Active
59	7.16667	8.20000	54	M	330003	Active
60	7.28571	7.42857	55	F	340004	Active
61	5.16667	4.00000	72	F	360019	Active
62	7.42857	6.28571	60	F	360023	Active
63	4.20000	6.85714	75	M	360033	Active
64	6.20000	2.42857	37	F	360046	Active
65	4.14286	2.00000	61	M	480003	Active
66	7.42857	6.14286	57	F	480008	Active
67	7.28571	8.14286	61	M	520002	Active
68	6.60000	5.85714	51	M	570009	Active
69	7.00000	7.14286	56	M	580001	Active
70	6.42857	3.00000	48	F	640003	Active
71	9.00000	7.85714	59	M	670002	Active
72	5.85714	5.00000	62	M	760002	Active
73	4.71429	0.00000	73	M	760012	Active
74	6.28571	6.00000	74	M	780004	Active
75	7.00000	6.83333	56	M	780009	Active
76	6.57143	5.66667	65	M	790010	Active
77	6.14286	0.00000	50	M	790021	Active
78	6.80000	2.85714	69	M	800003	Active
79	5.28571	5.42857	68	F	800005	Active
80	8.28571	7.00000	54	M	800014	Active
81	7.00000	1.14286	78	M	820007	Active

Appendix 5.2: Remdesivir for the Treatment of Severe COVID-19 (6-Category Scale Data)

base	trtan	result	count	day
2	1	1	0	28
2	1	2	0	28
2	1	3	0	28
2	1	4	0	28
2	1	5	0	28
2	1	6	0	28

(Continued)

base	trtan	result	count	day
3	1	1	90	28
3	1	2	10	28
3	1	3	9	28
3	1	4	2	28
3	1	5	2	28
3	1	6	10	28
4	1	1	9	28
4	1	2	1	28
4	1	3	6	28
4	1	4	0	28
4	1	5	0	28
4	1	6	10	28
5	1	1	0	28
5	1	2	0	28
5	1	3	0	28
5	1	4	0	28
5	1	5	0	28
5	1	6	0	28
6	1	1	0	28
6	1	2	0	28
6	1	3	0	28
6	1	4	0	28
6	1	5	0	28
6	1	6	0	28
2	0	1	2	28
2	0	2	0	28
2	0	3	1	28
2	0	4	0	28
2	0	5	0	28
2	0	6	0	28
3	0	1	40	28
3	0	2	3	28
3	0	3	10	28
3	0	4	1	28
3	0	5	2	28
3	0	6	7	28
4	0	1	4	28
4	0	2	0	28
4	0	3	1	28
4	0	4	1	28
4	0	5	0	28
4	0	6	3	28

(Continued)

base	trtan	result	count	day
5	0	1	0	28
5	0	2	0	28
5	0	3	0	28
5	0	4	0	28
5	0	5	1	28
5	0	6	0	28
6	0	1	0	28
6	0	2	0	28
6	0	3	0	28
6	0	4	0	28
6	0	5	0	28
6	0	6	0	28
2	1	1	0	21
2	1	2	0	21
2	1	3	0	21
2	1	4	0	21
2	1	5	0	21
2	1	6	0	21
3	1	1	72	21
3	1	2	7	21
3	1	3	27	21
3	1	4	3	21
3	1	5	3	21
3	1	6	10	21
4	1	1	4	21
4	1	2	2	21
4	1	3	8	21
4	1	4	4	21
4	1	5	1	21
4	1	6	8	21
5	1	1	0	21
5	1	2	0	21
5	1	3	0	21
5	1	4	0	21
5	1	5	0	21
5	1	6	0	21
6	1	1	0	21
6	1	2	0	21
6	1	3	0	21
6	1	4	0	21
6	1	5	0	21
6	1	6	0	21

(Continued)

base	trtan	result	count	day
2	0	1	2	21
2	0	2	0	21
2	0	3	1	21
2	0	4	0	21
2	0	5	0	21
2	0	6	0	21
3	0	1	30	21
3	0	2	4	21
3	0	3	19	21
3	0	4	3	21
3	0	5	3	21
3	0	6	6	21
4	0	1	2	21
4	0	2	0	21
4	0	3	3	21
4	0	4	1	21
4	0	5	0	21
4	0	6	3	21
5	0	1	0	21
5	0	2	0	21
5	0	3	0	21
5	0	4	0	21
5	0	5	1	21
5	0	6	0	21
6	0	1	0	21
6	0	2	0	21
6	0	3	0	21
6	0	4	0	21
6	0	5	0	21
6	0	6	0	21
2	1	1	0	14
2	1	2	0	14
2	1	3	0	14
2	1	4	0	14
2	1	5	0	14
2	1	6	0	14
3	1	1	44	14
3	1	2	18	14
3	1	3	49	14
3	1	4	6	14
3	1	5	3	14
3	1	6	5	14

(Continued)

base	trtan	result	count	day
4	1	1	1	14
4	1	2	0	14
4	1	3	10	14
4	1	4	6	14
4	1	5	1	14
4	1	6	8	14
5	1	1	0	14
5	1	2	0	14
5	1	3	0	14
5	1	4	0	14
5	1	5	0	14
5	1	6	0	14
6	1	1	0	14
6	1	2	0	14
6	1	3	0	14
6	1	4	0	14
6	1	5	0	14
6	1	6	0	14
2	0	1	1	14
2	0	2	1	14
2	0	3	0	14
2	0	4	1	14
2	0	5	0	14
2	0	6	0	14
3	0	1	16	14
3	0	2	10	14
3	0	3	25	14
3	0	4	5	14
3	0	5	5	14
3	0	6	4	14
4	0	1	1	14
4	0	2	0	14
4	0	3	2	14
4	0	4	2	14
4	0	5	1	14
4	0	6	3	14
5	0	1	0	14
5	0	2	0	14
5	0	3	0	14
5	0	4	0	14
5	0	5	1	14
5	0	6	0	14

(Continued)

base	trtan	result	count	day
6	0	1	0	14
6	0	2	0	14
6	0	3	0	14
6	0	4	0	14
6	0	5	0	14
6	0	6	0	14
2	1	1	0	7
2	1	2	0	7
2	1	3	0	7
2	1	4	0	7
2	1	5	0	7
2	1	6	0	7
3	1	1	4	7
3	1	2	22	7
3	1	3	81	7
3	1	4	12	7
3	1	5	4	7
3	1	6	2	7
4	1	1	0	7
4	1	2	1	7
4	1	3	4	7
4	1	4	14	7
4	1	5	1	7
4	1	6	6	7
5	1	1	0	7
5	1	2	0	7
5	1	3	0	7
5	1	4	0	7
5	1	5	0	7
5	1	6	0	7
6	1	1	0	7
6	1	2	0	7
6	1	3	0	7
6	1	4	0	7
6	1	5	0	7
6	1	6	0	7
2	0	1	0	7
2	0	2	2	7
2	0	3	1	7
2	0	4	0	7
2	0	5	0	7
2	0	6	0	7

(Continued)

base	trtan	result	count	day
3	0	1	1	7
3	0	2	14	7
3	0	3	39	7
3	0	4	6	7
3	0	5	2	7
3	0	6	2	7
4	0	1	1	7
4	0	2	0	7
4	0	3	2	7
4	0	4	3	7
4	0	5	1	7
4	0	6	2	7
5	0	1	0	7
5	0	2	0	7
5	0	3	0	7
5	0	4	0	7
5	0	5	1	7
5	0	6	0	7
6	0	1	0	7
6	0	2	0	7
6	0	3	0	7
6	0	4	0	7
6	0	5	0	7
6	0	6	0	7
2	1	1	0	10
2	1	2	0	10
2	1	3	0	10
2	1	4	0	10
2	1	5	0	10
2	1	6	0	10
3	1	1	15	10
3	1	2	27	10
3	1	3	68	10
3	1	4	7	10
3	1	5	3	10
3	1	6	5	10
4	1	1	0	10
4	1	2	1	10
4	1	3	9	10
4	1	4	8	10
4	1	5	2	10
4	1	6	6	10

(*Continued*)

base	trtan	result	count	day
5	1	1	0	10
5	1	2	0	10
5	1	3	0	10
5	1	4	0	10
5	1	5	0	10
5	1	6	0	10
6	1	1	0	10
6	1	2	0	10
6	1	3	0	10
6	1	4	0	10
6	1	5	0	10
6	1	6	0	10
2	0	1	0	10
2	0	2	2	10
2	0	3	0	10
2	0	4	1	10
2	0	5	0	10
2	0	6	0	10
3	0	1	5	10
3	0	2	9	10
3	0	3	36	10
3	0	4	8	10
3	0	5	3	10
3	0	6	3	10
4	0	1	1	10
4	0	2	0	10
4	0	3	2	10
4	0	4	3	10
4	0	5	1	10
4	0	6	2	10
5	0	1	0	10
5	0	2	0	10
5	0	3	0	10
5	0	4	0	10
5	0	5	1	10
5	0	6	0	10
6	0	1	0	10
6	0	2	0	10
6	0	3	0	10
6	0	4	0	10
6	0	5	0	10

(Continued)

base	trtan	result	count	day
6	0	6	0	10
2	1	1	0	5
2	1	2	0	5
2	1	3	0	5
2	1	4	0	5
2	1	5	0	5
2	1	6	0	5
3	1	1	2	5
3	1	2	18	5
3	1	3	86	5
3	1	4	16	5
3	1	5	3	5
3	1	6	0	5
4	1	1	0	5
4	1	2	0	5
4	1	3	3	5
4	1	4	19	5
4	1	5	2	5
4	1	6	3	5
5	1	1	0	5
5	1	2	0	5
5	1	3	0	5
5	1	4	0	5
5	1	5	0	5
5	1	6	0	5
6	1	1	0	5
6	1	2	0	5
6	1	3	0	5
6	1	4	0	5
6	1	5	0	5
6	1	6	0	5
2	0	1	0	5
2	0	2	2	5
2	0	3	1	5
2	0	4	0	5
2	0	5	0	5
2	0	6	0	5
3	0	1	0	5
3	0	2	6	5
3	0	3	49	5
3	0	4	6	5

(Continued)

base	trtan	result	count	day
3	0	5	2	5
3	0	6	1	5
4	0	1	0	5
4	0	2	1	5
4	0	3	2	5
4	0	4	3	5
4	0	5	3	5
4	0	6	0	5
5	0	1	0	5
5	0	2	0	5
5	0	3	0	5
5	0	4	0	5
5	0	5	1	5
5	0	6	0	5
6	0	1	0	5
6	0	2	0	5
6	0	3	0	5
6	0	4	0	5
6	0	5	0	5
6	0	6	0	5
2	1	1	0	3
2	1	2	0	3
2	1	3	0	3
2	1	4	0	3
2	1	5	0	3
2	1	6	0	3
3	1	1	0	3
3	1	2	11	3
3	1	3	100	3
3	1	4	12	3
3	1	5	2	3
3	1	6	0	3
4	1	1	0	3
4	1	2	0	3
4	1	3	2	3
4	1	4	22	3
4	1	5	2	3
4	1	6	1	3
5	1	1	0	3
5	1	2	0	3
5	1	3	0	3

(Continued)

base	trtan	result	count	day
5	1	4	0	3
5	1	5	0	3
5	1	6	0	3
6	1	1	0	3
6	1	2	0	3
6	1	3	0	3
6	1	4	0	3
6	1	5	0	3
6	1	6	0	3
2	0	1	0	3
2	0	2	2	3
2	0	3	1	3
2	0	4	0	3
2	0	5	0	3
2	0	6	0	3
3	0	1	0	3
3	0	2	5	3
3	0	3	54	3
3	0	4	4	3
3	0	5	1	3
3	0	6	1	3
4	0	1	0	3
4	0	2	0	3
4	0	3	2	3
4	0	4	5	3
4	0	5	2	3
4	0	6	0	3
5	0	1	0	3
5	0	2	0	3
5	0	3	0	3
5	0	4	0	3
5	0	5	1	3
5	0	6	0	3
6	0	1	0	3
6	0	2	0	3
6	0	3	0	3
6	0	4	0	3
6	0	5	0	3
6	0	6	0	3

Note: base = baseline score; trtan = treatment group (1 = rem; 0 = plbo); result = score at the specific day; count = number of patients; day = day in the study.

Appendix 5.3: Logistic Regression Analysis Using SAS for Data in Appendix 5.2

```
data df; set lib.df;
if result<=2 then score=1;else score=0;
if base=6 then delete;
if count=0 then delete;
run;

/*. Creating Table 5.2

data day28; set df;
if day=28;
proc freq;
tables trtan*result / nopercent nocum nocol;
weight count;
run;

data day14; set df;
if day=14;
proc freq;
tables trtan*result / nopercent nocum nocol;
weight count;
run;

*/


/**------ Logistic Regression Analysis ------;*/

proc logistic order=data data=df;
freq count;
class base(ref='2') trtan(ref='0')/param=reference;
model score(event='1')=base trtan day trtan*day trtan*base;

contrast 'Day=14 Base=3 Trt=0' intercept 1 Day 14 base 1 0 0 /
estimate=prob;
contrast 'Day=14 Base=3 Trt=1' intercept 1 trtan 1 Day 14 base
1 0 0 trtan*day 14 trtan*base 1 0 0/ estimate=prob;

contrast 'Trt comparison 1 vs 0' trtan 1 trtan*day 14
trtan*base 1 0 0/ estimate=exp;

contrast 'Day=28 Base=3 Trt=0' intercept 1 Day 28 base 1 0 0 /
estimate=prob;
contrast 'Day=28 Base=3 Trt=1' intercept 1 trtan 1 Day 28 base
1 0 0 trtan*day 28 trtan*base 1 0 0/ estimate=prob;

contrast 'Trt comparison 1 vs 0' trtan 1 trtan*day 28
trtan*base 1 0 0/ estimate=exp;
```

```
contrast 'Day=14 Base=4 Trt=0' intercept 1 Day 14 base 0 1 0 /
estimate=prob;
contrast 'Day=14 Base=4 Trt=1' intercept 1 trtan 1 Day 14 base
0 1 0 trtan*day 14 trtan*base 0 1 0/ estimate=prob;

contrast 'Trt comparison 1 vs 0' trtan 1 trtan*day 14
trtan*base 0 1 0/ estimate=exp;

contrast 'Day=28 Base=4 Trt=0' intercept 1 Day 28 base 0 1 0 /
estimate=prob;
contrast 'Day=28 Base=4 Trt=1' intercept 1 trtan 1 Day 28 base
0 1 0 trtan*day 28 trtan*base 0 1 0/ estimate=prob;

contrast 'Trt comparison 1 vs 0' trtan 1 trtan*day 28
trtan*base 0 1 0/ estimate=exp;


run;
```

HOMEWORK 5.1

Appendix 5.1 lists a dataset from a randomized clinical trial to evaluate treatment effect on WAPS. There are two treatment groups, Control and Active, and two measures of the WAPS, at baseline (WK_0) and week 7 (WK_7). Patients' age and sex are also included in the list.

1. Use the WAPS at week 7 as the response variable and at baseline (WK_0) as the covariate. Carry out the ANCOVA. Is the parallel slope assumption satisfied? Test the treatment effect adjusted for the covariate. Obtain the adjusted means and associated 95% Cl for each treatment group. Repeat the adjusted analysis using age, sex, and baseline WK_0 as covariates.

2. Create a variable, Change in WAPS, and use it as the response variable. Include baseline WAPS, age, and sex as the covariates to carry out ANCOVA. Report the results and give your conclusions.

HOMEWORK 5.2

Stratified Analysis (Altman 1985)

1. Following the notation in Section 5.4, suppose that we have a well-balanced design by stratified randomization and obtained the following result (Table 5.4):

TABLE 5.4

Homework 5.2.1: Stratified Analysis

		Treatment Group (T)			Response Rate A vs. B	
		A	**B**	**Total**		
Factor (X)	"+"	40/50	32/50	72/100	80%	64%
	"–"	60/150	48/150	108/300	40%	32%
Total		100/200	80/200	180/400	50%	40%

Source: Altman, D. G., *The Statistician*, 34, 125, 1985. With permission.

   a. In terms of the notation in Table 5.1, what value is φ?

   b. Test the overall treatment effect first by the combined results (100/200 vs. 80/200), and then by the CMH test. Compare and comment. (You may need to create two 2×2 tables to carry out the CMH test or may need to use the PROC FREQ options in SAS.)

2. Without materially changing the response rates (A vs. B) in each stratum, suppose that there is imbalance in the distribution of factor X in treatment groups (A has more X = "+" and less "–" than B) as displayed in Table 5.5.

   a. Has φ changed?

   b. Use a chi-square test to check the distribution of X between treatment groups. What is the p-value? What does this p-value represent?

   c. Test the overall treatment effect first by the combined results (103/200 vs. 77/200), and then by the CMH test. Compare and comment.

3. Without materially changing the response rates (A vs. B) in each stratum, suppose that there is imbalance in the distribution of

TABLE 5.5

Homework 5.2.2: Stratified Analysis

		Treatment Group (T)			Response Rate A vs. B	
		A	**B**	**Total**		
Factor (X)	"+"	47/59	26/41	73/100	80%	63%
	"–"	56/141	51/159	107/300	40%	32%
Total		103/200	77/200	180/400	51.5%	38.5%

Source: Altman, D. G., *The Statistician*, 34, 125, 1985. With permission.

TABLE 5.6

Homework 5.2.3: Stratified Analysis

		Treatment Group (T)			Response Rate A	
		A	B	Total	vs. B	
Factor (X)	"+"	33/41	38/59	71/100	80%	64%
	"–"	64/159	45/141	109/300	40%	32%
Total		97/200	83/200	180/400	48.5%	41.5%

Source: Altman, D. G., The Statistician, 34, 125, 1985. With permission.

factor X in treatment groups (B has more X = "+" and less "–" than A), as displayed in Table 5.6.

a. Has φ changed?
b. Use a chi-square test to check the distribution of X between treatment groups. What is the p-value? What does this p-value represent?
c. Test the overall treatment effect first by the combined results (97/200 vs. 83/200), and then by the CMH test. Compare and comment.

HOMEWORK 5.3

Use the data in Appendix 5.2 and instruction in Appendix 5.3 to perform the cumulative logistic regression analysis and obtain odds ratio estimates similar to Table 5.3, assuming the proportional odds model.

References

Abeyasekera S. (1984). The desirability of covariance adjustments. *Journal of the Royal Statistical Society. Series C (Applied Statistics)* 33: 33–37.

Altman DG. (1985). Comparability of randomized groups. *The Statistician* 34: 125–136.

Cochran WG. (1954). Some methods for strengthening the common chi-square tests. *Biometrics* 21: 86–98.

Cochran WG. (1957). Analysis of covariance. Its nature and uses. *Biometrics* 13: 261–281.

Mantel N and Haenszel W. (1959). Statistical aspects of the analysis of data from retrospective studies. *Journal of the National Cancer Institute* 2: 719–748.

Mantel N. (1963). Chi-square tests with one-degree of freedom: extensions of the Mantel-Haenszel procedure. *Journal of the American Statistical Association* 58: 690–700.

McCullagh P and Nelder JA. (1989). *Generalized Linear Models*. London: Chapman & Hall.

Mehrotra DV, Lu X and Li X. (2010). Rank-based analyses of stratified experiments: Alternatives to the van Elteren test. *The American Statistician* 64:121–130.

Shih WJ, Shen X, Zhang P, Xie T. (2020). Remdesivir is effective for moderately severe patients: A Re-analysis of the first double-blind, placebo-controlled, randomized trial on remdesivir for treatment of severe COVID-19 patients conducted in Wuhan City. *Open Access Journal of Clinical Trials* 12: 15–21.

Shih WJ, Yao C, and Xie T. (2020). Data monitoring for the Chinese clinical trials of remdesivir in treating patients with COVID-19 during the pandemic crisis. *Therapeutic Innovation & Regulatory Science* 54: 1236–1255.

Wang Y, Zhang D, Du G, et al. (2020). Remdesivir in adults with severe COVID-19: A randomised, double-blind, placebo-controlled, multicentre trial. *Lancet* 395(10236): 1569–1578. doi: 10.1016/S0140-6736(20)31022-9.

Weisberg S. (1985). *Applied Linear Regression*. New York: Wiley.

6

Regression Analysis of Survival Data

As mentioned in Section 4.4, survival data analysis is a generic term of methods used for time-to-event endpoints. The outcome event of interest may be a clinically significant morbid event such as death, stroke, myocardial infarction, serious infection, a major organ failure, or tumor progression. It can also be a good event such as disease recovery. For example, the US NIH-sponsored trial to test remdesivir for the treatment of severe COVID-19 used time to clinical improvement of at least 2 points in an 8-point scale as the primary endpoint (Beigel et al. 2020). Time-to-event endpoint differs from the other continuous variable endpoints in that the time might be right-censored when subjects have not experienced the event of interest at the time of data analysis. We emphasized in Section 4.4 the importance of defining the outcome event of interest and distinguishing it from the censoring event clearly in the study protocol and examining the independence assumption of the censoring event with the primary event of interest. To start, we first study the basic data display and log-rank test with only one binary covariate (which is usually the treatment or dose group in clinical trials). We then continue this chapter with the analysis of covariate-adjusted treatment effect for survival endpoints.

6.1 Kaplan–Meier Estimate and Log-Rank Test for Unadjusted Treatment Effect

As patients usually have different follow-up times, the life-table method (with equal time intervals) and the Kaplan–Meier (KM) product-limit method (without time intervals) are featured techniques for survival data analysis. As indicated in Appendix 4.3, survival data are a set of n triplets (T_i, δ_i, X_i), $i = 1, ..., n$, where $T_i = \min(Y_i, C_i)$ is the observed event time, δ_i is the event/censoring indicator ($\delta_i = 1$ if $T_i = Y_i$), and X_i is a set of covariates (baseline prognostic factors) for the individual i. We frequently see in the medical literature that KM graphs are used to summarize survival data, especially for visualizing the comparison between cohorts of patients with or without a log-rank test. Let $t_1 < t_2 < ... < t_D$ be D distinct, ordered (observed) event times, d_l be the observed number of events at time t_l, and r_l be the number of subjects at risk just before t_l; $l = 1, ...,D$. The KM estimator of the survival function is the product of conditional proportions of survivals out of the risk sets: For $t_j \le t < t_{j+1}$,

$$\hat{S}(t) = \left(1 - \frac{d_1}{r_1}\right)\left(1 - \frac{d_2}{r_2}\right)\cdots\left(1 - \frac{d_j}{r_j}\right) \qquad (6.1)$$

The variance is estimated by Greenwood's formula:

$$\hat{V}\left(\hat{S}(t)\right) = \hat{S}(t)^2 \sum_{l=1}^{j} \frac{d_l}{r_l(r_l - d_l)}$$

The log-rank test statistic for two-sample case based on a series of hypergeometric 2-by-2 tables is constructed by summing over the differences in observed versus expected failures in group 1 over the D event times. Specifically, the test statistic is

$$X^2 = \frac{\left[\sum_{l=1}^{D}\left(O_{t_l} - E_{t_l}\right)\right]^2}{\sum_{l=1}^{D} V_{t_l}} \qquad (6.2)$$

where, at time t_l, $O_{t_l} = d_{1l}$ is the observed number of events in group 1, $E_{t_l} = n_{1l}\left(\dfrac{d_l}{n_l}\right)$ is the expected number of deaths in group 1, $V_{t_l} = d_l n_{1l}\left(\dfrac{n_l - n_{1l}}{n_l^2}\right)\left(\dfrac{n_l - d_l}{n_l - 1}\right)$ is the variance of the expected number of deaths in group 1, d_l is the total number of events, and n_l is the total number at risk. It is asymptotically of chi-square distribution with 1 degree of freedom. We usually take the positive square root and compare to the standard normal distribution quantiles to obtain the significance level.

The KM product-limit estimator of the survival function (6.1) and the log-rank test (6.2) are nonparametric and do not involve model assumptions such as proportional hazards. We have also used a parametric exponential or Weibull model to do sample size planning based on log-rank test for survival endpoints in Chapter 4. These methods do not adjust for covariates other than the treatment group. When other covariates are considered in data analyses, as we often do, the semi-parametric Cox regression and stratified Cox regression analysis are often the popular methods to use. We will discuss them in the following sections. We also discuss model assumptions, model diagnostics, and alternative methods when model assumption is violated.

Software and Example 6.1

Appendix 6.1 is a dataset from the Phase II portion of a trial (Tan 2008) to study the combination of letrozole and sorafenib as the first-line therapy in postmenopausal women with hormone receptor-positive locally advanced or metastatic breast cancer. We use part of the overall survival data from the study for illustration purpose. With dose group as the only covariate, the log-rank test and KM estimate of the survival function are available in SAS PROC LIFTEST. The KM graphs are created easily by the plot option in the model statement as shown in Appendix 6.2. In R, the *plot* function applied to a *survfit* object will generate a graph of the survival function versus the survival time as shown in Appendix 6.5 (Homework 6.1).

6.2 Cox Regression Analysis and Proportional Hazards Model

In Chapter 4 (Appendix 4.1), the mathematical form and clinical interpretation of hazard rate as a function of time t, $h(t)$, as the "instantaneous risk" at time t was introduced. With a given set of covariates $X = \{X_1, ..., X_K\}$, the probability that an individual i with covariates x_i develops an event ("failure") at time t_i given that one of the individuals in the risk set R_i just prior to t_i "fails" at this time is given by

$$Pr[\text{individual fails at } t_i \mid \text{one failure in risk set at } t_i]$$

$$= \frac{Pr(\text{individual fails at } t_i \mid \text{survival to } t_i)}{Pr(\text{one failure in risk set at } t_i \mid \text{survival to } t_i)}$$

$$= \frac{h(t_i \mid x_i)}{\sum_{j \in R_i} h(t_i \mid x_j)}. \tag{6.3}$$

The survival function is

$$S(t \mid X) = Pr(Y > t \mid X) = e^{-\int_0^t h(s|X)ds} \equiv e^{-H(t|X)} \tag{6.4}$$

where $H(t|X) = \int_0^t h(s|X)ds$ is the cumulative hazard function. The hazard rate at time t is expressed as a function of treatment group and other covariates as well. (All vectors are column vectors as our convention for notation.) In the natural log scale analogous to the case of odds in multiple logistic regression, Cox (1972) formulated the following regression model:

$$\log h(t \mid X) = \log h_0(t) + \beta_1 X_1 + ... + \beta_K X_K$$

Equivalently,

$$h(t \mid X) = h_0(t)e^{\beta_1 X_1 + \ldots + \beta_K X_K} \equiv h_0(t)e^{X'\beta} \tag{6.5}$$

where X' is the transpose of X and $\beta = (\beta_1, \ldots, \beta_K)$ is the column vector of unknown regression coefficients. The baseline hazard rate function $h_0(t)$ represents the hazard rate at time t for an individual whose covariate values are all 0. It is merely a reference point, not being important whether it may be unrealistic, analogous to the intercept in the linear regression model we previously used in Eq. (5.1).

For two individuals with sets of covariates x_1 and x_2, respectively, the ratio of their hazard rates is

$$\frac{h(t \mid x_1)}{h(t \mid x_2)} = e^{\left(x_1' - x_2'\right)\beta}$$

The above equation indicates the ratio of hazards (relative risk) is independent of time. Thus, Cox regression model is also known as proportional hazards model. It is convenient (often reasonable as well) to assume the relative risk of developing the event remain constant over time. That is, even if the hazard rates of the two individuals change over time, the ratio of the two hazard rates remains constant, independent of time.

The assumption of proportional hazards (PH) should be checked when performing the data analysis. We may check by plotting graphs of survival curves based on the following. If the PH model is correct, then

$$S(t \mid X) = e^{-\int_0^t h(s \mid X)ds} = e^{-\int_0^t h_0(s)e^{X'\beta}ds} = e^{-e^{X'\beta}\int_0^t h_0(s)ds} = (S_0(t))^{e^{X'\beta}} \tag{6.6}$$

where $S_0(t) = S(t \mid 0) = e^{-\int_0^t h_0(s)ds} \equiv e^{-H_0(t)}$. Taking natural log on both sides of (6.6), we get $\log S(t \mid X) = e^{X'\beta}\log S_0(t)$. Since $\log S(t;X)$ is a negative number, we first express $-\log S(t \mid X) = -e^{X'\beta}\log S_0(t)$. Then, taking another log on both sides, we have:

$$\log(-\log S(t \mid X)) = \log(-\log S_0(t)) + X'\beta \tag{6.7}$$

This equation implies that the log(–log) transformation of the survival times of the two groups should be parallel along time when the PH model holds. Therefore, the log(–log(S(t))) plot (also called clog-log plot) of the fitted survival function at the event occurring times against time or some monotonic transformation of time such as log(t) is useful as a visual diagnostic tool for PH assumption. The KM graphs that we created by the plot option in the model statement of PROC LIFETEST previously (Example 6.1) can also plot log(–log S(t)) versus log(time) easily as shown in Appendix 6.3. Notice that since $S(t \mid X) = e^{-H(t \mid X)}$ and $H(t \mid X) = H_0(t)e^{X'\beta}$, the above equation can also be expressed by the cumulative hazard function as

$$\log H(t \mid X) = \log H_0(t) + X'\beta. \tag{6.8}$$

This checking of proportionality process also reveals an important concept in the survival data analysis regarding the covariates. The covariates, as we alluded to in ANCOVA and in logistic regression, are all time-fixed, baseline demographics (gender, race, and age) and characteristics or measures including prior therapy, initial disease stage, and genetic biomarker status. The reason they may vary with time here is because the risk sets of patients vary with time—shrinking each time an event occurs. The hazard rate (instantaneous risk) is conditional on the risk set (see Eq. (6.3)). Thus, the term "time-dependent covariate" is special for survival data analysis, meaning that the covariate is sensitively related to the time-varying risk set along the time. Of course, there may be other covariates that are truly time-varying, but we need to be sure that their changes are not due to treatment effect; otherwise, they should be part of endpoints, not covariates.

The graphical method does not work well for continuous covariate or categorical covariates that have many levels because the graph becomes too cluttered. Furthermore, the curves are sparse when there are fewer time points and it may be difficult to gauge the closeness to being parallel. More model diagnostic tools based on residuals will be discussed in Section 6.6.

6.3 Interpretation of the Regression Coefficients

The most important aspect of the regression model concerns the regression coefficients. If β_1 is zero (insignificant), then the associated covariate is not related to survival or does not contain information on survival when adjustment is made for the other covariates included in the model. The interpretation of the magnitude of the regression coefficient is like that in the logistic regression. For a categorical covariate such as treatment group, e.g., let $x_{11} = 1$ for Group 1 and $x_{21} = 0$ for Group 2, and other covariates having equal values for the groups. Then,

$$\frac{h\left(t \mid x_1 = \left(1, x_{12, \ldots,} x_{1k}\right)\right)}{h\left(t \mid x_2 = \left(0, x_{22, \ldots,} x_{2k}\right)\right)} = e^{\beta_1}$$

So, β_1 is the log-hazard ratio of Group 1 versus Group 2, given all other covariates being equal (i.e., "treatment effect adjusted for other covariates"). For a continuous covariate (such as age), we compare one person with, e.g.,

$x_{12} = a+1$ to another person with one unit apart, $x_{22} = a$, and other covariates being equal. Then,

$$\frac{h\left(t \mid \mathbf{x}_1 = \left(x_{11},a+1, x_{13}, \ldots, x_{1k}\right)\right)}{h\left(t \mid \mathbf{x}_2 = \left(x_{21},a, x_{23}, \ldots, x_{2k}\right)\right)} = e^{\beta_2}$$

So, β_2 is the log-hazard ratio of being one unit greater, given all other covariates being equal. In case one unit seems to be small for being meaningful, then it may be preferred to report $m \times \beta_2$, which is the log-hazard ratio corresponding to an m units increase.

6.4 Inference on Regression Coefficients Based on Partial Likelihood

6.4.1 Partial Likelihood Function

Inference for the Cox PH model is based on the so-called partial likelihood as follows. Following Eq. (6.3) and under proportional hazards model,

Pr[individual fails at t_i | one failure in risk set at t_i]

$$= \frac{h\left(t_i \mid \mathbf{x}_i\right)}{\sum_{j \in R_i} h\left(t_i \mid \mathbf{x}_j\right)}$$

$$= \frac{h_0\left(t_i\right)e^{\mathbf{x}_i'\beta}}{\sum_{j \in R_i} h_0\left(t_i\right)e^{\mathbf{x}_j'\beta}}$$

$$= \frac{e^{\mathbf{x}_i'\beta}}{\sum_{j \in R_i} e^{\mathbf{x}_j'\beta}} \qquad (6.9)$$

where R_i is the set of all individuals at risk just prior to t_i. Let $t_1 < t_2 < \ldots < t_D$ denote the D distinct, ordered (observed) event times. Let Ω_i be the set of all individuals who have developed events at time t_i and $\#\{\Omega_i\} = d_i$ be the number of events at t_i, and let $\mathbf{s}_i = \sum_{j \in \Omega_i} \mathbf{x}_j$, sum of the covariate vectors $\mathbf{x}_j$ over all individuals in Ω_i. Breslow (1974) expressed the partial likelihood as

$$L(\beta) = \prod_{i=1}^{D} \prod_{j \in \Omega_i} \frac{e^{\mathbf{x}_j'\beta}}{\sum_{k \in R_i} e^{\mathbf{x}_k'\beta}}$$

$$= \prod_{i=1}^{D} \frac{e^{s'_i\beta}}{\left[\sum_{k\in R_i} e^{x'_k\beta}\right]^{d_i}} \tag{6.10}$$

Efron's version (1977) has a minor correction:

$$\prod_{i=1}^{D} \prod_{j\in\Omega_i} \frac{e^{x'_j\beta}}{\sum_{k\in R_i} e^{x'_k\beta} - \frac{j-1}{d_i}\sum_{j\in\Omega_i} e^{x'_j\beta}}$$

Both versions of the partial likelihood consider each of the d_i events at a given time as distinct, construct their contribution to the likelihood function based on Eq. (6.9), and multiply all events at t_i, for all the D event times. In short, the partial likelihood is the product of conditional likelihoods from distinct event times. It is not a likelihood in the usual sense since the baseline hazard function is unknown and left unspecified. (For this reason, the inference is semi-parametric.) Tsiatis (1981) and Andersen and Gill (1982) proved that the partial likelihood shares the asymptotic properties of a full likelihood. Point estimate of the coefficients and their standard errors are computed in the usual way (i.e., taking the first derivatives of the likelihood function, setting to zeros, and solving for unknown regression parameters; taking the second derivatives to obtain the Fisher's information for variance estimates), along with the usual tests such as Wald, score, and likelihood ratio. See, e.g., Collett (1994). We shall continue to look at this derivation process in Section 6.7.2 when we further discuss the topic on weighted Cox regression (WCR), for which the above is a special case. When treatment group is the only covariate the score test from the partial likelihood agrees with the log-rank test derived from combining series of hypergeometric 2-by-2 tables at event times. Hence, the score test from Cox PH model is also called log-rank test in practice.

Note that SAS PROC PHREG uses Breslow's likelihood as a default, while the R function *coxph* uses Efron's likelihood as a default. When ties are few, both likelihoods are quite close. When there is no tie in event times, $d_i = 1$ for all t_i, both versions reduce to

$$L(\beta) = \prod_{i=1}^{D} \frac{e^{x'_i\beta}}{\sum_{k\in R_i} e^{x'_k\beta}} \tag{6.11}$$

6.4.2 Log-Rank Test and Stratified Cox Regression Model

The (score) log-rank test is always a valid test of the null hypothesis that the survival functions of two cohorts are the same. That is, the type I error rate agrees with the nominal level of the test when the null hypothesis is true. The effectiveness of the test in detecting departures from the null hypothesis, however, depends on the form of the difference. The log-rank test, in some sense, is optimal when the PH model is true. Sometimes we need to restrict the time range for a given dataset such that this assumption is applicable. Another situation is when the hazards are not proportional for some specific discrete covariate. Then we can stratify the heterogeneous population by that discrete covariate and fit the PH model for other covariates within each stratum. Here the subjects in each stratum have an arbitrary baseline hazard function. This is called stratified Cox regression model. Usually, this should improve the proportionality. Specifically, for stratum j, $h_j(t \mid X) = h_{0j}(t)e^{X'\beta}$, $j = 1, \ldots, J$. In this model, the regression coefficients are assumed to be the same in each stratum although the baseline hazard functions may be different and completely unspecified. The inference based on the partial likelihood method follows as before, where the partial log-likelihood function is the sum of J partial log-likelihood functions, each stratum using data for the individuals in the specific stratum.

Software and Example 6.2

Appendix 6.6 refers to a study of 20 grade III glioma and 17 glioblastoma (GBM) patients treated by adjuvant treatment with radioimmunotherapy ($n = 18$) versus standard of care as control ($n = 19$) (Grana et al. 2002). The survival dataset of the study is available from the R package *coin* (Everitt and Hothorn 2010). Appendices 6.6 and 6.7, respectively, show the *coxph* function in R from the *survival* package and PROC PHREG of SAS to fit the Cox stratified regression model and to obtain the point estimates along with the standard errors and the tests for the coefficients (Homework 6.2).

6.5 Estimation of Baseline Cumulative Hazard and Fitted Survival

We previously discussed $\log(-\log(S(t)))$ versus time plot for checking the assumption of proportional hazards by using the KM estimate of survival. The method was limited to only one categorical covariate. To expand to PH models with other covariates, we shall use residual plots in Section 6.6. Toward this end, we first need to estimate the cumulative baseline hazard function and obtain the fitted survival times with covariates. (Recall that the baseline hazard function was totally ignorable when making inference on regression coefficients was the interest in Section 6.4.)

Following before, we have D distinct, ordered, event times $t_1 < t_2 < \ldots < t_D$ and d_i number of events at t_i. The estimated baseline hazard function at t_i is given by

$$\frac{d_i}{\sum_{j \in R_i} e^{x_j'\beta}} \tag{6.12}$$

where $\hat{\beta}$ is the partial likelihood estimator of β, which enjoys the good large sample properties of an MLE. The estimator of the cumulative baseline hazard function $H_0(t) = \int_0^t h_0(s)ds$ is given by

$$\hat{H}_0(t) = \sum_{t_i \le t}\left[\frac{d_i}{\sum_{j \in R_i} e^{x_j'\hat{\beta}}}\right] \tag{6.13}$$

Hence, $\hat{S}_0(t) = e^{-\hat{H}_0(t)}$. This is the estimated baseline survival function for individuals with covariates $X = 0$. For individuals with covariates X, the estimated or fitted survival function is given by

$$\hat{S}(t;X) = (\hat{S}_0(t))^{e^{X'\hat{\beta}}} \tag{6.14}$$

In SAS PROC PHREG, $X'\hat{\beta}$ is called *linear predictor* in model checking with residuals.

6.6 Residuals for Model Diagnostics

As in ordinary or logistic regression analysis, model diagnostic and influential observation or outlier detection (the so-called "case analysis") are essential parts of modeling. Some of the covariates used in the Cox regression model may need some transformation, or some regression coefficients may be time-varying to have a better fit or to satisfy the proportionality assumption. Residual analysis is an integral part of such model diagnostics and case analysis for modeling. A few residuals are implemented in SAS or R package for practitioners. Here we discuss two: (i) martingale residuals, which is useful for checking whether some covariates need transformation; and (ii) pseudo-residuals, which is useful for both checking covariate transformation and time-varying coefficients. The latter is also useful for applying the *restricted mean survival time* (RMST) analysis as one of the methods for dealing with non-proportional hazards that we shall discuss in Section 6.7.3.

6.6.1 Martingale Residuals

Using the notation in Appendix 4.3, survival data observations are triplets (T_i, δ_i, X_i), $i = 1, ..., n$. The martingale residual for the i-th observation is defined as

$$r_i = \delta_i - \hat{H}_0(T_i)e^{x_i'\hat{\beta}} \tag{6.15}$$

where $\hat{H}_0(T_i)$ is from (6.13), the estimator of the cumulative baseline hazard function at time T_i. The martingale residual is the difference between the outcome (event/censor status, 0 or 1) and its expected value under the model, given the follow-up time T_i of the individual. For large samples, these residuals are uncorrelated and have mean 0 if the model fits the data. Thus, they can be used for model diagnostics.

We can fit the PH model including the set $\mathbf{X}$ of all predetermined covariates and obtain the martingale residuals. We first plot them versus $\mathbf{X}'\hat{\beta}$ *linear predictor*. Suppose a trend exists and we suspect that a continuous covariate, say X_1, may need transformation. Let $\mathbf{X} = (X_1, \mathbf{X}^*)$, where X_1 is the covariate under consideration and $\mathbf{X}^*$ is the rest of the covariates, which are assumed independent of X_1. To find a transformation for X_1, denoting it $f(X_1)$, we fit the data with only $\mathbf{X}^*$ first (with corresponding β^*). Since

$$H(t;\mathbf{X}) = H_0(t)e^{\mathbf{X}^{*'}\beta^*}e^{\gamma f(X_1)}$$

we may obtain the martingale residues from fitting the Cox model including covariates $\mathbf{X}^*$. Then plot the residuals against X_1. (LOESS or LOWESS smoothing may be applied to see the trend better; see Cleveland (1979). The smoothing fits local polynomial regression, using PROC LOESS in SAS or the R routine *loess*.) If the trend is linear, then no transformation is needed. If there appears a threshold in the trend, then dichotomizing X_1 is suggested.

Another closely related residual is called *deviance residual* which is a transformation of the martingale residual:

$$d_i = \text{sign}(r_i)\sqrt{2\left[-r_i - \delta_i \log(\delta_i - r_i)\right]} \tag{6.16}$$

The log and square root functions make the deviance residuals more symmetric. A large deviance residual thus indicates an outlier or influential case. SAS PROC PHREG and R package provide martingale and deviance residuals (and other residuals as well).

Software and Example 6.3

Appendix 6.8 shows SAS steps to obtain martingale and deviance residuals and to plot the residuals against the linear predictor scores $\mathbf{X}'\hat{\beta}$ from the fitted model. One may verify the scatter plots using a linear regression analysis to verify the intercept and slope of each plot of martingale and deviance residuals versus the linear predictor scores (Homework 6.4). We may also examine the age covariate by plotting the martingale residuals from the PH model without age and using the LOESS smoothing fit to find whether a dichotomizing of age at 55 is suggested or helpful (Homework 6.5).

6.6.2 Pseudo-Observations and Pseudo-Residuals

Let $I(Y > t)$ be the survival indicator. $S(t) = \Pr(Y > t) = E[I(Y > t)]$. With right-censoring, $I(Y > t)$ is not always observed and the idea is then to replace $I(Y > t)$ by the *pseudo-observation*. For a sample of size n triplets $(T_i, \delta_i, \mathbf{X}_i)$, i=1, ..., n, the pseudo-observation i at time $t \geq 0$ for the survival indicator $I(Y_i > t)$ is the "leave-one-out" (jackknife) observation, defined as

$$S_i(t) \equiv n\hat{S}(t) - (n-1)\hat{S}_{-i}(t) \tag{6.17}$$

where $\hat{S}(t)$ is the KM estimate based on the whole sample of n (observed or censored) event times and $\hat{S}_{-i}(t)$ is the KM estimate computed based on the $n-1$ subjects by leaving out the individual i. Set $\hat{S}(t) = 0$ if t is greater than the largest time in the data. The pseudo-observation is defined for both uncensored and censored event times. Note that $E[S_i(t)] \approx nS(t) - (n-1)S(t) = S(t)$. These pseudo-observations can be used for performing regression analyses on RMST as well as the model checking (goodness-of-fit examinations) for hazard regression models. We discuss the model-checking part in the immediate following and regression analysis on RMST later in Section 6.7.3.

Let $\hat{S}(t \mid \mathbf{X}_i)$ be the Cox PH model-fitted outcome for the individual i. A raw residual is defined as $S_i(t) - \hat{S}(t \mid \mathbf{X}_i)$. The standardized pseudo-residual is obtained by dividing the raw residual by a simple version of estimate of what would be the standard error of $S_i(t)$ without censoring (Perme and Andersen 2008; Andersen and Perme 2010):

$$e_i(t) = \frac{S_i(t) - \hat{S}(t \mid \mathbf{X}_i)}{\sqrt{\hat{S}(t \mid \mathbf{X}_i)\left[1 - \hat{S}(t \mid \mathbf{X}_i)\right]}} \tag{6.18}$$

For checking a particular covariate X^*, the Cox PH model assumes that the coefficient β^* (i.e., effect X^*) is constant in time and the covariate effect is linear. We can plot $e_i(t)$ against X^* using scatter plot with a LOESS smoothing curve. If the model fits the data well, we expect no trends at any time point. When either of the two assumptions is not met, we then expect to see a certain trend. The pattern of the trend may indicate a form of non-linear transformation $g(X^*)$ on X^* if the linear effect does not fit. If we see a change of trend from some time point to time point, then the effect β^* should be $\beta^*(t)$, i.e., not constant. In practice, we shall select only few time points to do the residual plots with LOESS smoothing curve, such as time points corresponding to the 20th, 40th, 60th, and 80th percentiles of the event times.

6.7 Methods for Non-Proportional Hazards

As alluded to previously, the (score) log-rank test is always valid under the null hypothesis of equal survival, and it is optimal under the PH model but not necessarily effective in detecting difference between groups when PH does not hold. Non-proportional hazards (NPH) survival data have been more visible lately in immunotherapy trials on oncology when the treatment effect has a tendency of delay. See Cohen et al. (2018) and Burtness et al. (2019) for example. To cope with NPH data, there are several options: (a) stratification for discrete covariates and some transformation for continuous covariates, as we indicated previously. This option should always be considered first. (b) Limiting a period when PH regression is more appropriate. This option may be exploratory since the selection of period is post hoc. (c) Inclusion of parameters for time-dependent effects. This option adds more complexity to the model. (d) Changing to a different measure of treatment effect rather than the constant hazard ratio. (e) Weighted estimation or combination of different tests. In the following, we briefly discuss three methods: the max-combo test, the WCR for average hazard ratio, and the RMST approach. The max-combo test is considered as an (e) option above. The RMST approach is a (d) type of option. The weighted regression for average hazard ratio is sort of both (d) and (e) options. How to perform data monitoring with an interim analysis when NPH is a possibility is a current research topic. We leave this topic for readers to consult Huang (2021), where detailed discussions can be found.

6.7.1 Maximum of the Combination of G(ρ, γ) Family of Weighted Log-Rank Tests

With treatment group as the only covariate, Fleming and Harrington (1991) defined a class of the weighted log-rank statistics as a generalization of Eq. (6.2):

$$G(\rho,\gamma) = \frac{\left[\sum_{i=1}^{D} w_{t_i}\left(O_{t_i} - E_{t_i}\right)\right]^2}{\sum_{i=1}^{D} w_{t_i}^2 V_{t_i}} \tag{6.19}$$

The weight function in general is $w(t;\rho,\gamma) = \left[\hat{S}(t-)\right]^{\rho}\left[1-\hat{S}(t-)\right]^{\gamma}, \rho \geq 0, \gamma \geq 0$, where $\hat{S}(t-)$ is the left-continuous KM estimate of the pooled survival function at t. This is the so-called $G(\rho, \gamma)$ family of weighted log-rank tests. $G(0,0)$ is the log-rank test, which weighs all events equally along the time; $G(1,0)$ is the Peto–Peto version of the Wilcoxon–Mann–Whitney test (Peto and Peto 1972), which weighs early events more. In fact, when $\rho > 0$, $\gamma = 0$, these tests give the most weight to early departures between the hazards rates, whereas, when $\rho = 0$, $\gamma > 0$, these tests give most weights to late departures, and $G(1,1)$ gives most weights to departures which occur in the middle time. With no *a priori* knowledge of the shape of the hazard trends, as often is the case, Lin et al. (2020) constructed the *max-combo* test, which is the maximum of the combination of $\{G(0,0),\ G(1,0), G(0,1),\ G(1,1)\}$. The joint distribution under the null hypothesis of equal survival function is obtained by Karrison (2016), which gave the correlation structure needed to adjust for multiple tests and paved the calculation of the max-combo method.

Software and Example 6.4

Max-combo test can be readily accomplished by several steps in SAS PROC LIFTEST, as demonstrated by Knezevic and Patil (2020). For practice, we can use the dataset in Appendix 6.1 or a dataset downloaded from sashelp.bmt. An SAS macro is also available for download via GitHub: https://github.com/dreaknezevic/combo-wlr (Homework 6.6).

6.7.2 Average Hazard Ratio by Weighted Cox Regression

The $G(\rho,\ \gamma)$ family of weighted log-rank tests, on which the max-combo test is based, considers no covariate other than the treatment group. To include other covariate, probably time-dependent covariates, and to attempt an interpretation for the treatment effect on the NPH survival time adjusted by covariates, Schemper (1992), Sasieni (1993), and Schemper et al. (2009) suggested the concept of *average hazard ratio* (AHR) and inference procedure for Weighted Cox Regression (WCR). When the NPH is due to some prognostic factor whose effect on the event risk changes over time, WCR seems to be a parsimonious method without adding more parameters in the analysis model. We discuss the procedure and its limitations.

We start from the partial likelihood function (6.11) discussed earlier by taking log of it:

$$\log L(\beta) = \sum_{i=1}^{D} \left\{ x_i'\beta - \log\left[\sum_{k \in R_i} e^{x_k'\beta} \right] \right\} \equiv \sum_{i=1}^{D} l_i \qquad (6.20)$$

Taking the first partial derivatives with respect to β_j, $j = 1,\ldots, k$,

$$\frac{\partial \log L(\beta)}{\partial \beta_j} = \sum_{i=1}^{D} \left\{ x_{ij} - \frac{\sum_{k \in R_i} x_{kj} e^{x_k'\beta}}{\sum_{k \in R_i} e^{x_k'\beta}} \right\} \equiv \sum_{i=1}^{D} \left\{ x_{ij} - \bar{x}_{ij} \right\}$$

$$= \sum_{i=1}^{D} \frac{\partial l_i}{\partial \beta_j} \qquad (6.21)$$

where $\bar{x}_{ij}$ is the weighted mean of the j-th covariate values for subjects in the risk set at time t_i, weighted by the hazard ratios (see Eq. (6.9)). This is the score function as we have seen before. Setting the score function to zero yields the estimate of β by the Newton–Raphson or other iterative algorithm, as we have seen before in the method of logistic regression. The individual $\{x_{ij} - \bar{x}_{ij}\}$ plays an important part for forming the score residual and Schoenfeld residual that are provided in SAS and R, but we do not discuss them here. The information matrix is obtained via the negative of the second derivatives

$$\frac{-\partial^2 \log L(\beta)}{\partial \beta_j \partial \beta_r} = \sum_{i=1}^{D} \frac{-\partial^2 l_i}{\partial \beta_j \partial \beta_r} \text{ (detailed expansion omitted), for } j, r = 1,\ldots, k.$$

We now consider weighing the contributions of the (uncensored) event times differently to the partial likelihood by introducing the weighted score equations, for $j = 1,\ldots, k$,

$$\sum_{i=1}^{D} w(t_i) \frac{\partial l_i}{\partial \beta_j} = 0 \tag{6.22}$$

where $w(t_i)$ is the weight at each event time t_i. The robust sandwich estimator of the covariance matrix provided by Lin and Wei (1989) is algebraically the same as that obtained from using the weighted second derivatives of the log partial likelihood. We omit the details here. Obviously, $w(t_i) = 1$, i.e., equal weight for all event times, which is the unweighted Cox PH, is a special case. Recall that the weights in the $G(\rho, \gamma)$ family of weighted log-rank tests were $w(t; \rho, \gamma) = \left[\hat{S}(t-)\right]^{\rho}\left[1 - \hat{S}(t-)\right]^{\gamma}, \rho \geq 0, \gamma \geq 0$, when treatment group is the only covariate. The weighted score test based on the partial likelihood reduces to the $G(\rho, \gamma)$ log-rank test when the above weight function is used.

Schemper et al. (2009), however, preferred the weight function

$$w(t) = \hat{S}(t)\hat{U}(t)^{-1} \tag{6.23}$$

for WCR, where $\hat{U}(t)$ denotes the KM estimator of the censoring distribution, or equivalently, the potential follow-up distribution. $\hat{U}(t)$ is obtained by reversing the meaning of the censoring indicator δ used for $\hat{S}(t)$. Schemper et al. (2009) explained that putting $\hat{U}(t)^{-1}$ in the weight function is to compensate for the attenuation in the observed events due to early censorship: "In the presence of time-dependent effects from covariates, the magnitudes of contributions to the log partial likelihood vary for different t, and as censoring eliminates such contribution with increasing probability for progressing t, the reconstruction of an uncensored situation by means of $\hat{U}(t)^{-1}$ is required for estimates of the average hazard ratios (e^{β}) under censoring." They also suggested to limit the time range for analysis to a more compact follow-up, rather than by the last event, to have a more stable estimate of the regression coefficients. When relatively few individuals in the sample experience much longer follow-up (without events) than the rest of sample, the weight at these individuals' definite event times becomes large and thus will reduce the stability of the estimates.

Note that, when no censoring, $\hat{U}(t) = 1$ and $w(t) = \hat{S}(t)$. Moreover, in the case of no other covariates than the treatment group, this WCR score test for comparing treatment groups is the same as $G(1,0)$, the Peto–Peto version of the Wilcoxon–Mann–Whitney test, as alluded to before. With other covariates, under converging hazards, this WCR putting more weights on the early events will be more powerful to detect between-group difference with treatment effect diminishing over time. As the hazard ratio is not constant, the resulting $e^{\hat{\beta}}$ should be interpreted as the weighted average hazard ratio. However, the population definition of average hazard ratio is yet to be defined.

For two-treatment groups $i = 0, 1$, Schemper et al. (2009) favored a definition by Kalbfleisch and Prentice (1981):

$$\text{AHR} = \frac{\int \left(\frac{h_1(t)}{h(t)}\right) w(t)f(t)dt}{\int \left(\frac{h_0(t)}{h(t)}\right) w(t)f(t)dt} \tag{6.24}$$

with $h_i(t) = f_i(t)/S_i(t)$, $h(t) = h_0(t) + h_1(t)$, $f(t) = (f_0(t) + f_1(t))/2$, and $w(t) = (S_0(t)f_1(t) + S_1(t)f_0(t))/(f_0(t) + f_1(t))$. Equation (6.24) simplifies to

$$\text{AHR} = \frac{\int S_0(t)f_1(t)dt}{\int S_1(t)f_0(t)dt}$$

which can be rewritten to give a more intuitive interpretation:

$$\text{AHR} = \frac{\int \Pr(T_0 > t)f_1(t)dt}{\int \Pr(T_1 > t)f_0(t)dt}$$

$$= \frac{\Pr(T_0 > T_1)}{1 - \Pr(T_0 > T_1)} \tag{6.25}$$

The last quantity is the odds of $\Pr(T_0 > T_1)$, termed *odds of concordance* (OC) in Schemper et al. (2009), which does not require proportional hazards to be interpretable.

Despite the lack of a direct mathematical relationship between the AHR above and the asymptotic representation of $e^{\hat{\beta}}$ from the WCR, Schemper et al. (2009) investigated the alpha level, power of WCR test of the treatment effect based on $e^{\hat{\beta}}$ and the value of $e^{\hat{\beta}}$ as an estimate of AHR above, using simulations. Under several different scenarios of survival and hazard functions and degrees of censoring, the WCR with $\hat{S}(t)\hat{U}(t)^{-1}$ as the weight worked very satisfactorily in all the aspects of testing treatment effect and estimation of AHR.

Software and Example 6.5

An SAS macro WCM and an R package *coxphw* are available at www.muw.ac.at/msi/biometrie/programs. Also see: https://cemsiis.meduni-wien.ac.at/kb/wf/software/statistische-software/

The example dataset "gastric" shows a non-proportional hazards pattern after 1 year. Appendix 6.9 works through the example with the R package (Homework 6.7). The second dataset "biofeedback" as another example of NPH model fitting with a time-dependent covariate using *phcoxw* is shown in Appendix 6.10 (Homework 6.8).

6.7.3 Restricted Mean Survival Time (RMST) by GEE using Pseudo-Observations

Unlike the average hazard ratio analyzed by WCR discussed in the last section, the RMST is well defined and the inference procedure has been well established. We start from a basic parameter in survival data, which is the mean residual life at time t, mrl(t). It is defined as $E(Y - t \mid Y > t)$. For a person with age = t, this parameter represents the expected remaining lifetime. Mathematically, $\text{mrl}(t) = \dfrac{\int_t^\infty (y-t)f(y)dy}{S(t)}$. The mean life is $\mu = \text{mrl}(0) = E(Y) = \dfrac{\int_0^\infty yf(y)dy}{S(0)} = \int_0^\infty yf(y)dy = \int_0^\infty ydF(y) = \int_0^\infty S(y)dy$ using integration by parts. Therefore, the mean survival time (if it exists) is the area under the survival curve. However, due to the right-censoring, the mean survival time may often be ill-defined. Instead, the restricted mean survival time, $\mu(\tau)$, which is the mean of the survival time limited to some horizon $\tau > 0$, is more appropriate. It equals the area under the survival curve $S(t)$ from t = 0 to t = τ:

$$\mu(\tau) = E\big(\min(Y, \tau)\big) = \int_0^\tau S(t)dt \tag{6.26}$$

In confirmatory studies, the cut-off time should be predetermined. A clinically meaningful end-of-study time in the study design should be considered. It may be argued that the need to define a reference time point is, in fact, an advantage, since it explicitly incorporates the time dimension of the trial into the results, which is often part of the study design but neglected in data analysis; neither the median nor the hazard ratio considers this explicitly.

The RMST is a robust and clinically interpretable summary measure of the event time distribution that does not rely on the PH assumption as for the hazard ratio measure. Unlike the median survival time, which represents only a "snapshot," RMST is estimable even under heavy censoring and covers over the survival curve up to the time τ. Since it is applicable independent of the PH assumption, and the RMST estimate incorporates both the number of events and the exposure times, a test of the difference or ratio between the RMST for the treatment arm and control arm may be more appropriate to determine treatment effect with respect to the time-to-event endpoint (see, e.g., Uno et al. 2014). Moving beyond the hazard ratio in quantifying the between-group difference in survival analysis, simulation studies and analyses of real data in the literature had shown that RMST had excellent performance in all typical non-proportional models (Royston and Parmar 2011; Andersen, Hansen and Klein 2004). There are parametric and nonparametric approaches to estimating the RMST adjusted for covariates. The parametric approach is detailed in Royston and Parmar (2011). Here, we study two nonparametric approaches to handling censored observations: One is based on pseudo-observations due to Andersen, Hansen, and Klein (2004), and the other technique is to utilize the inverse probability of censoring weighting (IPCW) by Tian et al. (2014). Both nonparametric approaches have the advantage of using the well-established generalized linear models (GLMs) for robust inference. Moreover, the pseudo-observations have the by-products of pseudo-residuals, which are useful for model diagnostics as we discussed previously. The IPCW is $\hat{U}(t)^{-1}$, which appeared in the WCR as a component of the weight that we discussed in the previous section.

The parameter of interest to measure the treatment effect is the RMST, $\mu(\tau) = \int_0^\tau S(t)dt$, for which we have an approximately unbiased estimator $\hat{\mu}(\tau) = \int_0^{\tau_a} \hat{S}(t)dt$ by plugging in the KM estimate of $S(t)$. The pseudo-observation $S_i(t)$ for the survival function in Eq. (6.17) is then translated to the pseudo-value for the RMST by

$$\hat{\mu}_i(\tau) \equiv \int_0^\tau S_i(t)dt = n\int_0^{\tau_a} \hat{S}(t)dt - (n-1)\int_0^{\tau_a} \hat{S}_{-i}(t)dt$$

$$\equiv n\hat{\mu}(\tau) - (n-1)\hat{\mu}_{-i} \tag{6.27}$$

With given covariates $\mathbf{X}_i$, a regression model corresponds to a specification of how $\mu(\tau|\mathbf{X}_i)$ depends on $\mathbf{X}_i$. This is done via the GLM using the pseudo-values for the RMST, $\hat{\mu}_i(\tau)$, as the response variable with a link function to the covariates and a simple working variance = 1 for $\hat{\mu}_i(\tau)$. A link function g for $\mu(\tau|\mathbf{X}_i)$ is such that $g(\mu(\tau|\mathbf{X}_i)) = \mathbf{X}_i'\beta$. Note that in the GLM setting for RMST, the regression coefficients here have different meanings than that in the Cox PH regression model, and we need to add a column vector $\mathbf{1}$ to $\mathbf{X}$ corresponding to the intercept β_0.

Two typical choices of the link functions are log and identity functions. For log link, we have a log-linear model:

$$\log E\left[(\min(Y_i, \tau)\right] = \beta_0 + X_i'\beta$$

The covariates-adjusted treatment effect is the ratio of RMSTs, estimated by $e^{\hat{\beta}}$. For the identity link, we have a linear model

$$E(\min(Y_i, \tau)) = \beta_0 + X_i'\beta$$

The covariates-adjusted treatment effect is the difference of RMSTs, estimated by $\hat{\beta}$. The semi-parametric estimates of regression coefficients are obtained by solving generalized estimating equations (GEEs), and the standard errors of the GEE estimates of β can be obtained from the robust "sandwich estimator" (Zeger and Liang, 1986).

Software and Example 6.6

RMST analysis can be performed in SAS or R. In R, the pseudo-value regression method is available in the package *KMsurv*. Appendix 6.11 illustrates the IPCW method as implemented in the package *survRM2* using the biofeedback data (Homework 6.9). In Appendix 6.12, we demonstrate SAS PROC RMSTreg with the option of method = pv (for pseudo-value) or = IPCW (inverse probability of censoring weighting) in the model statement (Homework 6.10).

Appendix 6.1: Dataset sorafos

```
# Arm: A (Sorafenib high dose), B (Sorafenib low dose)
# censor:  0 (uncensored), 1 (censored)
# os:  overall survival in months
       arm      censor           os
1      A        0               51.8000
2      A        0               45.4000
3      A        1               54.9000
4      A        1               54.8333
5      A        0               25.7667
6      A        0               17.4667
7      A        1               62.3333
8      A        0               39.0333
9      A        0               55.5333
10     A        0               48.4667
11     A        0               53.7333
12     B        0               28.9333
13     B        0               25.7667
```

14	B	1	46.5000
15	B	0	0.7333
16	B	0	26.2667
17	B	0	3.3000
18	B	0	1.5000
19	B	1	0.9333
20	B	0	20.5000
21	B	0	13.0000
22	B	1	3.9000
23	B	1	36.5333
24	B	0	17.0333
25	B	1	35.3333
26	B	1	3.8333
27	B	0	28.9000
28	B	1	13.7333
29	B	1	4.0333
30	B	0	11.4333
31	B	1	1.0333
32	B	0	18.2667
33	B	0	13.9000
34	B	1	23.2333
35	B	1	21.6000
36	B	1	1.2667
37	B	1	20.6333
38	B	1	20.0667
39	B	1	18.8000
40	B	1	13.5667

Appendix 6.2: Using SAS PROC LIFETEST to Plot Kaplan–Meier Graph

```
proc lifetest data = sorafos plots =survival(test atrisk);
time os*censor(1);
strata arm;
run;
```

Appendix 6.3: Using SAS PROC LIFETEST to Plot log(−log S(t)) vs log(t) Graph

```
proc lifetest data = sorafos plots =(s lls);
time os*censor(1);
strata arm;
run;
```

Appendix 6.4: Exporting SAS Dataset to R

```
/*  In SAS to export the SAS dataset sorafos to mydata.xpt */
/*  Need to have the SAS dataset sorafos ready first.      */
    libname out xport 'D:\mydata.xpt';
    data out.mydata; set sorafos; Run;
#   In R to import the data mydata.xpt
#   Need to install the Hmisc package first.
    library(Hmisc)
    mydata <- sasxport.get("D:/mydata.xpt")
```

Appendix 6.5: Using R Function to Do Log-Rank Test and Plot Kaplan–Meier Graph

```
#  Need to install the package survival in R first.
   library("survival")
   survdiff(Surv(os, censor)~arm, data=mydata)
      Call:
      survdiff(formula = Surv(os, censor) ~ arm, data =
      mydata)
          N   Observed   Expected   (O-E)^2/E   (O-E)^2/V
      arm=A  11      3       10.56        5.41       16.6
      arm=B  29     16        8.44        6.76       16.6
      Chisq= 16.6  on 1 degrees of freedom, p= 5e-05
   plot(survfit(Surv(os, censor)~ arm, data = mydata),
          xlab="Time(months)", ylab="Survival Probability")
```

Appendix 6.6: Using R Package and Dataset to Perform Cox Regression Analysis by coxph and PH Model Checking by cox.zph

```
# Need to install the package coin in R first.
# Use R functions to obtain and study the dataset "glioma".
    data("glioma", package="coin")
    ??glioma
    summary(glioma)
    print(glioma)
# Fit a stratified PH model with age, sex, and group as
  covariates.
    fit <- coxph(Surv(time, event) ~ age + sex + group +
    strata(histology), data=glioma)
```

```
      print(fit)
#  The above only shows tables of coefficients
#  Check PH model:  coefficient constant or not?
      temp <- cox.zph(fit)
      print(temp)        # Also only see tables, we need to
      plot beta versus time:
      plot(temp, var="age")
      plot(temp, var="sex")
      plot(temp, var="group")
```

Note: The plot gives an estimate of the time-dependent coefficient beta(t). If the proportional hazards assumption holds, then the true beta(t) function would be a horizontal line. The table component provides the results of a formal score test for slope=0; a linear fit to the plot would approximate the test.

Appendix 6.7: Using SAS PROC PHREG to Perform Stratified Cox Regression Analysis

```
/* SAS automatically converts the event="true" (from R) to
   =1(uncensored) */
/* Also plot KM survival with confidence interval */
      proc phreg data=one plots(cl)=s;
      class group sex histology;
      model time*event(0) = age sex group;
      stratum histology;
      run;
```

Appendix 6.8: Using SAS PROC PHREG to Perform Residual Analysis by Plots and Test

```
proc phreg data=one noprint;
  class group sex histology;
  model time*event(0)= age sex group;
  stratum histology;
  output out=Outp xbeta=Xb resmart=Mart resdev=dev;
run;
*proc print data=outp;
run;

/*
The following statements plot the residuals against the
linear predictor scores:
```

```
*/
  title "Glioma Study";
  proc sgplot data=Outp;
     yaxis grid;
     refline 0 / axis=y;
     scatter y=Mart x=Xb;
  run;
  proc sgplot data=Outp;
     yaxis grid;
     refline 0 / axis=y;
     scatter y=Dev x=Xb;
  run;
/* Check age factor by leaving out age */
  data two; set surv.glioma;
  proc phreg data=two noprint;
     class group sex histology;
  model time*event(0)= histology sex group;
 *stratum histology;
  output out=Outp xbeta=Xb resmart=Mart resdev=dev;
run;
proc print data=outp;
run;
proc sgplot data=Outp;
  yaxis grid;
  refline 0 / axis=y;
  scatter y=Mart x=age;
run;
/* We can also use proc gplot or better yet, proc loess for
   smoothing fit of the martingale residual versus age   */
  proc gplot data=Outp;
  plot Mart*age;
  run;
  proc loess data=Outp;
  model mart=age;
  run;
/* Create a time dependent variable Aget inside PROC PHREG.
Use the test statement to test the time dependent covariate
Aget. */
  proc phreg data=one;
  class group sex histology;
  model time*event(0) = age sex group histology aget ;
  aget = age*log(time);
  proportionality_test: test aget;
  run;
```

Note: As demonstrated, it is possible to generate time-dependent covariates by creating interactions of the covariates and a function of survival time (such as log of time) and include them in the model and test all of them at once. If any of the newly created time-dependent covariates are significant, then those covariates are not proportional.

Appendix 6.9: Using R Package coxphw to Perform Weighted Cox Regression for NPH

```
# Need to install the package coxphw in R first.
# Use R functions to obtain and study the dataset "gastric".
 library("coxphw")
  data("gastric",package="coxphw")
  ?gastric
  summary(gastric)
  print(gastric)
# Do the KM estimate, log-rank test with PH model first.
# Notice the time in the dataset is in Days, not Yrs.
  survdiff(Surv(time, status)~radiation,data=gastric)
  plot(survfit(Surv(time/365, status)~ radiation, data =
  gastric),
       xlab="Time(yrs)", ylab="Survival Probability")
  coxph(Surv(time, status)~radiation, data=gastric)
# Examine the KM plot and notice the NPH phenomenon
#   To use a piecewise (unweighted) PH model (template="PH"
below) with cut-off at Day 365.
  fun <- function(t) as.numeric(t > 365)
  coxphw(Surv(time, status) ~ radiation + fun(time):radiation,
         data=gastric, template="PH")
# Or change time (in days) to time/365 (in yrs)
  fun <- function(t) as.numeric(t > 1)
  coxphw(Surv(time/365, status) ~ radiation +
  fun(time/365):radiation,
         data=gastric, template="PH")
```

Note: The variable "radiation" is binary (=0 if no radiation, i.e., chemotherapy only; =1 if treatment is chemotherapy plus radiation). The second term in the above model is the interaction of dichotomized time and radiation. The HR estimate (exp(coef)) of radiation, i.e., the effect of radiation compared to therapy without radiation, in the first period is 2.405, as in this period, fun(yrs) equals 0. The HR of fun(yrs):radiation must be interpreted as the ratio of the two HRs of both time periods of radiation: the HR of the second period divided by the HR of the first period. Thus, the HR of the second period follows as the product of the two HRs, $2.405 \times 0.227 = 0.546$, or, equivalently, as the exponentiated sum of the two regression coefficients, $\exp(0.8774 - 1.4826) = \exp(-0.6052) = 0.546$.

```
# If not to break to 2-pieces and to fit model by unweighted
# estimation (PH template):
    fit1 <- coxphw(Surv(time, status) ~ radiation +
    time:radiation, data = gastric, template = "PH")
      print(fit1)
     -0.002643*365
    [1] -0.964695
```

Note: The effect of radiation in prolonging survival time is seen by the first term with positive coefficient. The interaction term shows the hazard ratio (radiation plus chemo versus chemo alone) changes over time. The negative sign of the regression coefficient of this term shows the hazard ratio decreases over time. The non-proportional hazard can also be seen from the KM plot.

```
# Continue to use coxphw to do weighted Cox regression with
  average hazard ratio (AHR).
  fit2 <- coxphw(Surv(time/365, status) ~ radiation, data =
  gastric, template = "AHR")
  summary(fit2)
# To see how the weight function in (6.23), i.e.,
  template="AHR", run:
  plot(fit2)
```

Appendix 6.10: Using R Package coxphw to Perform Weighted Cox Regression with More Covariates than Treatment Group Exhibiting NPH

```
# Continue using the package coxphw with the dataset
  "biofeedback" (Denk and Kaider 1997).
# Obtain the data from the package and study it: bfb=1
  (biofeedback therapy), bfb=0 (standard therapy);
  thdur = therapy duration (days) from the start of bfb/
  standard therapy (after surgery)
  to "successfully swallowing rehabilitation";
  success =1 (event observed), =0 (censored).
# log2heal=log2 transformed time elapsing from surgery to
  start of therapy,
#  which is a healing process (confounding covariate).
# Notice the endpoint event is a "good" event, the shorter
  time the better.
    data("biofeedback",package="coxphw")
    ?biofeedback
    summary(biofeedback)
    print(biofeedback)
# Examine the KM plot and log-rank test with PH model only
  treatment group first.
    survdiff(Surv(thdur, success)~bfb, data=biofeedback)
    plot(survfit(Surv(thdur, success)~ bfb, data =
    biofeedback), xlab="Time(days)", ylab="Survival
    Probability")
    coxph(Surv(thdur, success)~bfb, data=biofeedback)
# Notice the KM plot showing some graphical evidence of NPH
  of bfb: early advantage of bfb therapy diminishing later.
    fit <- coxph(Surv(thdur, success) ~ log2heal + bfb,
    data=biofeedback)
```

```
      print(fit)
# Table shows covariate-adjusted treated effect.
#   Check PH model:  Are the coefficients constant or not?
      temp <- cox.zph(fit)
      print(temp)          # Also only see tables, we need to
      plot beta versus time:
      plot(temp, var="log2heal")
# Graph shows beta not constant.
      plot(temp, var="bfb")     # Graph shows beta not constant
# Addressing Non-constant beta (i.e., time-dependent
  effects of log2heal and bfb)
# First, still use coxph to do an extended Cox regression
  model adding the covariate log2heal and the interaction
  of log2heal with time.
#   tt(x) function is "time transformation of x"
#   cluster(id) is to evoke the robust sandwich estimator of
    the covariance matrix provided by Lin and Wei (1989).
      stage1 <- coxph(Surv(thdur, success) ~ bfb + log2heal +
      tt(log2heal) + cluster(id), data = biofeedback,
      tt = function(x, t, ...) x * log(t), method =
      "breslow")
      summary(stage1)
#   The stage 1 model improved fit.  We now do WCR by coxphw.
      fit<-coxphw(Surv(thdur, success) ~ bfb + log2heal +
      log(thdur):log2heal,
                          data = biofeedback, template = "AHR")
      summary(fit)
      plot(fit)
```

Note: The average HR of bfb when adjusted for log2heal and the interaction of log2heal with time, log(thdur):log2healis, is estimated as 1.86 (95% CI 0.89–3.89; p = 0.101). From the plot(fit) graph, we can see that the variability of the normalized total weights is sufficiently small in this example.

```
#   We output the biofeedback data to Excel to prepare for
    the next exercise.
  write.table(biofeedback,file="f:\\biofbk.csv",sep=",",col.
  names=NA)
  csvbiofbk<-read.table("f:\\biofbk.csv",header=TRUE,
  sep=",",row.names=1)
```

Appendix 6.11: Using Biofeedback Data and the R Package survRM2 to Perform RMST by the IPCW Method for NPH

```
# Need to install the package survRM2 in R first.
  library(survRM2)
# Read in the dataset
```

```
csvbiofbk<-read.table("f:\\biofbk.csv",header=TRUE,
sep=",",row.names=1)
summary(csvbiofbk)
head(csvbiofbk)
# Create time, status and group variables
    time = csvbiofbk$thdur
    status = csvbiofbk$success
    group = csvbiofbk$bfb
# Create the covariate matrix from the dataset
    x= csvbiofbk[,c(6)]
    head(x)
#   First do RMST without covariate (to see what tau might
    be set)
#   Use the max time as the default tau, which is 100 days
    obj=rmst2(time, status, group)
    plot(obj, xlab="Years", ylab="Probability")
# Now do RMST with covariate (and set Tau=85 days)
    rmst2(time, status, group, tau=85, covariates=x)
```

Appendix 6.12: Using SAS PROC RMSTreg to Perform RMST for NPH

```
/* Continue using the dataset "biofeedback" (from Appendix
   6.11);
/* Output the pseudo-values for model diagnostics;
   proc rmstreg data=biofbk tau=85 OUTPV=pseudov;
     class bfb;
     model thdur*success(0) = bfb log2heal / link=log
     method=pv;
   run;
/*  Fit with the IPCW method;
   proc rmstreg data=biofbk tau=85;
     class bfb;
     model thdur*success(0) = bfb log2heal / link=log
     method=IPCW;
   run;
```

HOMEWORK 6.1

Use the data in Appendix 6.1, and follow the instructions in Appendices 6.2–6.5 to obtain KM plots, the log(–log(t)) vs. log(t) plot, and the log-rank test in SAS and R. Is the proportional hazards assumption valid in this dataset?

HOMEWORK 6.2

Use the glioma dataset illustrated in Appendix 6.6. Follow the instruction to fit a stratified PH model with age, sex, and group as covariates. Interpret the result of each regression coefficient in terms of hazard ratio. Compare the results from coxph function in R (see Appendix 6.6) and the PROC PHREG of SAS (see Appendix 6.7).

HOMEWORK 6.3

Continue Homework 6.2 with model checking for each of the covariates using cox.zph in R. Discuss whether there is hint from the graphs that some time-varying covariate effect may exist on the survival time in the glioma data. Which covariate (sex, age, or group) violates the PH (constant regression coefficient) assumption?

HOMEWORK 6.4

Continue Homework 6.2, and follow Appendix 6.8 to plot the residuals against the linear predictor scores from the fitted model. Do you detect any trend? Verify the scatter plots with a linear regression analysis of residuals versus linear predictor scores. Report the intercept and slope of each plot (martingale and deviance residuals).

HOMEWORK 6.5

Continue Homework 6.4. Fit the PH model without the covariate age. Obtain the martingale residuals for this model, and plot them versus age (using both the scatter plot or gplot, and the LOESS plot). Is there any indication for transformation of age needed? Would a dichotomizing age at 55 helpful?

HOMEWORK 6.6

Follow the steps to obtain the dataset BMT2 from sashelp.bmt given in the reference Knezevic and Patil (2020) and to carry out the max-combo test.

HOMEWORK 6.7

Follow the steps in Appendix 6.9 to fit WCR using the dataset "gastric" from the R package *coxphw* given in reference Schemper et al. (2009). Check the KM plot and the log(–log S(t)) versus log(t) plot. Comment on the PH model assumption. Summarize and compare the hazard ratio estimates, 95% confidence intervals, and p-values for the following: (a) HR with Cox PH model (unweighted); (b) piecewise HR with cut-off at 1 year (365 days); (c) average HR using the AHR weight in Eq. (6.23).

HOMEWORK 6.8

Follow Appendix 6.10 to fit a WCR for the dataset "biofeedback," which has a time-dependent covariate, using the *phcoxw* package.

HOMEWORK 6.9

Follow Appendix 6.11 to perform RMST analysis using the R package *survRM2* by adding the interaction term of log2heal*log(t). Compare and interpret the results with Homework 6.8.

HOMEWORK 6.10

Continue Homework 6.9 using SAS PROC RMSTreg with the method of pseudo-values as well as the IPCW. Compare the results with Homework 6.9.

References

Andersen PK and Gill RD. (1982). Cox's regression model for counting process: A large sample study. *The Annals of Statistics* 10: 1100–1120.

Andersen PK and Perme MP. (2010). Pseudo-observations in survival analysis. *Statistical Methods in Medical Research* 19: 71–99.

Andersen PK, Hansen MG, Klein JP. (2004). Regression analysis of restricted mean survival time based on pseudo-observations. *Lifetime Data Analysis* 10: 335–350.

Beigel JH, Tomashek KM, Dodd LE, et al. (2020). Remdesivir for the Treatment of Covid-19 — Final Report. *The New England Journal of Medicine* 383: 1813–1826.

Breslow NE (1974). Covariance analysis of censored survival data. *Biometrics* 30:89–99.

Burtness B, Harrington KL, Greil R, et al. (2019). Pembrolizumab alone or with chemotherapy versus cetuximab with chemotherapy for recurrent or metastatic squamous cell carcinoma of the head and neck (KEYNOTE-048): a randomised, open-label, phase 3 study. *Lancet* 394: 1915–1928

Cleveland WS. (1979). Robust locally weighted regression and smoothing scatterplots. *J. of American Statistical Assoc.* 74: 829–836.

Cohen EEW, Soulières D, Le Tourneau C, et al. (2018). Pembrolizumab versus methotrexate, docetaxel, or cetuximab for recurrent or metastatic head-and-neck squamous cell carcinoma (KEYNOTE-040): a randomised, open-label, phase 3 study. *Lancet* 2018; published online Nov 30. http://dx.doi.org/10.1016/S0140-6736(18)31999-8 (with Supplement).

Cox DR. (1972). Regression models and life-tables (with Discussion). Journal of the Royal Statistical Society Series B 34: 187–220.

Denk DM, Kaider A (1997). "Videoendoscopic Biofeedback: A Simple Method to Improve the Efficacy of Swallowing Rehabilitation of Patients After Head and Neck Surgery." *Journal for Oto-Rhino-Laryngology, Head and Neck Surgery.* 59: 100–105.

Efron B. (1977). The Efficiency of Cox's Likelihood Function for Censored Data. *J. of American Statistical Assoc.* 72: 557–565.

Everitt BS and Hothorn T. (2010). *A Handbook of Statistical Analysis Using R.* Second edition. CRC Press. New York.

Fleming TR & Harrington DP. (1991). *Counting Processes and Survival Analysis.* New York, NY: John Wiley & Sons.

Grambsch P and Therneau T. (1994). Proportional hazards tests and diagnostics based on weighted residuals. *Biometrika* 81: 515–526.

Grana C, Chinol M, Robertson C, Mazzetta C, Bartolomei M, et al. (2002). Pretargeted adjuvant radioimmunotherapy with Yttrium-90-biotin in malignant glioma patients: A pilot study. *The British Journal of Cancer* 86: 207–212.

Harrington DP and Fleming TR. (1982). A class of rank test procedures for censored survival data. *Biometrika* 69: 553–566.

Huang J. (2021). Current topics on treatment comparison for survival endpoints with non-proportional hazards. Ph.D. Dissertation, Department of Biostatistics, Rutgers School of Public Health, Rutgers University, The State University of New Jersey.

Karrison T. (2016). Versatile tests for comparing survival curves based on weighted log-rank statistics. *The Stata Journal* 16: 678–690.

Klein JP, Gerster M, Anderse PK, Tarima S, Perme MP. (2008). SAS and R functions to compute pseudo-values for censored data regression. *Computer methods and programs in biomedicine* 89: 289–300.

Knezevic A and Patil S. (2020). Combination weighted log-rank tests for survival analysis with non-proportional hazards. SAS Global Forum 2020. Paper #5062-2020. https://www.sas.com/content/dam/SAS/support/en/sas-global-forum-proceedings/2020/5062-2020.pdf (last accessed on 1/3/2021).

Liang K-Y and Zeger S. (1986). Longitudinal data analysis using generalized linear models. *Biometrika* 73: 13–22

Lin RS, Lin J, Roychoudhury S, et al. (2020). Alternative analysis methods for time to event endpoints under non-proportional hazards: A Comparative analysis. *Statistics in Biopharmaceutical Research* 12: 187–198.

Parner ET, Andersen PK. (2010). Regression analysis of censored data using pseudo-observations. *The Stata Journal.* 10: 408–422.

Perme PM and Andersen PK. (2008). Checking hazard regression models using pseudo-observations. *Statistics in Medicine* 27: 5309–5328.

Peto R and Peto J. (1972). Asymptotically efficient rank invariant test procedures. *Journal of the Royal Statistical Society Series A* 135: 185–207.

Royston P and Parmar MKB. (2011). The use of restricted mean survival time to estimate the treatment effect in randomized clinical trials when the proportional hazards assumption is in doubt. *Statistics in Medicine* 30: 2409–2421.

Royston P and Parmar MKB. (2013). Restricted mean survival time: an alternative to the hazard ratio for the design and analysis of randomized trials with a time-to-event outcome. *BMC Medical Research Methodology* 13: 152.

Sasieni P (1993). Maximum weighted partial likelihood estimators for the Cox model. *Journal of the American Statistical Association* 88: 144–152.

Schemper M, Wakounig S, and Heinze G. (2009). The estimation of average hazard ratios by weighted Cox regression. *Statistics in Medicine* 28: 2473–2489.

Schemper M. (1992). Cox analysis of survival data with non-proportional hazard functions. *The Statistician* 41: 455–465.

Tan A. et al. (2008). Phase I/II Trial of Letrozole (Femara®) and Sorafenib (Nexavar®) as first-line therapy in postmenopausal women with hormone receptor-positive locally advanced or metastatic breast cancer. The Cancer Institute of New Jersey Oncology Group # NJ 1107 Local Protocol # 040706. ClinicalTrials.gov NCT00634634.

Therneau TM, Grambsch PM, Fleming TR. (1990). Martingale-based residuals for survival models. *Biometrika* 77: 147–160.

Tian L, Zhao L, Wei L-J. (2014). Predicting the restricted mean event time with the subject's baseline covariates in survival analysis. *Biostatistics* 15: 222–233.

Tsiatis AA. (1981). A large sample study of Cox's regression model. *The Annals of Statistics* 9: 93–108.

Uno H, Claggett B, Tian L, et al. (2014). Moving beyond the hazard ratio in quantifying the between-group difference in survival analysis. *Journal of clinical oncology* 32: 2380–2385.

Zhao L, Tian L, Uno H, Solomon SD, Pfeffer MA, Schindler JS, et al. (2012). Utilizing the integrated difference of two survival functions to quantify the treatment contrast for designing, monitoring, and analyzing a comparative clinical study. *Clinical Trials* 9: 570–7.

Zucker DM. (1998). Restricted mean life with covariates: Modification and extension of a useful survival analysis method. *Journal of the American Statistical Association* 93: 702–9.

7

Sequential Designs and Methods—Part I: Expected Sample Size and Two-Stage Phase II Trials in Oncology

In Chapter 4, we mainly considered the fixed sample size design, in which there is no interim analysis. As we alluded to in Chapter 1, however, clinical trials often require periodic monitoring and data analyses at interim stages, while patients are continuously enrolled. This monitoring and analysis is especially necessary for trials that involve life-threatening diseases, potentially toxic therapies, long-term follow-ups, or large sample sizes. In this chapter and in Chapters 8 and 9, we examine sequential designs and methods for clinical trials with interim stages, with special attention on oncology trials.

As we discussed in previous chapters, all considerations for making a fixed sample size trial valid and efficient are also pertinent to sequentially designed trials (or *sequential trials* for short). In sequential trials, we need to focus special attention on the control of the overall type I error rate (α) and the impact of the target study power ($1 - \beta$) with any interim analyses. We also need to carefully preserve the integrity of the trial as more issues emerge with the possibility to introduce bias, especially because the trial remains ongoing and thereby offers a chance to alter the process when results are being monitored. (For example, we would prohibit discontinuing sites with poor results.) In addition, we need to set up *decision rules* or *guidelines* for possible early termination or other modifications of the study in the protocol or the *data analysis plan*, or both.

7.1 Maximum Sample Size and Expected Sample Size

When we design a sequential trial with a total sample size N, this N is actually the final projected sample size, if the trial continues to the end. As a sequential trial, the study might be terminated early, for example, in the middle of accrual, and thus this N would not be achieved. Therefore, unlike a nonsequential (fixed sample size) trial, the sample size in a sequential trial is actually not a fixed number. The designed N in the sequential trials is the possible *maximum sample size* for the study. There is also a concept of *expected sample size* in trials with a sequential design.

DOI: 10.1201/9781003176527-7

In order to reach the same statistical power, a sequential trial would require a larger *maximum sample size* than the corresponding fixed sample size for a nonsequential design. Hence, in order to plan a sequential trial, we should first use the sample size formula we discussed and learned in Chapter 4 and then increase this sample size number to obtain a corrected sample size for the corresponding sequential study. This increase in the maximum sample size also reflects a potential cost for conducting the extra monitoring of the study. However, the expected sample size for a sequential trial would be smaller with the chance of an early termination.

To illustrate these points, let us consider the distinctive characteristics of the Phase II cancer trials in the following section.

7.2 One-Stage versus Two-Stage Cancer Phase II Trials

7.2.1 Introduction

The main objective of a Phase II cancer trial is to determine whether a new therapy (usually a combination of agents or treatment regimens and modalities) has sufficient activity against a specific type of tumor to warrant further (Phase III) development. A major difference between cancer Phase II trials and trials involving many other diseases is that the former are usually designed as a single-arm trial without a concurrent control. Instead, historical data controls are often considered for comparison. (Extensive epidemiologic data, literature review, and meta-analysis are crucial to the interpretation of a Phase II cancer trial using historical controls.) Sometimes we call these single-arm Phase II trials as Phase IIA to differentiate them from those Phase IIB trial which are randomized controlled trials. The primary endpoint for cancer Phase II trials is usually the tumor response rate as defined clinically, based on a combination of reduction in tumor size and/ or changes in biomarkers, and event-free (e.g., progression-free) survival at a fixed time point. For example, in the year 2000, an international committee standardized easily applicable criteria known as *Response Evaluation Criteria in Solid Tumors (RECIST)* for measuring solid tumor response using x-ray, CT, and MRI technology. *RECIST* is recommended for most US NCI-sponsored trials. When a single (overall) *response rate* is calculated, *complete* and *partial responses* (CR+PR) are usually pooled together, versus *progressive disease* and *stable disease* (PD+SD). In addition to the solid tumor's "*RECIST*" response definition, treatment for multiple myeloma (malignant plasma cells in bone marrow) also has standard definition for "response." See the reference of Montefiore-Einstein Phase II stem cell transplantation for multiple myeloma protocol in the next chapter. Recently, immune-related response criteria evaluation (ir-RCE) has also been often used. Sometimes investigators also collect data on survival by using "landmark" time point for the survival endpoint to become a binary variable, such as 1-year overall survival (OS) rate or 3-month PFS rate, but confidence intervals are usually very wide due to the small sample size.

Hypothesis testing for a Phase II trial is usually based on response rates, because the response facilitates the decision of whether or not to proceed to a Phase III trial. The therapy would be deemed uninteresting if the true response rate (π) were no more than a certain level (π_0). On the other hand, the therapy would be accepted for further investigation in larger groups of patients (i.e., Phase III studies) if the true response were greater than some target level (π_1). The level for the uninteresting response rate (π_0) would most likely be derived from the literature regarding the standard therapy. The target level of response rate (i.e., the alternative hypothesis, π_1) is usually set based on the investigator's expectation of the new therapy to be interesting for further study, but it should also be realistic and based on earlier or preclinical data. Typically, for ethical and practical considerations, a two- or three-stage design is used for these Phase II trials, so that an ineffective treatment can be dismissed early at the end of the first stage. In the early 1960s, when anticancer agents showed low activity, Gehan's (1961) two-stage design was used widely, in which π_0 was set to be zero. Later, Simon (1989) generalized π_0 and introduced *optimal* and *minimax designs*. The optimal design minimizes the expected sample size under the null hypothesis, and the minimax design minimizes the maximum of the total sample size.

7.2.2 Review of the Binomial Distribution and Sample Size Estimation for a One-Sample Case Using R Functions

Recall that the *binomial distribution table* in a fundamental statistics textbook was used when we applied the *sign test* in Homework 3.2 (Chapter 3) for analyzing paired data from a crossover study. We now use the functions in the R package to implement the calculations. First, the *binomial density function* is

$$b(x;n,\ \pi) = \binom{n}{x}\pi^x(1-\pi)^{n-x}$$

The probability of having x responses out of n patients (sample size) when the chance of response is π (prob) can be obtained by using the R function:

```
dbinom(x, size, prob)
```

Second, the *binomial cumulative probability* is

$$B(r;n,\ \pi) = \sum_{x=0}^{r}b(x;n,\ \pi)$$

The probability of having at most r responses (≤r) out of n patients when the chance of response is π can be obtained by using the R function:

```
pbinom(r, size, prob)
```

The hypotheses in a single-arm trial are H_0: $\pi = \pi_0$ and H_A: $\pi = \pi_1$, and the associated sample size with the type I (α) and type II (β) errors is

$$n = \frac{\left[z_\alpha \sqrt{\pi_0(1-\pi_0)} + z_\beta \sqrt{\pi_1(1-\pi_1)} \right]^2}{(\pi_1 - \pi_0)^2} \qquad (7.1)$$

The above notation is best illustrated with an example. The response rate for the standard therapy for refractory Hodgkin's disease is 50% (π_0). A new experimental combination therapy is to be tested, and the investigator expects a response rate of 80% (π_1) for the new therapy. Assume a fixed sample size design is conducted with n = 10 patients. Let X be the number of responses in the 10 patients. Suppose we design the trial with the following decision rule: Dismiss the drug if X ≤ 7 (i.e., accept H_0). Claim the drug is worthy of further study if X ≥ 8. We need to understand the *operating characteristics* of this rule.

The type I error rate is $\alpha = \Pr(X \geq 8 \mid n = 10, \pi = \pi_0 = 0.5) = 1 - \Pr(X \leq 7 \mid n = 10, \pi = \pi_0 = 0.5)$. With R, we obtain

```
1-pbinom(7,10, π = 0.5)
[1] 0.0546875
```

The type II error rate is $\beta = \Pr(X \leq 7 \mid n = 10, \pi = \pi_1 = 0.8)$. The power is $1 - \beta = 1 - \Pr(X \leq 7 \mid n = 10, \pi = \pi_1 = 0.8)$. For power, we obtain from R

```
1-pbinom (7,10, π = 0.8)
[1] 0.6777995
```

Investigators often monitor cancer trials as they are ongoing. For example, in the above trial, suppose that there are only three responses after the first five patients. An interesting question then is, should the trial be continued? Before we tackle this question in the next section, we should bear in mind that one should not do an unplanned sequential monitoring of a fixed sample size trial. If that were done, then the error rates would no longer be controlled at the nominal level. When it is desirable to have an interim analysis, then the study team should consider a two-stage design in the protocol.

7.2.3 Example of a Two-Stage Design

Suppose we alter the above example a little bit as follows.

- Stage I: Enter $n_1 = 5$ patients. If $X_1 \leq 3$ responses are observed, then stop the study and dismiss the drug. Otherwise, continue to the next stage.

- Stage II: Enter another $n_2 = 5$ patients. Out of the total $n = n_1 + n_2 = 10$, if $X = X_1 + X_2 \geq 8$ responses are observed, then reject the null hypothesis and claim the drug is worthy of further study.

In other words, we now add an interim stage to monitor the study. Note that the first stage only stops the trial for futility (i.e., when the response rate is poor). This approach is used to save resources, as well as to avoid giving additional patients an ineffective therapy. This approach does not stop the trial at the first stage when the response *appears* to be effective, because this is only a small Phase II study. When we successfully pass the interim target level, we continue the trial to its designed end. At the end of the study, we can either dismiss the drug from further (Phase III) testing (i.e., accept the null hypothesis) or permit the drug to be tested in further (Phase III) trials (i.e., reject the null hypothesis).

Given the above design configuration ($n_1 = 5$, $r_1 = 3$, $n = 10$, $r = 7$), we ask: What are the *operating characteristics* of this two-stage sequential design? Specifically, we calculate the type I error and type II error rates, the probability of early termination (PET), and the expected sample size.

The following basic rule of probability will be applied repeatedly in a sequential design:

$$\Pr(A \text{ and } B) = \Pr(B \mid A) P(A)$$
$$= \sum_a \Pr(B \mid A = a) \Pr(A = a) \tag{7.2}$$

- First, the type I error rate $\alpha = \Pr(\text{reject } H_0 \mid H_0) = \Pr(\text{pass the first stage, and then observe at least } r = 8 \text{ responses out of } n = 10 \text{ patients} \mid \pi = 0.5)$; while passing the first stage we need $X_1 \geq 4$ responses out of $n_1 = 5$. Therefore,
  $\alpha = \Pr(\text{get } X \geq 8 \text{ responses out of } n = 10 \text{ patients} \mid \text{already have 4 responses from } n_1 = 5 \text{ patients}, \pi = 0.5) \times \Pr(4 \text{ responses from } n_1 = 5, \pi = 0.5) + \Pr(\text{get } X \geq 8 \text{ responses out of } n = 10 \text{ patients} \mid 5 \text{ responses from } n_1 = 5, \pi = 0.5) \times \Pr(5 \text{ responses from } = 5, \pi = 0.5)$
  $= \Pr(\text{get } X_2 \geq 4 \text{ responses out of } n_2 = 10 - n_1 = 5, \pi = 0.5) \times 0.15625 + \Pr(\text{get } X_2 \geq 3 \text{ responses out of } n_2 = 5, \pi = 0.5) \times 0.03125 = 0.1875 \times 0.15625 + 0.5 \times 0.03125 = 0.0449$.
  The above calculation can be carried out in R:

```
(1-pbinom(3,5,0.5))*dbinom(4,5,0.5)+(1-pbinom
    (2,5,0.5))*dbinom(5,5,0.5)
[1] 0.04492188
```

- Next, the power is obtained similarly by

$1 - \beta = \Pr(\text{reject } H_0 \mid H_A) = \Pr(\text{pass the first stage, then observe at least}$
$r = 8$ responses out of $n = 10$ patients $\mid \pi = 0.8)$
   With R,

```
(1-pbinom(3,5,0.8))*dbinom(4,5,0.8)+(1-pbinom
    (2,5,0.8))*dbinom(5,5,0.8)
[1] 0.6106907
```

- Third, the PET. Early termination occurs when we observe $X_1 \leq 3$ responses out of $n_1 = 5$ patients at the first stage. There are actually two PETs to consider.
  PET under H_0: $\Pr(X_1 \leq 3; n_1 = 5, \pi = 0.5)$

```
pbinom(3,5,0.5)
[1] 0.8125
```

  PET under H_A: $\Pr(X_1 \leq 3; n_1 = 5, \pi = 0.8)$

```
pbinom(3,5,0.8)
[1] 0.26272
```

Note that PET under H_0 is much greater than PET under H_A. This fact is intuitive because, if the experimental therapy is not working as well as expected ($\pi = 0.5$ only), we would like to terminate the trial early.

- *Expected sample size.* The expected sample size is a weighted average of sample sizes of the stages. We also calculate two expected sample sizes following the two PETs. In general,

$$E(N) = \sum_k k \times \Pr(N = k) \tag{7.3}$$

In our situation, the total sample size $N = n_1 = 5$ if the trial stops after Stage I, or $N = 10$ if it does not stop after Stage I. We already calculated PET $= 0.8125$ under H_0 and PET $= 0.2627$ if H_A is true. Hence,

$$E(N \mid H_0) = 5 \times 0.8125 + 10(1 - 0.8125) = 5.94$$

$$E(N \mid H_A) = 5 \times 0.2627 + 10(1 - 0.2627) = 8.69$$

Note that, if the therapy does not work well ($\pi = 0.5$), we would expect the study to terminate earlier; hence, fewer patients are tested compared to when it works well (six versus nine). The expected sample size in both cases is less than the maximum sample size $N = 10$.

We summarize the above illustration in Table 7.1 with the following comparisons: A two-stage design requires the configuration of four parameters (such

TABLE 7.1

Two-Stage versus One-Stage Designs

	Two-Stage	One-Stage
α	0.045	0.055
$1-\beta$	0.611	0.678
E(N)	5.94 (under H_0)	10
	8.69 (under H_A)	

Note: $H_0: \pi = \pi_0 = 0.5$ and $H_A: \pi = \pi_1 = 0.8$.

as $n_1 = 5$, $r_1 = 3$, $n = 10$, and $r = 7$), as opposed to the one-stage fixed-size design, where only two parameters are needed (e.g., $n = 10$ and $r = 7$). To test the same hypotheses with the same maximum sample size ($n = 10$), we have seen that the one-stage design has a greater power (0.678) and a higher type I error rate (0.055), compared to the two-stage design (0.611 and 0.045, respectively). This is because the above two-stage design increases the chance of accepting the null hypothesis with an interim analysis for futility (i.e., increases type II error rate, and hence lowers the power). The decrease in the type I error rate in the above two-stage design is because the rejection of the null hypothesis can only occur at the final stage when the interim data have passed through from the first stage. Later when we discuss a general sequential design that also allows for early rejection of the null hypothesis at the interim stages, we find an increase in the type I error rate. In addition, note that the two-stage design has a smaller expected sample size, which is a major advantage of the sequential design.

The above example also illustrates how to obtain the statistical properties of a given two-stage design with a configuration represented by (n_1, r_1, n, r). These statistical properties include α, $1-\beta$, and E(N) (Homework 7.1). A natural question following this illustration is, with a given (α, β) for testing a specific H_0 (π_0) versus H_A (π_1), how do we find a design with a configuration (n_1, r_1, n, r) that indicates the maximum and interim sample sizes, decision rules, and E(N)? These topics are discussed in Section 7.3. Also note that one may also be interested in calculating the probability of dismissing the drug (Homework 7.2).

7.3 Simon's Two-Stage Designs

There are two kinds of designs proposed in Simon (1989): 1) optimal design and 2) minimax design. The optimal design is the one where the expected sample size under the null hypothesis is the smallest among all feasible designs. The minimax design is the one where the maximum sample size is the smallest one among all feasible designs. A design is feasible if the configuration satisfies the constraints of the type I and type II error rates. The algorithm to search and construct these two designs is described in Sections 7.3.1 and 7.3.2.

7.3.1 Optimal Design

For specified values $(\pi_0, \pi_1, \alpha, \beta)$, fix a large N (e.g., N = 55). All configurations with $n \le N$ are searched. For each n_1 in the range of (1, n–1), we determine the integer values of (r_1, r), with r_1 in $(0, n_1)$ and r in (r_1, n), so that the type I error rate is controlled at α and the type II error rate is controlled at β. (We demonstrated the calculation of α and β in the previous section.) Then from all the feasible solutions, we choose the one with the smallest $E(N \mid \pi = \pi_0)$. (We also demonstrated the calculation of the $E(N \mid \pi = \pi_0)$ in Section 7.2.) Note that $E(N \mid \pi = \pi_0)$ is chosen to reflect the goal of stopping early if the drug does not work (i.e., stopping due to futility).

7.3.2 Minimax Design

We start with the fixed sample size n given by Equation 7.1. Recall that a sequential design requires a larger maximum sample size than the fixed-size design. Thus, this n is our lower bound. If we find a solution, we stop and obtain (n_1, r_1, n, r); otherwise, we increase n to n+1 and repeat the algorithm. The algorithm of finding a solution is similar to that for the optimal design: For each n_1 in the range (1, n – 1), determine the integer values of (r_1, r), with r_1 in $(0, n_1)$ and r in (r_1, n) to satisfy the constraints of type I and type II error rates (α, β). Do this until we finish with n_2 for that n. Note that, because we started from the lower bound for n and increased to the next n+1, we stop when a solution is found. Thus, this process chooses a solution that has the smallest n, the maximum sample size of the study.

7.4 Discussion

7.4.1 Software

The paper by Simon (1989) contains tables for many commonly used design configurations. Computer programs are also available for calculating Simon's two-stage designs. For example, a website at the National Cancer Institute[*] and the NCSS/PASS site[†] can be used for this purpose. In addition, many NCI-designated cancer centers also have accessible computer

---

[*] NCI website: http://linus.nci.nih.gov/brb/samplesize/otsd.html
[†] NCSS/PASS website: http://www.ncss.com/

programs on their websites, such as the Vanderbilt-Ingram Cancer Center.[‡] Another useful resource is the Clinical Trial Design Systems (CTDSystems) at the Duke Cancer Institute.[*] The CTDSystems is especially useful because it also provides a graphical display of the optimal and minimax designs (Homework 7.3). References on the CTDSystems can be found in Jung et al. (2001, 2004, 2006) and Jung and Kim (2004).

7.4.2 P-Value

Following the notation in Section 7.2.3, we give the p-value for a study with Simon's two-stage design. (Note: The p-value is the probability of getting the same or a more extreme result as the observed value in the direction of the alternative under the null hypothesis.)

For a case in which the trial is stopped at the first stage due to futility, that is, $x_1 \leq r_1$, the p-value is given by

$$\Pr(X_1 \geq x_1 \mid n_1, \pi = \pi_0) = 1 - \Pr(X_1 \leq x_1 - 1 \mid n_1, \pi = \pi_0)$$

$$= 1 - B(x_1 - 1; n_1, \pi = \pi_0)$$

(7.4)

This can easily be obtained with the R function: $1 - \text{pbinom}(x_1 - 1, n_1, \pi = \pi_0)$.

For a case in which $x_1 > r_1$, the trial continues to the second stage with an additional n_2 patients and x_2 responses. The p-value is calculated by

$$\Pr(X_1 > r_1, X_1 + X_2 \geq x_1 + x_2 \mid n_1, n_2, \pi = \pi_0)$$

$$= \sum_{x=r_1+1}^{\min(n_1, x_1+x_2-1)} \Pr(X_1 = x \mid n_1, \pi = \pi_0) \Pr(X_1 + X_2 \geq x_1 + x_2 \mid X_1 = x, n_2, \pi = \pi_0)$$

$$= \sum_{x=r_1+1}^{\min(n_1, x_1+x_2-1)} \Pr(X_1 = x \mid n_1, \pi = \pi_0) \Pr(X_2 \geq x_1 + x_2 - x \mid n_2, \pi = \pi_0)$$

$$= \sum_{x=r_1+1}^{\min(n_1, x_1+x_2-1)} b(x; n_1, \pi_0) \left[1 - B(x_1 + x_2 - x - 1; n_2, \pi_0) \right]$$

(7.5)

(because X_1 and X_2 are independent cohorts of patients). It is obvious that $X_1 = x < n_1$, and that $x_1 + x_2 - x - 1 \geq 0$ and thus $x \leq x_1 + x_2 - 1$. Hence, the upper limit for x is $\min(n_1, x_1 + x_2 - 1)$ (Homework 7.4).

[‡] Vanderbilt-Ingram Cancer Center (2007). Available at http://www.vicc.org/biostatistics/ts/twostage.php

[*] Duke Cancer Institute. "Clinical Trial Design Systems," available at http://www.dukecancer institute.org/biostatistics/

7.4.3 Other Issues

A common issue of concern with Simon's design is its rigid rules. In practice, trials are often interrupted for additional review of the study status or end up with deviations from the original design, either fewer patients enrolled due to accrual shortage or more patients enrolled due to over-running. Koyama and Chen (2008) discussed proper inference when deviation occurs at the second stage, including p-value adjustment, point estimate, and confidence interval calculations for the response rate. Their software is available online (Homework 7.5).* Wu and Shih (2008) tackled the issue of redesign when interruption and deviation occur.

Another concern is on the uncertainty of setting the response rate π_1 in the alternative hypothesis. Sometimes an enthusiastic investigator may expect the response rate higher, while a prudent co-investigator may want to set it lower. Lin and Shih (2004) proposed a strategy for adaptive two-stage designs that uses the information at the first stage of the study to decide the target response rate for the alternative hypothesis.

HOMEWORK 7.1

How does the expected sample size E(N) relate to the PET (probability of early termination) in a two-stage design with n_1 in the first stage and total $n = n_1 + n_2$ at the end of the trial? For biostatistics students, give a precise mathematical expression.

HOMEWORK 7.2

Consider a single-arm, two-stage design for a Phase II cancer trial. We test H_0: $\pi = 0.5$ versus H_A: $\pi = 0.8$, where π is the response rate of the new compound. The two-stage design is as follows:

Stage I: Enter $n_1 = 5$ patients. If $X_1 \leq 3$ responses are observed, stop the study and dismiss the drug. Otherwise, continue to the next stage.

Stage II: Enter another $n_2 = 5$ patients. Out of the total $n = n_1 + n_2 = 10$, if $X \geq 8$ responses are observed, reject the null hypothesis and claim the drug is worthy of further study.

1. Calculate the probability that this compound will be dismissed from further studies if the true response rate is 0.5.

---

* Koyama, T., Chen, H., and Gray, W. (2009). "Proper Inference from Simon's Two-Stage Designs." Available at http://biostat.mc.vanderbilt.edu/wiki/Main/TwoStageInference

2. Calculate the probability of dismissing further studies if the true response rate is 0.8.

(Note: When a compound is dismissed from further study on the same indication, it may be investigated for other indications with regimen modification or combination with other agents.)

HOMEWORK 7.3

Read the following paper: "A Phase II Study of Sorafenib in Patients with Platinum-Pretreated, Advanced (Stage IIIb or IV) Non-Small Cell Lung Cancer with a KRAS Mutation" (Dingemans, A. M., et al., *Clinical Cancer Research*, 2013, 19(3): 743–51).

1. What was the primary endpoint of this study?
2. This study used Simon's two-stage optimal design. Find what the assumed parameters were for the design.
3. Check the design decision rules given in the paper with the software given in the chapter.
4. What would the decision rules have been if Simon's minimax design had been used instead? Discuss the merits of the optimal design versus the minimax design in this case.
5. Comment on the result of the study with regard to the primary endpoint as reported in the paper, compared with the design.
6. What would the sample size have been if a one-stage fixed sample size design were used instead, with the same hypotheses, type I error rate, and power? Compare it with the maximum sample size and expected sample size of the two-stage optimal design used by the study.

HOMEWORK 7.4

1. Write a program in R to calculate the p-value in Equation 7.5.
2. Calculate the p-value for a hypothetical scenario where $x_1 = 6$ and $x_2 = 4$ under the design ($n_1 = 7, r_1 = 4, n = 20, r = 13$) for testing $H_0: \pi = \pi_0 = 0.5$ versus $H_A: \pi = \pi_1 = 0.8$.

HOMEWORK 7.5

A Phase II clinical trial was conducted to determine the overall response (CR+PR) of a combination therapy with paclitaxel, 13-cis-retinoic acid, and interferon alfa-2b in women with Stage IVB or recurrent cervical cancer. The response rate was expected to be greater than that of paclitaxel alone in the referenced historical studies of 18%. The combination therapy was considered clinically interesting if the response rate was greater than 30%. Simon's two-stage optimal design was applied, with type I error rate = 0.10 and power = 0.80.

1. Verify that the optimal design's solution is $(n_1, r_1, n, r) = (27, 5, 66, 15)$, and interpret this configuration.

2. It turned out that there were $x_1 = 9$ responders (CR+PR) during the first stage and the study continued to the second stage. However, because of slow accrual, the protocol was closed after only 6 additional patients were accrued. In the second stage, 1/6 patients had a partial response. Use the method and software of Koyama and Chen (2008) to obtain the p-value, the median estimate, and the 90% confidence interval of the response rate (CR+PR). Comment on whether the p-value and the confidence interval give the same conclusion or not.

References

Dingemans AM, Mellema WW, Groen HJ, van Wijk A, Burgers SA, Kunst PW, and Thunnissen E. (2013). A Phase II study of Sorafenib in patients with platinum-pretreated, advanced (Stage IIIb or IV) non-small cell lung cancer with a KRAS mutation. *Clinical Cancer Research* 19: 743–751.

Gehan, EA. (1961). The determination of the number of patients required in a preliminary and a follow-up of a new chemotherapeutic agent. *Journal of Chronic Disease* 13: 346–353.

Jung SH, Carey M, and Kim KM. (2001). Graphical search for two-stage phase II clinical trials. *Controlled Clinical Trials* 22: 367–372.

Jung SH and Kim KM. (2004). On the estimation of the binomial probability in multistage clinical trials. *Statistics in Medicine* 23: 881–896.

Jung SH, Lee TY, Kim KM, and George S. (2004). Admissible two-stage designs for phase II cancer clinical trials. *Statistics in Medicine* 23: 561–569.

Jung SH, Owzar K, George SL, and Lee TY. (2006). P-value calculation for multistage phase II cancer clinical trials (with discussion), *J Biopharmaceutical Statistics* 16: 765–783.

Koyama T and Chen H. (2008). Proper inference from Simon's two-stage designs. *Statistics in Medicine* 27: 3145–3154.

Lin Y and Shih WJ. (2004). Adaptive two-stage designs for single-arm phase IIA cancer clinical trials. *Biometrics* 60: 482–490.

Simon, RM. (1989). Optimal two-stage designs for Phase II clinical trials. *Controlled Clinical Trials* 10: 1–10.

Wu Y and Shih WJ. (2008). Approaches to handling data when a Phase II trial deviates from the pre-specified Simon's two-stage design. *Statistics in Medicine* 27: 6190–6208.

8

Sequential Designs and Methods—Part II: Monitoring Safety and Futility

8.1 Monitoring Safety

We started with a definition of a clinical trial in Chapter 1, which led to the immediate concern of conducting experiments with human beings. We further highlighted ethics and regulations regarding the trial participant's right to privacy, information on risk and benefit, and safety protection. In order to remain ethically compliant with these intents, we must monitor and protect the subject's safety periodically throughout the trial. When the risks of continuing the trial outweigh the potential benefits, the trial should be modified or even stopped to protect the safety of those already in the trial, as well as to prevent exposure to the risk for those who are yet to be recruited. Similarly, if early superiority (efficacy) is clearly demonstrated, modification or even early termination of the trial should be considered, because it is unethical to continue subjects on the inferior arm. Stopping or modification for efficacy is discussed in Chapter 9.

8.1.1 Adverse Events

An *adverse event* (AE) is any untoward medical occurrence in a subject participating in a clinical study who is administered a medical (investigational or noninvestigational) product. An AE may not necessarily relate causally to the treatment. An AE can therefore be any unfavorable and unintended sign (including an abnormal laboratory finding), symptom, event, or disease temporally associated with the use of the product, whether or not it is related to that product or device (EMA 1995, NCI 2009). An AE in a clinical trial is commonly classified based on the investigator's judgment on the following:

- *Relationship* to the study medication, as definitely, probably, possibly related, or not likely related. Another system of treatment relationship is simply the binary judgment: related or not related, which has been adopted by some countries recently.
- *Severity*, as mild, moderate, or severe intensity. Another system of severity is by grade: Grade 1 to Grade 5; Grade 5 being death.

DOI: 10.1201/9781003176527-8

- *Seriousness*, as yes or no. A serious AE (SAE) is any adverse experience that (i) results in death; (ii) is life-threatening; (iii) requires inpatient hospitalization or prolongation of existing hospitalization; (iv) results in persistent, permanent, or significant disability/incapacity; (v) is a congenital anomaly/birth defect; (vi) is a suspected transmission of any infectious agent via a medicinal product; or (vii) is judged medically important for expedited reporting and/or emergent intervention to prevent one of the outcomes listed above (such as suicide attempt) (EMA 1995).

All AEs should be reported in the case report form (CRF). The accompanying information also includes the AE start date and time (to determine whether the AE is "treatment emergent"), duration, action taken, and the outcome—whether recovered/resolved, worsened, improved, or continuing on the day of the report. AEs are identified by clinical history, physical examinations, and laboratory tests. The US FDA and other regulatory agencies require that all AEs, regardless of how remotely they are considered to be related, be collected and reported. An example of this might be illustrated in reporting (severe) traffic accidents following therapy, with the idea that some extremely remotely associated events might, if seen with some frequency, actually have a relationship with the treatment. Some AE may be a pre-existing condition that worsened after treatment. To avoid confusion with progression of the disease under study, the term "treatment emergent adverse event" (TEAE) is used in data analysis to exclude disease progression as an AE.

Clinical AEs are further grouped according to the body system and organ class involved (cardiac, eye, hepatobiliary, infections and infestations, gastrointestinal, musculoskeletal and connective tissue, nervous system, psychiatric, renal and urinary, respiratory, thoracic, skin, etc.).

Laboratory AEs are measured by urine and blood tests. ECG, *vital signs* (blood pressures, pulse rate, weight, height, and perhaps body temperature and respiratory rate for some lung studies), and physical examination findings are also analyzed. It is more meaningful to analyze the laboratory data and vital signs by comparing changes from baseline with regard to the *normal ranges* rather than calculating the mean or median. For multicenter trials, a central laboratory should be used to standardize the tests and normal ranges, especially for any tests that are new or not part of the standardized tests monitored by laboratory-accrediting agencies such as the American College of Pathology. In data analyses, the laboratory values are classified as below, within, or above the normal ranges—sometimes twice or three times the upper or lower limits of the normal ranges (ULN and LLN, respectively). For example, for drugs that may induce liver injury, Hy's law specifies that subjects with any elevated AT (AST or ALT) of $>3 \times \text{ULN}$ and ALP $<2 \times \text{ULN}$, associated with an increase in bilirubin $\geq 2 \times \text{ULN}$, should be examined with special attention (FDA 2007). So, for statisticians this can become a 3×3 pre- versus post-treatment ordinal categorical data problem, testing for symmetry versus asymmetry within each treatment group. Shih (1987) presented a method for square tables that discussed such an analysis.

For data analyses, issues with multiple tests arise when many routine laboratory tests and clinical examinations are performed. Some prefer conservativeness for safety without any adjustment of the p-values. Some advocate for a tier system prioritizing the tests and examinations for a predefined set of AEs that are known to occur with other drugs of the same class, such as GI bleeding for NSAIDs, cardiac events for COX-II inhibitors, thrombocytopenia (low blood platelet count) for sulfa-containing antibiotics and anticonvulsants (e.g., heparin), vomiting and hair loss for certain cancer treatments, and hypoglycemia for antidiabetic drugs. Special attention should be paid to this predefined set of AEs (called AEs of special interest) and "suspected unexpected serious AEs" (SUSA or SUSAR), which are usually documented in the investigator's brochure (IB) and defined in the data analysis plan for confirmatory trials. Routine laboratory tests and examinations are generally analyzed for exploratory purposes.

8.1.2 Monitoring SAEs Using Bayesian Methods

As discussed above, except for the prespecified treatment-class-related AEs, it is usually not appropriate to use significance tests for monitoring safety endpoints due to the issue of multiplicity. Other methods may be more suitable for answering clinical questions. In this chapter, a basic Bayesian method is introduced that has been used for trials involving chemotherapy, immunotherapy, and peripheral stem cell transplantation in treating patients with *multiple myeloma.*

With high-dose chemotherapy and autologous stem cell transplantation for patients with multiple myeloma, risks of severe myelotoxicity, mucositis, life-threatening infections, and early mortality are all prominent complications. Furthermore, for allogeneic transplantation following chemoimmunotherapy, early allogeneic graft failure and severe acute graft-versus-host disease (GVHD) after treatment regimen are additional serious concerns (Eastern Cooperative Oncology Group 2001). In these scenarios, it is desirable to have a close monitoring plan as each patient is treated in the trial. This is known as *continuous monitoring* (as opposed to group sequential monitoring, discussed in the next chapter), which is only suitable for an *immediate response* type of endpoint. If a critical number of predefined serious events are reached, the study should be stopped. Otherwise, the study may continue. The question is, what is that critical number?

8.1.3 The Beta-Binomial Model

The monitoring process can be formulated as follows. The event rate associated with the tested treatment is denoted by θ. Let θ^* be a predefined threshold value (e.g., 0.15). When (x, n) is observed, where x is the number of events out of n treated patients, we calculate the *posterior probability* of the event rate exceeding the threshold: p=Pr(θ>θ* | x out of n). The study is stopped if p is very high, say 80%. Otherwise, the study may continue. In a Bayesian framework, the event rate θ is regarded as a random variable with a probability distribution, not as a fixed parameter. For any given θ, "X out of n" follows the binomial distribution, that is, X~binom(n; θ). Recall that in Chapter 7 we used its pdf and cdf in R:

```
dbinom(x, size, prob)
pbinom(x, size, prob, lower.tail=TRUE)
```

The fundamental *Bayes theorem* is the following probability relationship:

$$Pr(A\,|\,B) = \frac{Pr(B\,|\,A)Pr(A)}{Pr(B)} \tag{8.1}$$

This rule is very useful when we want to know the *conditional or posterior probability* of A given B, but what we have is the reverse information: the conditional probability of B given A. However, we also need the *marginal probability* of A, which is the *prior* probability in the Bayesian framework. The denominator Pr(B) is a normalization constant because we are conditioning on B.

Incidentally, the Bayes theorem is also the basis for calculating information regarding diagnosis of a disease with a medical device. In such a situation, the Bayes rule expresses

$$\begin{aligned}&Pr(\text{true disease | observed symptom})\\ &= \frac{Pr(\text{symptom | disease})\,Pr(\text{disease})}{Pr(\text{symptom})}\end{aligned}$$

where Pr(true disease status | observed symptom) is commonly known as the *positive predictive value* (PPV), Pr(symptom | disease) is the *sensitivity* of the diagnostic device, and Pr(disease) is the *prevalence* of the disease. These are familiar terms in a public health context.

When there are n patients being treated, we evaluate

$$Pr(\theta > \theta^* \,|\, x \text{ out of } n) = \int_{\theta^*}^{1} f(\theta\,|\,x,n)d\theta \tag{8.2}$$

by applying the Bayes rule to the posterior pdf

$$f(\theta\,|\,x,n) = \frac{f(x\,|\,\theta,n)\,f(\theta)}{f(x\,|\,n)} \tag{8.3}$$

The posterior pdf is viewed as a function of θ for the given data (x, n). The marginal pdf in the denominator is the normalization constant of the posterior pdf, and it does not include θ. To find the posterior distribution with a *conjugate prior*, it often suffices to write

$$f(\theta \mid x,n) \propto f(x \mid \theta,n)\, f(\theta) \qquad (8.4)$$

In other words, the posterior is proportional to the product of the likelihood of the data and the prior distribution.

The beta-binomial relationship is a convenient model for binary endpoints, because the beta distribution is the conjugate prior of the binomial distribution. It works as follows. With f(x $\mid$ θ, n) as a binomial pdf binom(x, n, θ) $\propto \theta^x (1-\theta)^{n-x}$ for a given (θ, n), the corresponding conjugate distribution as a function of θ is the beta distribution with shape parameters (a, b) with pdf beta(a, b)$\propto \theta^{a-1}(1-\theta)^{b-1}$. Following Equation 8.4, the posterior f(θ $\mid$ x, n)$\propto \theta^{a+x-1}$ $(1-\theta)^{b+n-x-1}$ has the form of a beta distribution with parameters (a+x, b+n−x). In the context of the data (x, n), the (hyper)parameters (a, b) for the beta distribution can be interpreted as, prior to observing the data, "a" being the number of events out of "a+b" hypothetical subjects. The *beta-binomial model* containing a beta posterior with parameters (a+x, b+n−x) indicates that, after getting the data, the numbers of events and subjects become a+x and a+b+n, respectively. The choice of parameters of the prior distribution will determine how much influence the "prior knowledge" will contribute to the final (posterior) result, when paired with the observed data. The *uniform distribution* with domain (0, 1) is a special case of the beta distribution with a=b=1. In this case, with the prior sample size a+b=2, the data (x, n) will be the dominating factor for the posterior, and the prior is called a *flat, vague, or noninformative prior* in the Bayesian framework. We review more properties of the beta distribution and how to elicit the (a, b) hyperparameters from the investigator in Section 8.1.4.

For a given set of shape parameters (a, b), the probability $\Pr(\theta > \theta^* \mid x$ out of n) in Equation 8.2 can be obtained by using the R function pbeta(q, shape1, shape2). To find the usage and a numerical example, simply type the following in R:

```
> help(pbeta)
```

Example 8.1

Continuing to use the stem cell transplantation trial in Section 8.1.2 as an example, let $\theta^* = 0.15$ be the predefined threshold value. We would like to evaluate the risk of early mortality for the therapy at an interim stage when data (x, n) are available by calculating the (posterior) probability $p = \Pr(\theta > 0.15 \mid (x, n))$ and comparing it against a threshold, say 80%. Suppose that we have no prior information regarding the death rate of the tested stem cell transplantation therapy. This translates to the noninformative prior, that is, beta(1, 1). After experimenting on n=5 patients, x=1 early death occurred. The posterior (θ $\mid$ x, n)~beta(a+x, b+n−x)=beta(2, 5). Calculate $p = \Pr(\theta > 0.15 \mid x=1, n=5)$ in R:

```
1-pbeta(0.15, 2, 5)
[1] 0.7764843
```

Because this answer is lower than 80%, we do not stop the study at this interim stage. (However, we would stop the study if the threshold were 0.75. For safety analysis, there is no general rule for choosing a threshold.) Note that, for a nonstatistician, 1 death out of 5 patients seems greater than a rate of 0.15. However, the calculation of probability takes into account random variation and clinicians' prior beliefs. When the trial continues, the current posterior beta(2, 5) will then become the prior with (a=2, b=5) for the next evaluation when a different cohort of (x, n) is available. We can also use the same noninformative prior and accumulate the new data (x, n) instead of (a=2, b=5).

Figure 8.1 illustrates the noninformative prior beta(1, 1)=U(0, 1) modified by the point mass data (concentrated at the point 1/5) leading to the posterior beta(2, 5).

8.1.4 Elicitation of the Shape Parameters (a, b) of Beta Distribution

When the investigator has prior information on the event rate from the beginning of the trial, the noninformative prior is no longer suitable. Some eliciting methods to obtain the appropriate hyperparameters (a, b) are given by Wu, Shih, and Moore (2008). It is useful to plot the pdf $f(\theta; a, b)$ of beta(a, b), $0 \leq \theta \leq 1, a > 0, b > 0$, for several possible values of (a, b) and use them during the elicitation discussion with the investigator. As an illustration, the pdf $f(\theta; a, b)$ of beta(a, b) for a=5, b=11 can easily be graphed in R by entering

```
t=seq(0, 1, by=0.01)
pdf=dbeta(t, 5, 11)
plot (t, pdf, type="l", xlab="Theta", ylab="Beta density",
   lwd=2)
```

Note that the mean of beta(a, b) is $a/(a+b)$ and the mode $m=(a-1)/(a+b-2)$. For $1 < a < b$, the pdf skews to the left, such that the mode is less than the mean and both are less than 0.5 (see the example plot in Figure 8.2).

Wu, Shih, and Moore (2008) recommended two eliciting methods to obtain the appropriate hyperparameters (a, b): Method A is a "location and interval" method, and Method B is a "percentiles only" method. For both methods, we draw some rough beta distributions (pdf) during the discussion with the investigator about his/her prior beliefs (or available prior data) by performing the following:

- Method A: Elicit from the investigator the mode m (the location); select the highest density interval (r_1, r_2), and ask the investigator for the coverage probability u (area) under the pdf curve between (r_1, r_2).

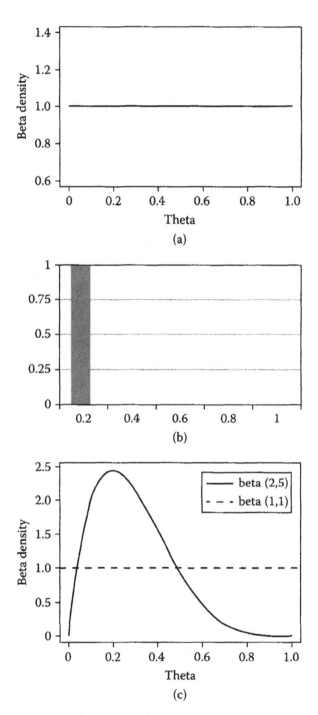

FIGURE 8.1
Posterior (c) is prior (a) modified by the data (b).

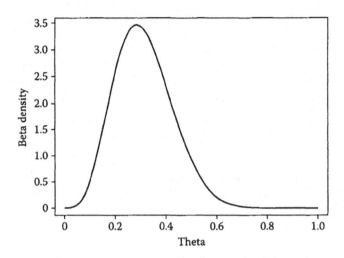

FIGURE 8.2
Density function of a beta distribution.

Given the above information, we are able to determine the parameters (a, b) of the beta prior by solving the following two equations:

$$\frac{a-1}{a+b-2} = m$$

and

$$\int_{r_1}^{r_2} f(r; a, b) dr = u \tag{8.5}$$

where $f(r; a, b) = \dfrac{\Gamma(a+b)}{\Gamma(a)\Gamma(b)} r^{a-1} (1-r)^{b-1}$ is the pdf of beta(a, b). For Method A (mode and interval), $a > 1$, $b > 1$ and $r_1 < m < r_2$. An R function, MI(m, r1, r2, u), is provided in Appendix 8.1 for obtaining the parameters (a, b).

- Method B: Give a lower percentile K_1 (100 μ_1%) and an upper percentile K_2 (100 μ_2%), and elicit from the investigator the values μ_1 and μ_2, respectively. With the information of two percentiles, K_1 and K_2, accompanying the corresponding probabilities, μ_1 and μ_2, the beta parameters can then be obtained from the numerical solution of

$$\int_0^{K_1} f(r; a, b) dr = \mu_1$$

and

$$\int_0^{K_2} f(r;a,b)dr = \mu_2 \qquad (8.6)$$

For Method B (percentiles only), $a \geq 1$. An R program, PO(K1, u1, K2, u2), is provided in Appendix 8.2 for obtaining the parameters (a, b).

Wu, Shih, and Moore (2008) found that when the misspecification error in judging the mode is mild, Method A is favored over Method B. The reverse is true when the error is severe.

8.1.5 Discussion

Using the posterior probability is a Bayesian approach, which enables us to incorporate expert opinion (or prior data) when making inferences and decisions. Of course, this capability is not limited to monitoring SAEs. The method can also be used for monitoring other types of events, including efficacy events (see Homework 8.1).

Some trials incorporate prior information, but utilize it in a different way. For example, one multiple myeloma trial (Montefiore-Einstein Cancer Center 2011) has the following monitoring design described in its protocol (p. 49):

> The anticipated treatment related mortality with the proposed regimen is less than 5% based on previous studies… We will consider a 30-day mortality of more than 5% as unacceptable. The 30-day mortality will be evaluated after the first 20 patients have been enrolled. If no more than 1 patient suffers a mortality within 30 days … we will continue to accrue… If 2 or more patients suffer a mortality … within 30 days of treatment, we will suspend accrual….

Apparently, this study set a stopping rule of $1/20 = 0.05$ as compared to the threshold based on the literature for monitoring the study, instead of using the literature to construct a prior distribution. The monitoring design thus failed to consider any variability associated with the observed data. Furthermore, with the concern of an SAE, such as 30-day mortality, a continuous monitoring plan, for example every 5 patients, seems to be more desirable than waiting for a decision when $n = 20$. As a homework assignment, we ask the readers to use the Bayesian approach to develop a continuous safety monitoring plan (Homework 8.2).

8.1.6 Monitoring Rare Serious Events by Gamma–Poisson Distribution

The monitoring of treatment-related 30-day mortality in the multiple myeloma trial discussed above (Montefiore-Einstein Cancer Center 2011) might also be considered in another framework as a rare but serious event, if the event rate is measured in terms of per patient-month (or other continuous timescale). When using events per patient-time for a rare event, or when counting event episodes that may happen more than once in subjects with different follow-up time, the sampling distribution for the number of events would follow a *Poisson distribution* with a mean rate parameter (say λ), rather than a binomial distribution. Assuming subject i to have x_i number of events or event episodes observed within t_i follow-up time, the pdf of Poisson with mean rate (in unit time) of λ is

$$f(x_i;\lambda) = \frac{e^{-(\lambda t_i)}(\lambda t_i)^{x_i}}{x_i!}$$

With n subjects, the likelihood function is

$$L(\lambda; x_i, i = 1,\ldots,n) = \prod_{i=1}^{n}\frac{e^{-(\lambda t_i)}(\lambda t_i)^{x_i}}{x_i!} = [e^{-\lambda\left(\sum_{i=1}^{n}t_i\right)}](\lambda^{\sum_{i=1}^{n}x_i})\prod_{i=1}^{n}\frac{t_i^{x_i}}{x_i!}$$

$$\propto \lambda^k e^{-\lambda T},$$

$\lambda > 0$, $T > 0$, $k = 0,1,2,\ldots$, where $k = \sum_{i=1}^{n}x_i$ is the total number of events and $T = \sum_{i=1}^{n}t_i$ is the total patient-time of the sample of n subjects. The conjugate prior for λ in the Bayesian analysis would be a gamma distribution, gamma(a, b). The gamma distribution is a two-parameter family of continuous probability distributions with a shape parameter "a" and a rate parameter "b" (both>0). The pdf is:

$$f(\lambda;a,b) = \frac{b^a}{\Gamma(a)}\lambda^{a-1}e^{-\lambda b} \qquad \lambda > 0$$

where $\Gamma(a)$ is the *gamma function*. A gamma density can easily be graphed by the R function *dgamma*; for example (Figure 8.3),

```
t = seq(0, 1, by = 0.01)
pdf = dgamma(t, shape = 5, rate = 100)
plot(t, pdf, type="l", xlab="Lambda", ylab="Gamma density",
lwd = 2)
```

To find the prior parameters, we can elicit the prior by using the values of the mean and variance:

$$E(\lambda) = a / b$$

$$Var(\lambda) = a / b^2$$

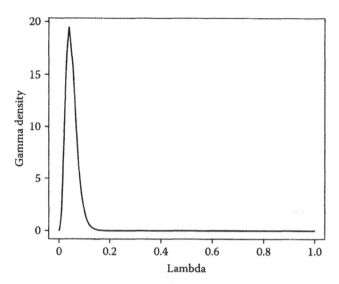

FIGURE 8.3
Density function of a gamma distribution.

or by methods similar to Method A ("location and interval" method) or Method B ("percentiles only" method), which were discussed for the beta distribution case. The parameter "a" represents the number of events, and "b" represents the total patient-time.

The posterior distribution is, thus, the gamma(k+a, T+b) distribution, whose pdf is proportional to

$$\lambda^{k+a-1} e^{-\lambda(T+b)}$$

We can then set a cut-off rate, λ^*, to stop the trial for safety when the posterior probability meets a threshold level of the SAE rate, for example 80%:

$$\Pr\left(\lambda \geq \lambda^* \mid k, T, a, b\right) \geq 80\%$$

Example 8.2

A completed suicide event rate in a population suffering from major depression is estimated at about 2%. In conducting a trial with a similar population, the investigator would like to stop the study if the investigational treatment group demonstrates a (true) completed suicide rate greater than 2%. The prior was determined using the data from a previous study, which had four events out of 200 patient-months. In the current ongoing trial, there are two events out of 50 patient-months: should the study be stopped?

By using the Poisson–gamma model, the estimates of prior parameters are $a=4$ and $b=200$; the current data are $k=2$ and $T=50$. The posterior is gamma(λ; 6, 250). We calculate the posterior probability $\Pr(\lambda>0.02 \mid k+a=6, T+b=250)$ by the R function:

```
1-pgamma(0.02, shape=6, rate=250)
[1] 0.6159607
```

Depending on the prespecified threshold level, the study may be stopped (say for a threshold of 60%) or not stopped (say for a threshold of 80%).

8.2 Monitoring Futility with Conditional Probability

The Bayesian posterior probability is a conditional probability given the data. With the assistance of a prior distribution, we used the Bayesian approach to monitor the safety without using significance tests. In this section, we discuss the use of conditional probability to monitor the possible *futility* of a study without a prior distribution or a p-value.

In Chapter 7, we discussed two-stage Simon's designs, where a Phase II cancer trial may be stopped at the first stage if the result is not as good as expected (desired). In that scenario, we accepted the null hypothesis and dismissed the compound from further testing to save resources and prevent more patients from being treated by an ineffective therapy. This is also known as "stopping the trial for futility." In Simon's design, the consideration was to use a least sample size while preserving the type I and type II error rates. The following conditional probability approach, on the other hand, is a monitoring tool, which does not necessarily control the type I and type II error rates.

8.2.1 Two-Stage Monitoring Process

Monitoring futility can be performed by the conditional probability (CP) method in a (classical) non-Bayesian fashion. The idea is illustrated as follows: Suppose that our final analysis is a z-test based on a total of N observations ($n=N/2$ in each treatment group for equal allocation), denoted as Z_N for the test statistic. Suppose at the end of the trial we compare it to the critical value 1.96, which is the critical value for the significance level of 0.025 for a one-sided z-test. At the interim stage, we have a total of $N_1 = 2n_1$ observations and obtain Z_{N_1}. We then (naturally) ask, what will be the probability of having the final test $Z_N>1.96$? That is, we would like to evaluate the conditional probability, $\Pr(Z_N>1.96 \mid Z_{N_1})$. If this probability is low, then we might stop the trial for futility.

For example, suppose we plan a trial with a total sample size of $N = 100$. When we have data for 50 patients, we calculate the z-test based on the results of these 50 patients and get $Z_{50} = 1.0$. What is $Pr(Z_{100} > 1.96 \mid Z_{50} = 1.0)$? It turns out that the answer depends on certain factors, as follows:

Let the information time (fraction) be $t = N_1/N$. For the two-sample case, following the setting in Chapter 4 (Section 4.2), $H_0 : \delta = \mu_1 - \mu_2 = 0$, and assuming known equal within-group variance, it is straightforward to derive that

$$Z_N = \sqrt{t}\, Z_{N_1} + \sqrt{1-t}\, Z_{N-N_1} \tag{8.7}$$

(see Appendix 8.3.1). That is, we decompose the final test statistic into two parts, one test statistic based on the samples of the first stage and one based on the rest. Note that Z_N is a weighted average of two independent normal random variables. (A linear combination of normal random variables is still normal.) The weights correspond to the square root of the sample size fraction, t, contained in each Z statistic. Specifically,

$$Z_{N_1} = \sqrt{\frac{N_1}{4\sigma^2}}\,\hat{\delta} = \frac{\sqrt{N_1}\,\hat{\delta}}{2\sigma} \sim N\!\left(\frac{\sqrt{N_1}\,\delta}{2\sigma}, 1\right) \tag{8.8}$$

$$Z_{N-N_1} \sim N\!\left(\frac{\sqrt{N-N_1}\,\delta}{2\sigma}, 1\right)$$

and

$$Z_N \sim N\!\left(\frac{\sqrt{N}\,\delta}{2\sigma}, 1\right) \tag{8.9}$$

We then use the decomposition (Equation 8.7) to calculate the CP:

$$Pr\!\left(Z_N > 1.96 \mid Z_{N_1}\right)$$

$$= Pr\!\left(\sqrt{t}\, Z_{N_1} + \sqrt{1-t}\, Z_{N-N_1} > 1.96\right)$$

$$= Pr\!\left(Z_{N-N_1} > \frac{1.96 - \sqrt{t}\, Z_{N_1}}{\sqrt{1-t}}\right)$$

$$= Pr\!\left(Z_{N-N_1} - \frac{\sqrt{N-N_1}\,\delta}{2\sigma} > \frac{1.96 - \sqrt{t}\, Z_{N_1}}{\sqrt{1-t}} - \frac{\sqrt{N-N_1}\,\delta}{2\sigma}\right)$$

$$= 1 - \Phi\left(\frac{1.96 - \sqrt{t}\ Z_{N_1}}{\sqrt{1-t}} - \frac{\sqrt{N - N_1}\ \delta}{2\sigma} \right) \tag{8.10}$$

From Equation 8.10 we can see that the CP of the one-sided final test being significant at the 0.025 level depends not only on the interim result Z_{N_1}, but also on when the interim analysis is performed in terms of t and the true treatment effect, δ/σ. There are many possibilities for the δ. A pessimistic estimate of the CP is to adopt the null hypothesis, $\delta=0$. An optimistic estimate is to adopt the alternative hypothesis, δ^*, for which the study is powered. Somewhere in between the null and alternative hypotheses is the point estimate of δ based on the interim data and the assumption that the current trend will continue to the end of the trial. Another estimate may be the upper or lower limits of a confidence interval. Moreover, one can make a weighted average of the above choices. If we place a (prior) distribution for δ, with a certain degree of variability centered at the point estimate and, for example, averaging Equation 8.10 with respect to this (prior) distribution, we then obtain a predictive probability of the one-sided final test being significant.

The point estimate of δ with the interim data is seen in Equation 8.8:

$$\hat{\delta} = \frac{2\sigma}{\sqrt{N_1}} Z_{N_1} \tag{8.11}$$

Thus, set $\delta = \hat{\delta}$ in (8.10) and, since $\dfrac{N - N_1}{N_1} = \dfrac{1-t}{t}$, we obtain

$$CP\left(Z_{N_1}, t, \text{current trend} \right) = 1 - \Phi\left(\frac{1.96 - \sqrt{t}\ Z_{N_1}}{\sqrt{1-t}} - \frac{\sqrt{1-t}}{\sqrt{t}} Z_{N_1} \right)$$

$$= \Phi\left(\frac{Z_{N_1}}{\sqrt{t(1-t)}} - \frac{1.96}{\sqrt{1-t}} \right) \tag{8.12}$$

Equation 8.12 can also be derived from the familiar regression formula of a bivariate normal distribution; see Appendix 8.3.3. Continuing the example where we supposed $Z_{N_1} = 1.0$ at $t=50/100=1/2$, under the current trend, $CP = \Phi\left(2 - 1.96\sqrt{2} \right)$ by the R function:

```
pnorm(2-1.96*sqrt(2))
[1]  0.2200991
```

If the threshold for the CP is set at 0.25 in the monitoring plan, then the study would be considered to stop for futility. There is also another topic of possible increase in sample size to rescue a trial when the conditional power is low as revealed in an interim analysis as above. We will discuss this topic in Chapter 10.

In-Class Exercises

1. What would be the CP if the same Z-value $\left(Z_{N_1} = 1.0\right)$ was observed at an earlier or later information time fraction, say $t = 1/3$ or $2/3$?
2. What Z-value would one need to have at an interim analysis for the CP to be at least 50%, assuming that the current trend will continue? The answer should be a function of t.

8.2.2 Discussion

Some points with regard to early termination require further attention. First, stopping the study for futility means that the compound (or concept) is dismissed from further testing in this study. This action does not necessarily mean that the sponsoring company or the investigator would abandon the compound completely. The compound may be modified for the dose regimen or route of administration, combined with other compounds, or studied for other indications with other populations.

Second, performing an interim analysis affects the type I error rate. As we previously demonstrated with Simon's two-stage design, when the interim analysis stops the trial only for futility, the type I error rate will be deflated, as also shown algebraically: Let P_0 mean "probability under the null hypothesis,"

$$\alpha = P_0\left(\text{Reject } H_0\right)$$

$$= P_0\left(\text{Not stop at } t < 1 \text{ then, reject } H_0 \text{ at } t = 1\right)$$

$$< P_0\left(\text{reject } H_0 \text{ at } t = 1\right)$$

$$= P_0\left(Z_N > 1.96\right) = 0.025$$

Normally, this suggests that one can set the critical value less than 1.96 for the final analysis to be significant at the 5% level for a two-sided test or the 2.5% level for a one-sided test, which is quite a gain. However, this is not a practice permitted by the US FDA for Phase III pivotal studies in the NDA or BLA setting, because the regulatory agency (rightly) regards the futility rule as not enforceable, that is, non-binding to the company. Provided that it is not a safety issue, the company may not adhere to the futility rule and still continue the study despite the low CP, which, although unwise, is nevertheless a possible business decision.

Third, futility (regarding efficacy) and safety are often tied together in decision making since they are the components of the whole risk/

benefit package. From the role of a *data and safety monitoring committee* (DSMC) –
see Chapter 9 – usually it is the safety issue arising first and then indicating and
leading to the futility analysis during the trial monitoring. A recent example
is the KEYNOTE-598 study of pembrolizumab plus ipilimumab, which ended
early for patients with metastatic non-small cell lung cancer (Boyer et al. 2021).
According to the findings from an interim analysis, this combination demonstrated no incremental benefit compared with pembrolizumab monotherapy in
terms of either overall survival or progression-free survival, which were the co-
primary endpoints of the study, and the combination crossed futility boundaries. In fact, the external data and safety monitoring committee recommended
that the study be stopped for futility and that participants discontinue ipilimumab and placebo since the committee was concerned that adding ipilimumab
to pembrolizumab did not improve efficacy but was associated with greater toxicity than pembrolizumab monotherapy.

Appendix 8.1: R Function for Obtaining Parameters of Prior Distribution Beta(a, b) Based on Method A

Gives the mode (m) and the coverage probability (u) of an interval (r1, r2).

The R Function MI (Mode and Interval Method)

```
# programmed by Yujun Wu; see Wu, Shih and Moore (2008)
# r1 < m < r2
###########################################################
# Method A: Location (mode) and Interval
# Elicitation information: (1) mode m
#                          (2) Pr(r1<r<r2) = u
###########################################################

MI <- function(m, r1, r2, u) {

    S <- function(x){
       (pbeta (r2, x [1] ,x[2] ) -pbeta (r1, x [1] ,x[2] ) -u)
^2 + ( (x[1] -1) /
              (x [1] +x [2] -2) -m) ^2
    }
    obj = constrOptim(c(2,2), S, NULL, ui =
rbind(c(1,0),c(0,1)),
          ci = 0(1,1), mu = 1e-100, outer.eps = 1e-100)
    obj $par
}
# Example:
MI(0.05,0.01,0.10,0.8)
```

Appendix 8.2: R Function for Obtaining Parameters of Prior Distribution Beta(a, b) Based on Method B

Gives the lower (100u1%) percentile (K1) and the (100u2%) percentile (K2).

The R Function PO (Percentiles Only Method)

```
# programmed by Yujun Wu; see Wu, Shih and Moore (2008)
# K1 < K2
############################################################
# Method B: percentiles only
# Elicitation information: (1) K1 : Pr(r<K1) = u1
#                          (2) K2 : Pr(r<K2) = u2
############################################################

PO <- function(K1,u1,K2,u2) {

    S <- function(x){
        (pbeta(K1, x [1],x[2])-u1)^2 +(pbeta(K2,x[1],x[2])-u2)^2
    }
    obj = constrOptim(c(2,2), S, NULL, ui =
rbind(c(1,0),c(0,1)),
        ci = 0(1,1), mu = 1e-100, outer.eps = 1e-100)
    obj $par
}
# Example:
PO(0.05, 0.90, 0.15, 0.99)
```

Appendix 8.3: Notes on the Two-Stage Monitoring Process

Appendix 8.3.1

Any process S_m that is a sum of m identically independently distributed (iid) random variables W_i (i=1 to m), $S_m = \sum_1^m W_i$, can also be written as a sum of two independent partial sums, $S_m = S_{m_1} + S_{m-m_1}$ for $m_1 < m$. Furthermore, with the assumption of finite variances for W_i, by the Central Limit Theorem, $\sqrt{m}(S_m / m)$ is asymptotically normally distributed and so are the component partial sums with sample sizes m_1 and $m - m_1$, respectively. Hence, without loss of generality, we consider the z-test statistics for comparing two treatment groups with equal sample size and common within-group variance σ^2 and equal accrual rate, and express the following for any independent partial sum process. Let n=N/2 and $n_1 = N_1 / 2$.

Specifically, for testing difference in means, let

$$\bar{X}_n \sim N(\mu_X, \sigma^2/n), \bar{Y}_n \sim N(\mu_Y, \sigma^2/n), Z_N = \frac{1}{\sigma\sqrt{2}}\sqrt{n}(\bar{X}_n - \bar{Y}_n), \text{ and}$$

$$Z_{N_1} = \frac{1}{\sigma\sqrt{2}}\sqrt{n_1}(\bar{X}_{n_1} - \bar{Y}_{n_1}). \text{ Then}$$

$$Z_N = \frac{1}{\sigma\sqrt{2}}\frac{1}{\sqrt{n}}\left(\sum_{i=1}^n X_i - \sum_{i=1}^n Y_i\right)$$

$$= \frac{1}{\sigma\sqrt{2}}\frac{1}{\sqrt{n}}\left[\sqrt{n_1}\left(\frac{\sum_1^{n_1} X_i - \sum_1^{n_1} Y_i}{\sqrt{n_1}}\right) + \sqrt{n-n_1}\left(\frac{\sum_{n_1+1}^n X_i - \sum_{n_1+1}^n Y_i}{\sqrt{n-n_1}}\right)\right]$$

$$= \sqrt{N_1/N}\, Z_{N_1} + \sqrt{(N-N_1)/N}\, Z_{N-N_1}$$

$$= \sqrt{t}\, Z_{N_1} + \sqrt{1-t}\, Z_{N-N_1}$$

with $t = N_1/N = n_1/n$. (This is Equation 8.7.)

Notice that $E(Z_N) = \sqrt{n/2}\delta/\sigma$, $E(Z_{N_1}) = \sqrt{n_1/2}\delta/\sigma$, $Var(Z_N) = Var(Z_{N_1})$ $= 1$ and $Cov(Z_N, Z_{N_1}) = Cov(\sqrt{t}\, Z_{N_1} + \sqrt{1-t}\, Z_{N-N_1}, Z_{N_1}) = \sqrt{t}$. These characterize the joint distribution of (Z_N, Z_{N_1}), and are used in Appendix 8.3.3.

Appendix 8.3.2

The above equation $Z_N = \sqrt{t}\, Z_{N_1} + \sqrt{1-t}\, Z_{N-N_1}$, for $t = N_1/N = n_1/n$, can be generalized to $Z_w = w_1 Z_{N_1} + w_2 Z_{N-N_1}$ for any weights $(w_1, w_2) > (0, 0)$ with $w_1^2 + w_2^2 = 1$. We can also express the Z statistic by its corresponding p-value: $Z_w = \Phi^{-1}(1-p) = w_1\Phi^{-1}(1-p_1) + w_2\Phi^{-1}(1-p_2)$. Hence, a further extension of the final test is to combine the p-values (p_1, p_2) of the two stages: $1-p = \Phi\left[w_1\Phi^{-1}(1-p_1) + w_2\Phi^{-1}(1-p_2)\right]$. The advantage of this extension is that the p-values of the two stages can be obtained by different tests or different endpoints when necessary and sensible. For example, the first endpoint for an interim analysis could be a surrogate endpoint, and the final test could be based on a clinical endpoint. When there is a multiple comparison situation, the p-values at the two stages could also be the adjusted p-values. The generalization to more than two stages is also apparent. However, if the weights are too arbitrary or weigh too differently for observations at different stages, the weighted test Z_w can lose efficiency or even become peculiar. More on multiple tests and adaptive designs are discussed in later chapters.

Appendix 8.3.3

In this section, we review the basic formulas for the bivariate normal distribution, simple linear regression, and application to the derivation of the CP (Equation 8.10). Let (X, Y) have a bivariate normal distribution, with $E(Y)=\mu_Y$, $E(X)=\mu_X$, $Var(Y) = \sigma_Y^2$, $Var(X) = \sigma_X^2$, and $Corr(Y, X)=\rho$, $0< |\rho| <1$. The simple linear regression has $E(Y \mid X) = \mu_Y - \rho \dfrac{\sigma_Y}{\sigma_X}(X - \mu_X)$, and $Var(Y \mid X) = \sigma_Y^2(1 - \rho^2)$. Therefore,

$$E(Z_N \mid Z_{N_1}) = E(Z_N) - \sqrt{t}(Z_{N_1} - E(Z_{N_1}))$$

$$= \sqrt{n/2}\,\delta/\sigma - \sqrt{t}\left(Z_{N_1} - \sqrt{\frac{n_1}{2}}\,\delta/\sigma\right)$$

and

$$Var(Z_N \mid Z_{N_1}) = 1 - t.$$

When we substitute the estimate $\hat{\delta} = \dfrac{2\sigma}{\sqrt{N_1}}Z_{N_1} = \dfrac{\sqrt{2}\sigma}{\sqrt{n_1}}Z_{N_1}$ (as Equation 8.11) for δ, we have

$$E(Z_N \mid Z_{N_1}) = \sqrt{n/n_1}\,Z_{N_1} - \sqrt{t}(Z_{N_1} - Z_{N_1}) = \sqrt{1/t}\,Z_{N_1}$$

Therefore,

$$Pr(Z_N > 1.96 \mid Z_{N_1}, \text{current trend})$$

$$= 1 - \Phi\left(\frac{1.96 - \sqrt{1/t}\,Z_{N_1}}{\sqrt{1-t}}\right)$$

$$= \Phi\left(\frac{Z_{N_1}}{\sqrt{t(1-t)}} - \frac{1.96}{\sqrt{1-t}}\right)$$

HOMEWORK 8.1

A pilot study was conducted to evaluate the impact of green tea extract in patients with indolent chronic lymphocytic leukemia (CLL) or low-grade non-Hodgkin's lymphoma (NHL) who are not receiving cytotoxic therapy (Strair et al. 2005). The primary endpoints were toxicity and disease impact. The protocol described the following monitoring plan: Patients are monitored every 4 months while taking green tea extract, and each clinical evaluation will be scored as stable disease, clinically improved (complete response+partial response), or progressive disease. The study will accrue up to 24 patients. It will be discontinued if the investigating team is at least 80% certain that fewer than 15% of patients have a clinically improved response (futility) or if the team is at least 90% certain that more than 30% of patients will progress within 1 year (toxicity and futility). You are asked to formulate a statistical strategy to set up the stopping rule when patients are sequentially observed over the study period.

> Make two tables of posterior probabilities that display the stopping rule. The tables can be made with spreadsheets: The rows are numbers of patients (sample size at the time of monitoring) and the columns are numbers of patients with event. Inside the tables, display the posterior probabilities. Use a noninformative prior distribution. (Writing an SAS or R program will make your job much easier.)
>
> After constructing the tables, make clear instructions and highlight the tables (e.g., with shade or color) to direct the team regarding the stopping rule.

HOMEWORK 8.2

For the multiple myeloma trial (Montefiore-Einstein Cancer Center 2011), use the Bayesian approach to develop a continuous safety monitoring plan. For determining the beta prior distribution on the treatment-related 30-day mortality rate, let the mode be 0.05 and the probability of mortality rate falling between 0.01 and 0.15 be 80%. Use the R program in Appendix 8.1 to find the beta parameters. Construct a table of posterior probabilities that displays the stopping rules up to $n=40$. Repeat the same exercise if we narrow the interval of mortality rate to 0.01 and 0.10 for coverage probability of 80%.

References

Boyer M, Şendur MAN, Rodríguez-Abreu D, Park K, Lee DH, Çiçin I. (2021). Pembrolizumab Plus Ipilimumab or Placebo for Metastatic Non–Small-Cell Lung Cancer With PD-L1 Tumor Proportion Score ≥ 50%: Randomized, Double-Blind Phase III KEYNOTE-598 Study. doi:10.1200/JCO.20.03579 Journal of Clinical Oncology. Published online January 29, 2021. PMID: 33513313.

Eastern Cooperative Oncology Group. (2001). Chemotherapy and Peripheral Stem Cell Transplantation in Treating Patients with Multiple Myeloma. ClinicalTrials. gov Identifier: NCT00014508.

EMA (European Medicines Agency). (1995). ICH Topic E 2 A: Clinical Safety Data Management: Definitions and Standards for Expedited Reporting. http://www. ema.europa.eu/docs/en_GB/document_library/Scientific_guideline/2009/09/ WC500002749.pdf

FDA (US Department of Health and Human Services Food and Drug Administration). (2007). *Guidance for Industry*, Drug-Induced Liver Injury: Premarketing Clinical Evaluation Oct 2007.

Montefiore-Einstein Cancer Center. (2011). A Phase II Study Assessing the Efficacy and Toxicity of PK-Directed Intravenous Busulfan in Combination with High-Dose Melphalan and Bortezomib as Conditioning Regimen for First-Line Autologous Hematopoietic Stem Cell Transplantation in Patients with Multiple Myeloma, Albert Einstein Cancer Center, NY. https://clinicaltrials. gov/identifier: NCT01605032.

NCI (National Cancer Institute). (2009). Common Terminology Criteria for Adverse Events. http://evs.nci.nih.gov/ftpl/CTCAE/CTCAE_4.03_2010–06–14_Quick Reference_5x7.pdf (accessed March 18, 2014).

Shih WJ. (1987). Maximum likelihood estimation and likelihood ratio test for square tables with missing data. *Statistics in Medicine* 6: 91–97. www.ncbi.nlm.nih.gov/ pubmed/3554443.

Strair R, Rubin A, Bertino J, Schaar D, Gharibo M, Goodin S, Krimmel T, et al. (2005). *Green Tea for Patients with Indolent Non-Hodgkin's Lymphoma or Chronic Lymphocytic Leukemia not Receiving Cytotoxic Therapy*. The Cancer Institute of New Jersey, New Brunswick, NJ.

Wu Y, Shih WJ, and Moore DF. (2008). Elicitation of a beta prior for Bayesian inference in clinical trials. *Biometrical Journal* 50: 212–223.

9

Sequential Designs and Methods—Part III: Classical Group Sequential Trials

In Chapters 7 and 8, we discussed two-stage designs. Group sequential design is a generalization for multi-stage designs. The classical group sequential procedure (design, monitoring, and analysis) is probably the most commonly applied method to facilitate the conduct of interim analysis in clinical trials, especially trials with mortality or severe or irreversible morbidity as the primary endpoints. In clinical trials with such endpoints, the fundamental consideration is an ethical obligation to modify or terminate the study at the earliest opportunity to prevent administration of a less favorable (for efficacy or toxicity) therapy to additional patients. Conducting these clinical trials in stages, with group evaluation sizes predetermined by a certain schedule, provides logistical feasibility over fully sequential methods, because the endpoint in these trials can often take a long time to occur. However, the advantage of reducing the average sample number still applies. Many different methods for group sequential procedures are available and include different stopping boundaries, different type I error spending/use functions, conditional or predictive power approaches, and Bayesian methods. These procedures are based on a *fixed maximum sample size*. We call them *classical group sequential methods* to distinguish them from the more recent development in using *adaptive group sequential methods*, in which one can extend the maximum sample size or modify other design specifications, such as study population or endpoint, as the trial is ongoing. With more flexibility and potential of introducing bias by monitoring interim data, regulatory authorities have developed strict guidance, particularly for group sequential trials. The logistics of a group sequential trial are also complicated and require careful planning and execution.

9.1 Regulatory Requirements and Logistical Considerations for Trial Monitoring

The International Conference on Harmonization *Guidelines for Industry* (ICH 1998) discuss regulatory requirements on interim analyses in general (E3, Section 11.4.2.3) and group sequential procedures in particular, regarding data monitoring and early stopping (E9, Sections 3.4 and 4.1–4.6). The following is a summary (Shih 2000):

- All interim analyses should be carefully planned in advance and fully described in the protocol. Unplanned interim analyses should be avoided if at all possible. In the event that an unplanned interim analysis was conducted, a protocol amendment describing the interim analysis should be completed prior to unblinded access to treatment comparison data. In addition, the study report should also explain the necessity of the interim analysis and the degree to which the blindness was broken, and provide an assessment of the potential magnitude of bias introduced as well as the impact on the interpretation of the results.

- The schedule of analyses, or at least the considerations that will govern the generation of the interim analysis, should be stated in the protocol or amendment before the time of the first interim analysis; the stopping guidelines and their properties should also be clearly stated there.

- The procedure plan should be written or approved by the data monitoring committee (DMC), when the trial has one.

- Any changes to the trial and any consequent changes to the statistical procedures should be specified in an amendment to the protocol at the earliest opportunity.

- The procedures selected should always ensure that the overall probability of the type I error is controlled.

- The execution of an interim analysis must be a completely confidential process when unblinded data and results are potentially involved. All staff involved in the conduct of the trial should remain blinded to the results of such analyses. Investigators should only be informed about the decision to continue or discontinue the trial, or to implement modifications to trial procedures.

- Any interim analysis planned for administrative purposes only should also be described in the protocol and subsequently reported. Examples include speeding up recruitment and updating trial progress for stakeholders. The specific purposes should be clearly stated and should specifically exclude any possibility of early stopping. In these circumstances, the blinding should not be broken.

The organization of a trial conduct and data monitoring is an important part of the study design. Figure 9.1 illustrates the four components of a trial organization, involving the trial sponsor (e.g., industry/company, NIH/branch, academia/university department); investigators; contract research organization (CRO), which manages the database and issues reports to the DMC

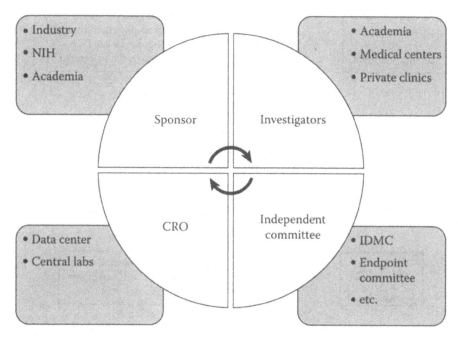

FIGURE 9.1
Four components of a trial organization.

according to an agreed schedule; and external independent committees, including a data monitoring committee (DMC or IDMC) and, if necessary, an endpoint adjudication committee (EAC). The separation of these components is specifically designed to install checks and balances to prevent potential operational bias.

Read the article in Homework 9.1 for an example of a trial with detailed organization and study schedules in the design section.

The primary obligation of the DMC is to protect the safety of the patients in the trial. In many trials, the DMC is also charged with monitoring the efficacy of the study medications according to the DMC charter. Safety must ultimately be monitored with respect to the risk–benefit ratio; thus, efficacy cannot be ignored in the whole picture of the DMC's function. In addition, the DMC often also focuses on ongoing accrual and the trial and data integrity as a service to those subjects who enrolled themselves in anticipation of completing and answering the study question. Usually, the DMC is organized with members from institutions external to the sponsor and investigators; it is supposed to make independent recommendations to the sponsor through an executive committee or sponsor committee; thus, it is also known as an independent DMC or IDMC. The DMC also includes an independent statistician and sometimes a patient advocate. A functional flowchart of the DMC is illustrated in Figure 9.2. A good discussion on IDMC is given by Ellenberg (2001) and Herson (2017).

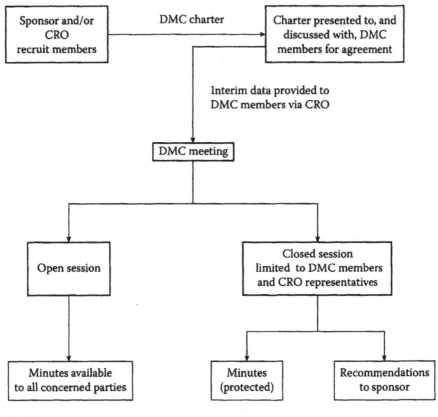

FIGURE 9.2
IDMC's process.

9.2 Statistical Methods

9.2.1 Fundamentals

Let us start by considering the design of a clinical trial with a plan of monitoring the data at calendar times ct_1, ct_2, ..., ct_K for some fixed $K > 1$. For example, a trial monitoring committee might plan to meet every April 1 and October 1 for the first 2 years and then every June 15 for the rest of the trial duration. The amount of information at the calendar time provided by the data can be considered as an idea of *generalized sample size*. Mathematically, it refers to the (observed) *Fisher information* and it is used for obtaining the statistic in the *score test*. (See Appendices 4.2–4.5 of Chapter 4.) In estimation, the variance of an estimator is the inverse of the Fisher information, and vice versa. For continuous and binary endpoints, the information is proportional to the subject count (what we called sample size before).

This is seen by using $\bar{X}_n - \bar{Y}_n$ to estimate the treatment mean difference δ. With $\mathrm{Var}\left(\bar{X}_n - \bar{Y}_n\right) = \dfrac{2\sigma^2}{n}$, the information equals $\dfrac{n}{2\sigma^2}$. Appendices 4.1–4.4 of Chapter 4 also showed that, for time-to-event (survival) endpoints, the information is proportional to the event count. By a similar derivation with likelihood functions, we can show that, for a longitudinal analysis, the information is proportional to the number of visits (e.g., subject-months for calculating the exposure experience), which is a special case of correlated (clustered) data in general. From Chapter 4, Section 4.5, we can see that for clustered data, the information is proportional to the subunit and whole-unit counts together. When we are dealing with a process with time, we then denote the information at calendar time ct_i as I_i and the fixed total (maximum) information at ct_K as I_{max}. The corresponding $t_i = I_i / I_{max}$ at ct_i, $i = 1, \ldots,$ K, are the information times (or *information fractions*). Note that $t_K = 1$. When the information is proportional to the sample size, then $t_i = \dfrac{I_i}{I_{max}} = N_i / N_{max}$. This coincides with the notation we previously used in Chapter 8, where we only considered two stages. Because the information time is just a rescaled calendar time, we sometimes write $I(t_i) = I_i$ for convenience.

At information time t_i, $i = 1, \ldots, K$, standardized Z-statistics, Z_{t_1}, Z_{t_2}, $\ldots$, Z_{t_K} are calculated based on the accumulated data for testing hypotheses about the treatment effect represented by a parameter θ. A focal statistical problem of the group sequential procedures is to find critical values to satisfy certain desirable operational characteristics. These critical values are termed *group sequential boundaries*. For example, for a one-sided hypothesis with the decision options being "either reject H_0: $\theta = 0$ or continue at the interim stages," and "reject or accept H_0 at the final stage," the problem is to find values $b_1, b_2, \ldots, b_K$ such that the overall type I error rate α is maintained at a prespecified level α:

$$P_{H_0}\left(\text{Reject } H_0\right) = P_{H_0}\left(Z_{t_1} \geq b_1 \text{ or } Z_{t_2} \geq b_2 \text{ or}\ldots Z_{t_K} \geq b_K\right) = \alpha \qquad (9.1)$$

Finding the critical values $b_1, b_2, \ldots, b_K$ is necessary because, for example, Armitage, McPherson, and Rowe (1969) showed that for K > 1, if the critical values at the interim stages remain at 1.96, then

$$P_{H_0}\left(Z_{t_1} \geq 1.96 \text{ or } Z_{t_2} \geq 1.96 \text{ or}\ldots Z_{t_K} \geq 1.96\right) > 0.025$$

Table 9.1 gives more cases of inflation of type I error rate by repeated testing of H_0 with the same critical value without proper adjustment for the nominal level of error rate at $\alpha = 0.01, 0.02,$ or 0.05.

Equation 9.1 uses a one-sided test for easy illustration. For a corresponding two-sided hypothesis test, a symmetric boundary would replace α with

TABLE 9.1

Inflation of Type I Error Rate Occurs by Repeated Testing of H_0 with the Same Critical Value without Proper Adjustment

K	Nominal 0.05	Nominal 0.02	Nominal 0.01
1	0.05	0.02	0.01
2	0.0831	0.0345	0.0177
3	0.1072	0.0456	0.0237
4	0.1262	0.0545	0.0286
5	0.1417	0.0620	0.0327
10	0.1933	0.0877	0.0474
20	0.2479	0.1163	0.0640

2α and then apply the one-sided boundary symmetrically to the lower boundary. Asymmetric boundaries have also been proposed in the literature (e.g., DeMets and Ware 1982); however, they are seldom used in a regulatory NDA/BLA or MAA setting. In the following, we consider several commonly cited group sequential boundaries.

9.2.2 Equally Spaced Group Sequential Boundaries

Suppose that the information times are equally spaced: $t_1 = 1/K$, $t_2 = 2/K$, ..., $t_K = K/K = 1$. In the 1970s, Haybittle (1971), Peto et al. (1976), Pocock (1977), and O'Brien and Fleming (1979) proposed different boundaries as follows:

- Haybittle–Peto: Find $b_i = c$ for $i = 1,..., K-1$ and $b_K = z_\alpha$ such that

$$P_{Ho}\left(Z_{t_1} \geq c \text{ or } Z_{t_2} \geq c \text{ or} ... Z_{t_K} \geq z_\alpha\right) \approx \alpha \qquad (9.2)$$

For example, if we set $\alpha = 0.025$ and $K = 5$, then $c = 3.291$. The boundaries are (3.291, 3.291, 3.291, 3.291, 1.960). Notice the approximation of α in (9.2) since it is mathematically impossible to exactly equal α when the last boundary value is z_α.

The rationale for the Haybittle–Peto boundary was to let the critical value of the final test be z_α, as if it were for a fixed sample size trial, to alleviate the perception of "alpha punishment" from clinical colleagues. However, when the final test is at the same level as the fixed-size design, the overall type I error rate must be inflated by tests at the interim stages. Hence, the above example cannot be exactly correct. One can only say that the last critical value resembles the fixed sample size design. Thus, Pocock (1977) proposed a corrected solution as follows:

- Pocock: Find $b_i = c$ for $i = 1, ..., K$ such that

$$P_{Ho}\left(Z_{t_1} \geq c \text{ or } Z_{t_2} \geq c \text{ or}...Z_{t_K} \geq c\right) = \alpha \qquad (9.3)$$

For example, if we set $\alpha = 0.025$ and $K = 5$, then $c = 2.413$. The boundaries are (2.413, 2.413, 2.413, 2.413, 2.413).

The rationale for the Pocock boundary was to simplify the monitoring process by having a constant (same) critical value for all the tests. However, this convenience ignores the fact that early tests are based on less information than later tests. We often desire to protect the trial from being stopped too early, unless the evidence in the data is tremendously convincing, or we are monitoring a safety endpoint. This led to the following O'Brien–Fleming (OBF) boundary.

- OBF: Find c such that

$$P_{Ho}\left(Z_{t_1} \sqrt{t_1} \geq c \text{ or } Z_{t_2} \sqrt{t_2} \geq c \text{ or}...Z_{t_K} \sqrt{t_K} \geq c\right) = \alpha \qquad (9.4)$$

For $\alpha = 0.025$ and $K = 5$, $c = 2.04$. Hence, $b_i = 2.04 / \sqrt{t_i} = 2.04 / \sqrt{i/5}$. The boundaries are (4.562, 3.226, 2.634, 2.281, 2.040).

Note that in Equation 9.4, it is the $Z_{t_i} \sqrt{t_i}$, not the Z-statistics themselves, that we compare to the same critical value throughout the study, in order to account for the increasing cumulative information in the dataset as time goes on. The quantity $Z_{t_i} \sqrt{t_i}$ is known as the *B-value* (B for *Brownian motion*) by Lan and Wittes (1988).

Figure 9.3 depicts the above b_i boundaries for the z-tests for a two-sided hypothesis. For a one-sided hypothesis H_A: $\theta > 0$, there should not be a lower boundary; only the upper boundary (with alpha = 0.025) applies. We can still use Figure 9.3, but the area below the lower boundary will then be interpreted as acceptance of H_0: $\theta \leq 0$ for considering futility with a symmetric boundary. The boundary shape shows that the OBF boundary has the characteristic that the critical value starts high in the beginning and then lowers toward the end of the trial. Therefore, it is the most stringent boundary for early interim analyses among the three. The choice of boundary, however, should depend on the purpose or intention of using a design with early stopping rules. The calculation of the boundaries requires iterative numerical integrations.

At the design stage, it may be reasonable to plan for a fixed number of K analyses at equally spaced information times. However, when the trial is ongoing and being monitored, operational changes often occur. Interim analyses might not necessarily follow the preplanned schedule, and the frequency of the analyses, K, may also change. This situation requires a more flexible procedure. Slud and Wei (1982) and Lan and DeMets (1983) developed the *type I error spending/use function* (or called *alpha-spending function*) approach to meet this need.

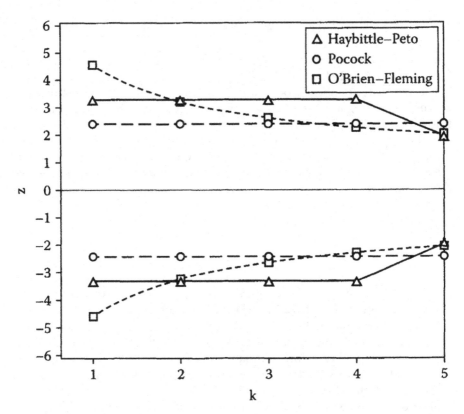

FIGURE 9.3
Three classical sequential boundaries with five analyses at equally spaced intervals, two-sided alpha = 0.05.

9.2.3 Type I Error Spending/Use Function Approach

The idea of the type I error spending/use function as an approach can be illustrated as follows: We first untie the fixed K in the expression in Equation 9.1 and decompose the rejection region, R, into disjointed regions as follows:

$$R = \{Z_{t_1} \geq b_1 \text{ or } Z_{t_2} \geq b_2 \text{ or } Z_{t_3} \geq b_3 \ldots\}$$

Let $R_1 = \{Z_{t_1} \geq b_1\}$. Thus, $\{Z_{t_1} \geq b_1 \text{ or } Z_{t_2} \geq b_2\} = \{Z_{t_1} \geq b_1\} \cup \{Z_{t_1} < b_1,$ $Z_{t_2} \geq b_2\} \equiv R_1 \cup R_2,$ and $\{Z_{t_1} \geq b_1 \text{ or } Z_{t_2} \geq b_2 \text{ or } Z_{t_3} \geq b_3\} = (R_1 \cup R_2) \cup,$ $\{Z_{t_1} < b_1, Z_{t_2} < b_2, Z_{t_3} \geq b_3\} \equiv (R_1 \cup R_2) \cup R_3$ and so on. Hence,

$$P_{Ho}(R) = P_{Ho}(R_1 \cup R_2 \cup R_3 \cup \ldots)$$
$$= P_{Ho}(R_1) + P_{Ho}(R_2) + P_{Ho}(R_3) + \ldots = \alpha$$

At t_1, we specify a value of $\alpha(t_1) = P_{Ho}(R_1)$ and solve for b_1. At t_2, specify

$$\alpha(t_2) = P_{Ho}(R_1 \cup R_2) = P_{Ho}(R_1) + P_{Ho}(R_2) \ \left(\text{due to disjointed regions}\right)$$

$$= \alpha(t_1) + P_{Ho}(R_2)$$

This leads to $P_{Ho}(R_2) = \alpha(t_2) - \alpha(t_1)$, and we can solve for b_2, since b_1 is already known from the first stage. Similarly, at t_3, specify

$$\alpha(t_3) = P_{Ho}(R_1 \cup R_2 \cup R_3) = \left(P_{Ho}(R_1) + P_{Ho}(R_2)\right) + P_{Ho}(R_3)$$

$$= \alpha(t_2) + P_{Ho}(R_3)$$

Therefore, $P_{Ho}(R_3) = \alpha(t_3) - \alpha(t_2)$. We then solve for b_3, because b_1 and b_2 were already solved in the previous steps. The process continues.

Note that, when solving for b_2, we only need the joint distribution of $\left(Z_{t_1}, Z_{t_2}\right)$. In Appendix 8.3 of Chapter 8, we introduced the idea of decomposing a sum process into two independent partial sums and derived formulas for calculating the conditional probability. Here, we generalize that idea with the generalized sample size, that is, statistical information. In a generalized term, for a *partial sum process* with *independent increments*, where we can write the score test statistic as $Z_{t_i} = \dfrac{S(t_i)}{\sqrt{I(t_i)}}$ with the numerator being the cumulative sum of the observations (iid variates with mean θ) and the denominator being the square root of the cumulative statistical information in estimating θ at time t_i, the correlation is then

$$\rho(t_1,\ t_2) = \text{Corr} = \text{Cov}\left(Z_{t_1},\ Z_{t_2}\right) = \text{Cov}\left(\frac{S(t_1)}{\sqrt{I(t_1)}},\ \frac{S(t_2)}{\sqrt{I(t_2)}}\right)$$

$$= \text{Cov}\left(\frac{S(t_1)}{\sqrt{I(t_1)}},\ \frac{S(t_1) + \left(S(t_2) - S(t_1)\right)}{\sqrt{I(t_2)}}\right)$$

$$= \frac{1}{\sqrt{I(t_1)I(t_2)}}\text{Var}\left(S(t_1)\right) = \sqrt{\frac{I(t_1)}{I(t_2)}} = \sqrt{\frac{I(t_1)/I(t_K)}{I(t_2)/I(t_K)}} = \sqrt{\frac{t_1}{t_2}}$$

where $t_i = I(t_i)/I(t_K) = I_i/I_{max}$, as noted previously in Section 9.2.1.

Other time point boundaries follow similarly. When the information is proportional to the sample size, then $\rho(t_1, t_2) = (N_1/N_2)^{1/2} = (t_1/t_2)^{1/2}$. Therefore, the joint distribution only involves the ratio of information at the current stage and before, not the later time points. This approach allows for a great deal of flexibility when monitoring trials, because there is no requirement for K, the total number of analyses, nor is there the "equally spaced t_i" restriction.

All that is needed is $\alpha(t_1) < \alpha(t_2) < \ldots < \alpha(1) = \alpha$, a strictly increasing function $\alpha(t)$, known as the *type I error (alpha)-spending/use function*, prespecified in the study design protocol.

Example 9.1: Two-Stage Design (One Interim and One Final Analyses) With Symmetric Boundaries

Specify the overall type I error $\alpha = 0.05$ (two-sided test) and the *linear (uniform) alpha-spending function* as $\alpha(t) = \alpha t$. Suppose we conduct an interim analysis when $t_1 = 1/2$; then $\alpha(t_1 = 1/2) = 0.025$. The corresponding boundary point at $t_1 = 1/2$ is $b_1 = 2.2414$. This leaves $\alpha - \alpha(t_1 = 1/2) = 0.025$ to be spent at the final stage $t_2 = 1$. Solving $\Pr\{|Z_{t_1}| < 2.2414, |Z_{t_2}| \geq b_2\} = 0.025$ given that the correlation of the bivariate normal distribution is $\sqrt{t_1 / t_2} = \sqrt{1/2}$, we obtain $b_2 = 2.1251$. (An R function to do this calculation is given in Appendix 9.1.) Note that at the final stage $\alpha_2 \equiv \Pr(|Z| \geq 2.1251) = 0.0336$. That is, with this linear/uniform spending function, $\alpha(t) = \alpha t$, if an interim testing is to be conducted in the middle of the trial, the p-value at the final stage has to be less than 0.034, instead of the 0.05 level, to be significant. This requirement often feels like a "penalty" to some clinical investigators. On the other hand, because there was $\alpha(t_1 = 1/2) = 0.025$ spent for the interim analysis, the remaining alpha available for the final analysis is $0.05 - 0.025 = 0.025$, but due to the correlation of Z_{t_1} and Z_{t_2}, the critical region for the analysis actually corresponds to an alpha level of $0.0336 > 0.025$.

Following this example, a natural question arises: What kind of alpha-spending function would describe the Pocock boundary and the OBF boundary in Section 9.2.2? We look at the following example in search for an answer.

Example 9.2

$K = 5$, $\alpha = 0.025$, Pocock boundary: (2.413, 2.413, 2.413, 2.413, 2.413).

1. With the first critical value, we can find the corresponding alpha spent at the first stage $P_{Ho}(Z_{t_1} \geq 2.413) = 0.0079$. Therefore, $\alpha(t_1 = 1/5) = 0.0079$. Next, we continue to calculate for the second stage.

2. The cumulative alpha at the second stage is $P_{Ho}(Z_{t_1} \geq 2.413$ or $Z_{t_2} \geq 2.413)$
$= P_{Ho}(Z_{t_1} \geq 2.413) + P_{Ho}(Z_{t_1} < 2.413, Z_{t_2} \geq 2.413)$
$= 0.0079 + 0.0059$
$= 0.0138$. Therefore, $\alpha(t_2 = 2/5) = 0.0138$

3. The cumulative alpha at the third stage is $P_{Ho}(Z_{t_1} \geq 2.413$ or $Z_{t_2} \geq 2.413$ or $Z_{t_3} \geq 2.413)$

$= P_{Ho}\left(Z_{t_1} \geq 2.413 \text{ or } Z_{t_2} \geq 2.413\right) + P_{Ho}\left(\left(Z_{t_1} < 2.413, Z_{t_2} < 2.413\right),\right.$
$\left. Z_{t_3} \geq 2.413\right)$
$= 0.0138 + 0.0045$
$= 0.0183$. Therefore, $\alpha(t_3 = 3/5) = 0.0183$. Note that we add 0.0045, the incremental alpha, to the second-stage alpha 0.0138.

4. Following similar steps, we obtain for the fourth-stage cumulative alpha: $P_{Ho}\left(Z_{t_1} \geq 2.413 \text{ or } Z_{t_2} \geq 2.413 \text{ or } Z_{t_3} \geq 2.413 \text{ or } Z_{t_4} \geq 2.413\right)$
$= \ldots$ (similar steps)
$= 0.0183 + 0.0036$
$= 0.0219$. Hence, $\alpha(t_4 = 4/5) = 0.0219$

5. The final-stage alpha would be the total alpha ($= 0.025$ in this case), as shown:
$P_{Ho}\left(Z_{t_1} \geq 2.413 \text{ or } Z_{t_2} \geq 2.413 \text{ or } Z_{t_3} \geq 2.413 \text{ or } Z_{t_4} \geq 2.413 \text{ or }\right.$
$\left. Z_{t_5} \geq 2.413\right)$
$= \ldots$ (similar steps)
$= 0.0219 + 0.0031$
$= 0.0250$. Thus, $\alpha(t_5 = 1) = 0.0250$.

We can graph (0, 0.0079, 0.0138, 0.0183, 0.0219, 0.0250) versus (0, 0.2, 0.4, 0.6, 0.8, 1) to find this (discrete) cumulative alpha-spending function. The continuous alpha-spending function is discussed in the next section.

Example 9.3

$K = 5$, $\alpha = 0.025$, OBF boundary: (4.562, 3.223, 2.634, 2.281, 2.040).
Following similar steps as done previously, we can obtain the (discrete) type I error spending function $\alpha(t_1 = 1/5) = 0.0000$, $\alpha(t_2 = 2/5) = 0.0006$, $\alpha(t_3 = 3/5) = 0.0045$, $\alpha(t_4 = 4/5) = 0.0128$, and $\alpha(t_5 = 1) = 0.0250$ (Homework 9.2).

9.2.4 Pocock-Type, OBF-Type, and Other Continuous Boundaries

Removing the restriction of a fixed K and equally spaced $t_i = i/K$, Lan and DeMets (1983) gave the continuous alpha-spending function for the general Pocock-type boundary as

$$\alpha_{Pocock}(t) = \alpha \ln\left[1 + (e - 1)t\right] \tag{9.5}$$

and for the general OBF-type boundary as

$$\alpha_{OBF}(t) = 2\left[1 - \Phi\left(\frac{Z_{\alpha/2}}{\sqrt{t}}\right)\right] \tag{9.6}$$

where $\Phi(\cdot)$ is the cdf of the standard normal distribution.

The boundaries corresponding to the continuous alpha-spending functions are approximately close to the original, discrete, equally spaced boundaries. The *x-type boundary* describes the fact that these continuous boundaries differ from, but follow closely, the characteristics of the original Pocock boundary, being flat with constant critical values throughout the study, and that of the original OBF boundary, being very stringent in the beginning of the trial and then decreasing as information is gathered.

Other continuous type I error rate spending functions have also been proposed in the literature. Kim and DeMets (1987) studied certain members of the *power family*

$$\alpha(t) = \alpha t^c, \ c > 0$$

The power $c = 1$ corresponds to the linear or uniform spending, and $c = 3$ closely resembles the OBF type.

The landmark clinical trial Scandinavian Simvastatin Survival Study (4S) in heart disease (1993) (mentioned in Chapter 2), the breakthrough immunotherapy KEYTRUDA® trials KN-040 in head and neck cancer (Cohen et al. 2019), and KN-042 in non-small cell lung cancer (Mok et al. 2019) all used a member of the *truncated exponential distribution family* of alpha-spending functions proposed by Hwang, Shih, and DeCani (1990):

$$\alpha(\gamma, t) = \alpha \left[\frac{1 - e^{-\gamma t}}{1 - e^{\gamma}} \right], \quad \gamma \neq 0 \quad \text{for } 0 \leq t \leq 1 \tag{9.7}$$

$$= \alpha t, \qquad \qquad \gamma = 0$$

We can see here that $\gamma = 0$ is the uniform spending, $\gamma > 0$ is the concave spending, and $\gamma < 0$ is the convex spending of the type I error rate. Concave spending of alpha is suitable for short-term trials with an immediate response, such as single-dose analgesic studies, where accelerated early stopping is desirable in early phases of drug development; usually, $1 \leq \gamma \leq 4$. Convex spending of alpha is suitable for large trials in chronic diseases where patient recruitment is slow and staggered and follow-up is long, so that very early termination with limited samples is not encouraged; usually, $-5 \leq \gamma \leq -1$. For example, the 4S trial and KN-040 trial used $\gamma = -4$. KN-042 trial used $\gamma = -0.9023$.

The (continuous) Pocock-type boundary is included in Equation 9.7, with $\gamma = 1$; the (continuous) OBF-type boundary is also a member of Equation 9.7, with approximately $\gamma = -4$ or -5; the *power family* member $\alpha(t) = \alpha t^{3/2}$ is closely approximated by $\gamma = -1$, and $\alpha(t) = \alpha t^2$ is approximated by $\gamma = -2$. See Hwang, Shih, and DeCani (1990) for a graph of alpha-spending rate and table of boundaries of this general family of alpha-spending functions.

Software and In-Class Exercise:

The calculation of the boundaries requires iterative numerical integrations. SAS and R, as well as some commercial software, are available for obtaining the boundaries; for example, the SEQDESIGN and SEQTEST procedures of SAS and the R package "gsDesign". Preference here is given to the software provided by the University of Wisconsin, which can be acquired by following the steps. A reference for this software is given in Reboussin et al. (2000).

Go to the following University of Wisconsin web page to download the Lan-DeMets software to your computer step by step and perform the practice sessions in this chapter.

- https://biostat.wiscweb.wisc.edu/resources/software/
- Under the heading "Programs for Computing Group Sequential Boundaries Using the Lan-DeMets Method," click on the Download link for Windows to download WinLD.exe, or download the MSDOS executable ld98.exe. Unzip the file and install.
- The WinLD.chm file is the user manual; it contains some good examples.

Practice 9.1: Run the Lan-DeMets software. Under Compute, select Bounds.

1. Design boundaries (set up to plan a trial protocol)
   Compute the boundaries of the Pocock and OBF types and the power family with appropriate power parameters to match the Hwang, Shih, and DeCani (HSD) truncated exponential family with appropriate parameters. Compare them with the discrete, equally spaced Pocock and OBF boundaries in Section 9.2.2 (for K = 5).
   For example, the upper two-sided $\alpha = 0.05$ symmetrical, discrete, equally spaced Pocock boundary for K = 5 is (2.413, 2.413, 2.413, 2.413, 2.413). In contrast, the Pocock-type boundary based on Equation 9.5 is not exactly as flat as that, but is (2.4380, 2.4268, 2.4101, 2.3966, 2.3859).

2. Updating boundaries when monitoring a trial
   Suppose that the trial initially used K = 5 with a (continuous) equally spaced OBF-type boundary in the design. Consider the two scenarios:
   The first scenario: At the first interim analysis, the actual information time turns out to be $t_1 = 0.3$ (as opposed to planned = 0.2), and the trial design is now rescheduled to $t_2 = 0.75$ and $t_3 = 1$ for the next interim and final analyses. Compute the revised OBF-type boundary.
   The K = 5 equally spaced, upper two-sided $\alpha = 0.05$ symmetrical OBF-type boundary is (4.8769, 3.3569, 2.6803, 2.2898, 2.0310). The revised schedule (0.3, 0.75, 1.0) leads to a different boundary (3.9286, 2.3403, 2.0118).
   The second scenario: After the first interim analysis (at $t_1 = 0.2$), the trial continues, but the schedule of subsequent interim analyses has been changed to $t_2 = 3/5$, followed by the final analysis at $t_3 = 1$. The revised schedule (0.2, 0.6, 1.0) leads to the boundary: (4.8769, 2.6686,

1.9809). It is quite clear that the first critical value (4.8769) remains unchanged as planned, because it has already been used by the first interim analysis at the planned time ($t_1 = 0.2$).

In both scenarios, for the subsequent changes of frequency and schedule, we have to make sure that these changes are due to administrative reasons (e.g., the enrollment rate has been slower or faster than expected), not prompted by the interim result of the first analysis. Thus, it is obvious that the DMC needs to be independent from the trial sponsor and that the trial sponsor should not be provided with the interim unblinded data.

9.3 Power, Information, and Drift Parameter

Group sequential methods provide a chance for early termination of a trial by rejecting H_0 in such a way that the overall type I error rate is maintained. The trade-off, however, is some loss of power, because the tests at early stages involve smaller sample sizes, and the rejection regions are tighter at later stages, both resulting in lower power. In order to maintain the same power as the fixed-size design, a group sequential trial would require a larger *maximum* information/sample size, but the *average* (expected) information/sample size would be smaller (under H_A). The maximum information/sample size is a function of the type I and type II errors, the number of analyses, and the strategy of spending α (i.e., the boundaries for the interim and final analyses).

• Given $b_1, b_2, ..., b_K$ (determined by the alpha-spending strategy),

$\text{Power} = 1 - \beta = P_{H_A}\left(\text{Reject } H_0\right) = P_{H_A}\left(Z_{t_1} \geq b_1 \text{ or } Z_{t_2} \geq b_2 \text{ or}...Z_{t_K} \geq b_K\right)$ as a function of the treatment effect (expressed in terms of the *drift* parameter; see Equation 9.8 below).

• Conversely, given power (by the fixed sample size design), we can calculate N_{max} (or, in general, I_{max}) for a group sequential design (specified by the boundary) through the calculation of the *drift* parameter, as explained in the following paragraphs.

It is helpful to start with a fixed sample size and adjust it to obtain the maximum sample size for the sequential design. From the sample size calculation in Equation 4.6 (Chapter 4) for a fixed sample size design (with equal treatment group allocation, n subjects per group), we saw the basic relationship

$E(Z \mid H_A) = z_{\alpha/2} + z_\beta$, where $Z = \sqrt{\dfrac{n}{2}} \dfrac{\bar{X}_n - \bar{Y}_n}{\sigma}$. Denote $\varphi_f \equiv E(Z) = \sqrt{\dfrac{n}{2}} \dfrac{\delta}{\sigma}$, which is the *noncentrality parameter* of the fixed-size z-test under H_A that pivots the power of the test (see Equation 4.6). Note that $\varphi_f^2 \propto n$. (The subscript f in φ_f emphasizes that this is for fixed sample size design.)

For a sequential design, the interim stage sample size at a given time $t = n/n_{max}$ is $n = n_{max}t$, and the final $N_{max} = 2n_{max}$ is the *maximum* sample size at $t = 1$. The test statistic of the interim analysis, $Z(t)$, is based on the interim sample size n (per group). The sample size of the fixed-size design (without any interim analysis) corresponds to the (final) maximum sample size of the sequential design. Thus,

$$EZ(t) = \sqrt{\frac{n}{2}}\frac{\delta}{\sigma} = \sqrt{t}\sqrt{\frac{n_{max}}{2}}\frac{\delta}{\sigma} = \sqrt{t}\varphi \tag{9.8}$$

where $\varphi \equiv EZ(t = 1) = \sqrt{\frac{n_{max}}{2}}\frac{\delta}{\sigma}$ is called the *drift* parameter in the Lan-DeMets program for the sequential design. It corresponds to the noncentrality parameter φ_f for the fixed-size design.

Recall that, when using $\bar{X}_n - \bar{Y}_n$ to estimate the treatment mean difference $\delta = \mu_X - \mu_Y$, $\text{var}(\bar{X}_n - \bar{Y}_n) = \frac{2\sigma^2}{n}$, $I_n = \frac{n}{2\sigma^2}$. Therefore, in a sequential trial, Equation 9.8 can also be written as

$$EZ(t) = \sqrt{\frac{n}{2}}\frac{\delta}{\sigma} = \sqrt{I_n}\delta = \sqrt{tI_{max}}\delta \tag{9.9}$$

Hence,

$$\varphi = EZ(t = 1) = \sqrt{I_{max}}\delta \tag{9.10}$$

Next, we set up the maximum information of a sequential design from the corresponding fixed-size design. We see from Equation 9.10 that $\varphi^2 \propto I_{max}$. Without interim analyses, recall that for $Z \sim N(E(Z), 1)$, $\varphi_f = E(Z) = z_{\alpha/2} + z_\beta$ is the drift parameter for the fixed-size design. For example, $\alpha/2 = 0.025$, $1 - \beta = 0.90$, implying that $\varphi_f = 1.96 + 1.28 = 3.24$. With $K = 5$ equally spaced interim analyses, using the OBF-type boundary, we get $\varphi = 3.2788$ from the Lan-DeMets program. Therefore, $(\varphi/\varphi_f)^2 = (3.2788/3.24)^2 = 1.024$. The maximum information of a sequential design requires 1.024 times the corresponding information of the fixed-size design. The size inflation of 2.4% may not seem a lot for a small study, but it may mean a lot for a large trial. In general, for boundaries such as those of the OBF type, when the final critical value is close to $z_{\alpha/2}$, the sample size inflation factor is not large. For the Pocock-type boundary, it can be substantial. However, in all cases, the expected information required for a sequential trial would be less than the fixed-size design due to the possibility of early termination.

TABLE 9.2

Drift Parameter of the Score Test

Comparison	Drift Parameter	Note
Normal means	$\sqrt{n_{max}}\sqrt{1/2\sigma^2}\left(\mu_x - \mu_y\right)$	n = per group size
Binomial probabilities	$\sqrt{n_{max}}\sqrt{1/2\bar{\pi}(1-\bar{\pi})}\left(\pi_x - \pi_y\right)$	n = per group size $\bar{\pi} = \left(\pi_x + \pi_y\right)/2$
Survival distributions (log-rank test)	$\sqrt{D_{max}}\sqrt{1/4}\log(\mathrm{HR})$	D = total deaths HR = hazard ratio

The drift parameters derived from the score (asymptotic) z-tests for comparing two normal means, two binomial probabilities, and two survival distributions (with the log-rank test) are listed in Table 9.2.

In-Class Exercise

Practice 9.2: For two-sided $\alpha = 0.05$, $1 - \beta = 0.90$, with $K = 5$ equally spaced interim analyses, using the OBF-type boundary, use the Lan-DeMets program (via Compute Drift) to calculate the drift parameter to get $\varphi = 3.2788$ and calculate the sample size inflation factor.

9.4 P-Value When Trial Is Stopped

At each time t, we calculate the z-test value, z(t), and the predefined boundary. When the test value crosses the boundary, we have the stopping time (τ). When we observe (t, $z(\tau)$) and stop the trial, we need to report the *p-value*. The p-value is the probability under the null of obtaining a result that is at least as extreme as the observed one, that is (t, $z(\tau)$). Therefore, we need to incorporate *order* for the two-dimensional summary statistic values (t, z(t)). There are different ways of ordering in this two-dimensional space. The most commonly used one is the following *stage-wise ordering*:

$$\left(\tau_2,\ z(\tau_2)\right) < \left(\tau_1,\ z(\tau_1)\right) \text{ if and only if } \tau_2 < \tau_1 \text{ or when } \tau_2 = \tau_1,\ z(\tau_2) \geq z(\tau_1)$$

$$(9.11)$$

That is, we compare the stopping time first. An earlier stopping time is more extreme than a later stopping time. With the same stopping time, a larger test statistic value is more extreme. Hence, with the stage-wise ordering, for outcome ($\tau = t_j$, $Z(t_j) = z_j$), more extreme outcomes are those pairs that either have the test statistic crossing the boundary at an earlier time $t = 1, ..., j - 1$, or stop at $t = j$ but with a larger statistic than the observed z_j. Thus, the p-value is calculated by the following probability under the null hypothesis

$$p = \Pr\left(\bigcup_{i=1}^{j-1}\left(Z(t_i) \geq b_i\right) \cup \left(Z(t_j) \geq z_j\right)\right) \qquad (9.12)$$

We can see that the interim analysis-adjusted p-value only depends on boundaries before the stopping time and the observed z-value at the stopping time. (When using the Lan-DeMets program, one may put arbitrary boundaries after j, as the calculation of the cumulative exit probability will only be up to j.) The adjusted p-value in Equation 9.12 is approximately equal to the unadjusted p-value $\Pr(Z(t_j) \geq z_j)$ for large b_i, $i < j$. Large boundary values make early stopping more difficult; hence, the adjustment of the p-value is negligible. For example, for the OBF-type boundaries, the adjusted p-value is close to the unadjusted p-value.

In-Class Exercise

Practice 9.3: We are monitoring a trial that is designed with five equally spaced interim analyses by the OBF-type boundary z-values: 4.88, 3.36, 2.68, 2.29, 2.03. After observing $(0.6, Z(0.6) = 2.94)$, since $2.94 > 2.68$, the trial stops at $t = 0.6$. The p-value $= \Pr(Z(0.2) \geq 4.88$ or $Z(0.4) \geq 3.36$ or $Z(0.6) \geq 2.94) = 0.00183$ by numerical integration. Note that the unadjusted $\Pr(Z \geq 2.94) = 0.00164$.

In the Lan-DeMets program, select Compute Probability and User Input to specify the boundaries. Input boundaries $(b_1, b_2, ..., b_{j-1}, z_j) = (4.88, 3.36, 2.94)$ and arbitrary boundaries after 2.94. After clicking Calculate, read the *cumulative exit probabilities* up to $\tau = 0.6$.

9.5 Estimation of Treatment Effect

Not only do we need to report the p-value, we also should, and often, need to estimate the treatment effect after the trial stops. The drift parameter (see Table 9.2) is also used for estimating the (standardized) treatment effect after we observe (τ_{obs}, z_{obs}). For example, for the difference of means, we calculate the $100(1-\alpha)\%$ confidence interval (φ_L, φ_U) from

$$P_{\varphi_L}\left\{(\tau, Z(\tau)) > (\tau_{obs}, z_{obs})\right\} = \alpha/2$$

and

$$P_{\varphi_U}\left\{(\tau, Z(\tau)) < (\tau_{obs}, z_{obs})\right\} = \alpha/2$$

Then, convert (φ_L, φ_U) to the treatment effect via the relationship $\varphi = \sqrt{n_{max}} \sqrt{1/2\sigma^2} (\mu_X - \mu_Y)$. Other scenarios are given in Table 9.2.

In-Class Exercise

Practice 9.4: This comes from the help manual (WinLD.chm) of the Lan-DeMets program.

Select "Compute Confidence"; set $K = 6$ and information times: 0.23, 0.33, 0.44, 0.58, 0.71, 0.83. (In User Input, feed the information times. Notice that the last time point is not necessarily 1.)

Specify two-sided symmetric bounds by using the linear spending function (with Function: Power family with Phi = 1)

Standardized statistic value: $z = 2.82$

Confidence level: 0.95

Calculate: $(\varphi_L, \varphi_U) = (0.19, 4.94)$ and the boundary

- Convert to CI of $(\mu_X - \mu_Y)$ with the values of n, σ
- Convert to CI of $(\pi_X - \pi_Y)$ with the values of n, $\bar{\pi}$
- Convert to CI of log(HR) with the value of D.

The upper bounds are displayed: 2.527, 2.616, 2.562, 2.473, 2.426, 2.388. (Note that the boundary has a hump at the second time point.) Because $z = 2.82$, this indicates that the study would be stopped at the first interim analysis when $t = 0.23$.

Practice 9.5: The study in Proschan, Lan, and Wittes (2006, page 129) is summarized as follows:

- Weight change (kg) over 3 months in n = 200 (per arm).
- Planned $K = 4$, equal intervals, with the OBF-type boundary.
- Actual $t_1 = 0.22$, $t_2 = 0.55$ (not 0.25, 0.5 as planned).
- At the third look, the mean weight losses in the two groups are $\bar{x}_{152} = 8.1$ kg and $\bar{y}_{144} = 6.0$ kg (subscript indicates sample size on which the sample mean is based).
- Hence, $t_3 = (152 + 144)/400 = 0.74$.
- The pooled sd = 4.8 kg, so $z = 3.76$.
- We want to report the p-value and 95% CI of $\delta = \mu_X - \mu_Y$.

Answer: Use the Lan-DeMets program to perform the following steps:

1. For p-value: Select Compute Probability
   - $K = 4$, User Input t: 0.22, 0.55, 0.74, 1
   - Two-sided symmetric, OBF spending function ($\alpha = 0.05$)

- Calculate to get boundaries at t_1 (4.64) and t_2 (2.81)
- Change Determine Bounds to User Input and fill in the following: 4.64, 2.81, 3.76 (= z), 1 (arbitrary)
- Calculate to obtain exit probability = 0.005 (two-sided p-value). (Note: The unadjusted p-value is $Pr(|Z| > 3.76) = 0.0002$.)

2. For CI: Select Compute Confidence (Interval)
   - $K = 4$, User Input t: 0.22, 0.55, 0.74, 1
   - Two-sided symmetric, change Determine Bounds to User Input and fill in the following:
     4.64, 2.81, 3.76 (= z), 1 (arbitrary)
   - Standardized statistic value: 3.76
   - Confidence level: 0.95
   - Calculate to obtain $(\varphi_L, \varphi_U) = (1.106, 5.536)$
   - Convert to CI for $\delta = \mu_X - \mu_Y$ with $n = 200$, $\sigma = $ pooled sd = 4.8 by using

$$\varphi = \sqrt{n_{max} / 2\sigma^2} \left(\mu_X - \mu_Y\right)$$

to get $(\delta_L, \delta_U) = (0.531, 2.657)$.

Appendix 9.1: R Function *qfind* for Calculating the Critical Value (Boundary) of the Second (Final) Analysis

This function is suitable for a two-stage design with any spending of alpha < 0.05 at the first (interim) stage, at any information time < 1. No specification of an alpha-spending function is required.

Assumptions include overall alpha = 0.05, two-sided, and symmetric boundaries.

```
# First, install package mvtnorm

library(mvtnorm)
# Input: p1 = interim alpha spent, p2 = 0.05-p1;
# tfrac =interim information fraction
# return: (c1, c2) = critical values of the two stages;
# alpha2= nominal alpha for c2
qfind <-
function(p1 = 0.01, p2 = 0.04, tfrac = 0.5, tol = 1e-10)
{
            c1 <- qnorm(1 - p1/2)
            low <- 0
            upp <- 4
```

```
                mid <- (low + upp)/2
                val <- pbvn(c1, mid, tfrac)
while(abs(val - p2) > tol) {
if(val > p2)
low <- mid
else upp <- mid
mid <- (low + upp)/2
val <- pbvn(c1, mid, tfrac)
}
a2 <- 2 * pnorm(- mid)
out <- c(c1, mid, a2, val)
names(out) <- c("c1", "c2", "alpha2", "p2")
return(out)
}
pbvn <- function(x, y, tfrac = 0.5)
{
2*(pmvnorm(c(-x, -Inf), c(x, -y), corr =
matrix(c(1,sqrt(tfrac),
     sqrt(tfrac),1),nrow = 2))[[1]])
}
# Try the default
qfind()
# Example - find the two-sided critical values from a
one-sided alpha spent
p1 = 0.002578977
qfind(p1 = 0.002578977*2, p2 = (0.025-p1)*2, tfrac = 0.5)
```

Appendix 9.2: A Further Note on the Partial Sum Process with Independent Increments

For immediate responses, either continuous or binary, cumulative sums of the independent random variables from time to time are easily seen to have independent increments. The usefulness of this "partial sum with independent increments" property is illustrated in Section 9.2.3. An important development was made by Tsiatis (1981, 1982), who showed that the log-rank statistic computed over time behaves like a partial sum of independent normal random variables. This result extended the use of group sequential methods to clinical trials with survival data. Jennison and Turnbull (1997) provided a unified theory that explains the "independent increments" structure commonly seen in group sequential test statistics. Scharfstein, Tsiatis, and Robbins (1997) demonstrated that all sequentially computed Wald statistics based on efficient estimators, for example, MLEs of the parameter of interest, will under mild regularity conditions have the asymptotic multivariate normal distribution similar to the earlier setup. Hence, the group sequential procedure extends to more complicated situations such as the proportional hazards model (Sellke and Siegmund 1983) and correlated observations including longitudinal data with random effects model

(Wei, Su, and Lachin 1990; Lee and DeMets 1991) or with distribution-free analyses (Lachin 1997), which includes the Wilcoxon–Mann–Whitney rank-sum test (Spurrier and Hewett 1976) that is useful for ordered categorical endpoints. An application of stratified WMW test used in a group sequential design is given in Shih, Chen, and Xie (2020) for the first placebo-controlled, double-blind, randomized trial of remdesivir for the treatment of severe COVID-19 patients, as mentioned in Chapter 5.

Appendix 9.3: Information Time/Fraction and Maximum-Duration Trial versus Maximum-Information Trial

Taking statistical information as the inverse of the variance of the parameter estimate, Lan and Zucker (1993) defined the *information time/fraction* as the amount of information accrued by calendar time divided by the total information at the scheduled end of the trial. We have seen that the information time played an essential role in the type I error spending function approach. Depending on the statistics used (Lan, Reboussin, and DeMets 1994), a whole unit information can be approximated by either a subject (for comparing means) or an event (for comparing survival distributions). In either case, the total information must be known. If not known, as is often the case, then the information time/fraction can only be estimated. For example, in the time-to-event case, Tsiatis (1981) showed that the variance of the log-rank statistics, when calculated over time, grows proportionally to the number of events observed. Hence, the information time is equal to the proportion of the maximum number of events expected by the end of a study, with the numerator being the observed number of events at the (calendar) time of interim analysis. For a maximum-information trial, the maximum number of events expected by the end of a study is chosen in advance to achieve a desired power, given other design parameters. However, for a maximum-duration trial, that is, when the maximum trial duration is fixed, the maximum information is random. In such a trial, the denominator of the information time can be estimated under either the null or the alternative hypothesis, or by other means of projection, thus leading to different information timescales.

A natural compromise to overcome this difficulty of uncertain information timescale is to first choose an estimate of the maximum information, say either "under the null" or "under the alternative" hypothesis. Then set the information time to be 1 if the proportion exceeds 1 or if the current analysis is the last analysis and the proportion has not yet reached 1. The consequence of this compromise is that the type I error spending function will be altered from the original one that was prespecified in the design. A simple example that illustrates this can be found in Kim, Boucher, and Tsiatis (1995). In real applications, we can only hope that the alpha-spending function will not be altered as much as in this illustrative example. A real example is the pembrolizumab KEYNOTE-604 trial; see Homework 9.8.

Example 9.4: Over-Running and Under-Running Change the Alpha-Spending Function

Suppose $K = 2$ analyses were planned for a trial where the one-sided significance level of 0.05 was specified in the protocol. At the design stage, the uniform (linear) type I error spending function, $\alpha(t) = 0.05t$, was chosen for monitoring. The expected total number of events is 200 under the null hypothesis, but is 100 under the alternative (Figure 9.4). Suppose that there are 50 events at the first analysis. If we have chosen the information timescale based on the null hypothesis, then $t_1 = 50/200 = 0.25$, and $\alpha(t_1) = 0.0125$. The group sequential boundary b_1 such that $\Pr\{Z_{t_1} \geq b_1\} = 0.0125$ is $b_1 = 2.24$. Suppose at the final analysis, the number of events is truly 200, as expected under the null hypothesis, the correlation between Z_{t_1} and Z_{t_2} is $(t_1/t_2)^{1/2} = (0.25)^{1/2} = 0.5$. Thus, the group sequential boundary b_2 such that $\Pr\{Z_{t_1} < 2.24, Z_{t_2} \geq b_2\} = 0.05 - 0.0125 = 0.0375$ is $b_2 = 1.74$.

However, if the realized number of events at the final analysis turns out to be 100 instead (i.e., an under-running situation), then the "true" t_1 should be $50/100 = 0.5$ and we should have spent $\alpha(t_1) = 0.025$. But we cannot go back in time, because we have already adopted $b_1 = 2.24$ for the test at the first analysis. What we can do is to recognize that (a) at $t_1 = 0.5$ (not 0.25), we used $\alpha(t_1) = 0.0125$ and (b) the correlation between Z_{t_1} and Z_{t_2} is $(t_1/t_2)^{1/2} = (0.5)^{1/2}$. Thus, the group sequential boundary b_2 such that $\Pr\{Z_{t_1} < 2.24, Z_{t_2} > b_2\} = 0.0375$ is $b_2 = 1.70$. From the fact that $\alpha(0.5) = 0.0125 < 0.025$, we see that the type I error spending function was no longer the uniform (linear) spending function. Instead, it is a convex function, running under the uniform (linear) spending function. The risk of under-running is losing study power and potentially confusing with early stopping.

The over-running case is the opposite, when 100 events under the alternative hypothesis were used to estimate $t_1 = 50/100$, but 200 events occurred at the final analysis. The consequence is that the linear spending function is altered to a concave function, running over the uniform (linear) spending function. The final critical value b_2 is calculated based on the correlation between Z_{t_1} and Z_{t_2}, which is $(t_1/t_2)^{1/2} = (t_1/1)^{1/2} = (50/200)^{1/2} = (1/4)^{1/2}$. Note that we may still use the original denominator 100 in the design for timescale, $t_1 = 50/100$. Then $t_2 = 200/100 = 2$. The correlation between Z_{t_1} and Z_{t_2} is still $(t_1/t_2)^{1/2} = (1/4)^{1/2}$, and we still obtain the same b_2. However, beware that most software do not accept $t > 1$, since in the alpha-spending function the information time/fraction is defined between 0 and 1. This approach (letting $t > 1$) is not recommended since it does not reveal the alteration of the alpha-spending function.

The use of an alpha-spending function is a way to define how the type I error may be spent during the trial when interim analyses are conducted so that there is no ambiguity on the control of the overall type I error rate. The control of the overall alpha level can be taken care of at the final analysis when the actual total information is observed by finding the correct critical value for the final test. A potential risk for the over-running case, as illustrated above, is that we might have already spent too much alpha at the interim analyses (due to severe under-estimation

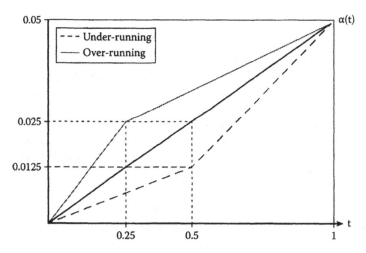

FIGURE 9.4
The alpha-spending function is altered when under-running or over-running of a trial occurs.

of the total information in a maximum duration trial.) A convenient way to mitigate the "over-spending" problem is to not use the projected information fraction (as it can be wrong in this case) but to use another scale (such as relative calendar time) to spend the alpha. For example, if the trial is planned to end and final analysis conducted at "300 total deaths or 36 months after the first subject is enrolled, whichever is later", then we have two possible scales to spend the alpha. We may use the *minimum* of the two scales to avoid over-spending alpha at the interim analyses. Again, the final analysis should always use the right scale, which is the information fraction, that relates to the correlation of the test statistics, for calculating the final critical value to control the overall type I error rate.

HOMEWORK 9.1

Read the article "Sorafenib in Advanced Hepatocellular Carcinoma" (Llovet, J. M., et al., *New England Journal of Medicine*, 2008, 359(4): 378–390), and identify the trial organization and study monitoring schedules.

HOMEWORK 9.2

Work out the steps of constructing the alpha-spending function for the equally spaced K = 5 OBF boundary, and plot it against the alpha-spending function of the Pocock boundary.

HOMEWORK 9.3

For the article "Sorafenib in Advanced Hepatocellular Carcinoma" (Llovet, J. M., et al., *New England Journal of Medicine*, 2008, 359(4): 378–390), do the following:

1. Describe the study design and endpoints of the trial.
2. Determine approximately how much alpha was "spent" at each analysis (two interim and one final) for each endpoint. (Note: The proportion of information at any particular time can be assumed to be roughly approximated by the number of deaths that occurred out of what was expected.)
3. Compare your answer from part (2) to the amount of the type I error that would have been "spent" if a Pocock boundary had been assumed.
4. Give a very brief summary of the results including the stopping decision.
5. Based on Figure 2 of this paper:
   a. Compare between treatments with respect to the 25th, 50th, and 75th percentiles for each endpoint.
   b. Compare across treatments with respect to the probability of survival, the probability of symptomatic progression, and the probability of radiologic progression at 9 months.

HOMEWORK 9.4

Read the article "Efficacy of everolimus in advanced renal cell carcinoma: a double-blind, randomised, placebo-controlled phase III trial" (*Lancet* 2008, 372: 449–56 by Motzer, Escudier, Oudard, et al. for the RECORD-1 Study Group). Do the following:

1. Describe the study design, identify the trial organization, study endpoints, and monitoring schedules.
2. Describe the interim analysis plan and actual monitoring on the alpha spending. Approximately how much alpha was "spent" at each analysis (interim and final) for each endpoint.
3. Verify the boundary values, and final confidence interval estimate of the treatment effect in terms of PFS.

HOMEWORK 9.5

Read the article "Efficacy and safety of sunitinib in patients with advanced gastrointestinal stromal tumour after failure of imatinib: a randomised controlled trial" (Lancet 2006, 368: 1329–38 by Demetri GD, van Oosterom AT, Garrett CR, et al.). Do the same 1–3 as the above homework.

HOMEWORK 9.6

Read the article "Early versus standard antiretroviral therapy for HIV-infected adults in Haiti" (N *Engl J Med* 2010, 363: 257–65 by Severe, Juste, Ambroise et al.). Do the same 1–3 as the above homework.

HOMEWORK 9.7

Read the article "Phase III randomized clinical trial comparing tremeli-mumab with standard-of-care chemotherapy in patients with advanced melanoma" (*J Clin Oncol* 2013, 31: 616–622 by Ribas, Kefford, Marshall, et al.). Do the same 1–3 as the above homework.

HOMEWORK 9.8

Read the article "Pembrolizumab or placebo plus etoposide and platinum as first-line therapy for extensive-stage small-cell lung cancer: randomized, double-blind, phase III KEYNOTE-604 study" (*Journal of Clinical Oncology* 2020, 38: 2369–2379 by Rudin, Awad, Navarro, et al.) Comment on the over-running issue of the overall survival (OS) endpoint, and discuss how it affects the information time/fractions of the interim analyses and the boundary value of the final analysis.

References

Armitage P, McPherson CK, and Rowe BC. (1969). Repeated significance tests on accumulating data. *Journal of the Royal Statistical Society, Series A* 132: 235–244.

Cohen EEW, Soulières D, Le Tourneau C, et al. for the KEYNOTE-040 investigators. (2019). Pembrolizumab versus methotrexate, docetaxel, or cetuximab for recurrent or metastatic head-and-neck squamous cell carcinoma (KEYNOTE-040): a randomised, open-label, phase 3 study. *Lancet* 12;393(10167): 156–167.

Demetri GD, van Oosterom AT, Garrett CR, et al. (2006). Efficacy and safety of sunitinib in patients with advanced gastrointestinal stromal tumour after failure of imatinib: a randomised controlled trial. *Lancet* 368: 1329–1338.

DeMets DL and Ware JH. (1982). Asymmetric group sequential boundaries for monitoring clinical trials. *Biometrika* 69: 661–663.

Ellenberg SS. (2001). Independent data monitoring committees: rationale, operations and controversies. *Statistics in Medicine* 20: 2573–2583.

FDA (US Department of Health and Human Services, Food and Drug Administration). (2006). *Guidance for Clinical Trial Sponsors: Establishment and Operation of Clinical Trial Data Monitoring Committees*. http://www.fda.gov/AboutFDA/CentersOffices/OfficeofMedicalProductsandTobacco/CDER/ManualofPoliciesProcedures/ (accessed on 2/17/2014).

Haybittle JL. (1971). Repeated assessment of results in clinical trials of cancer treatment. *British Journal of Radiology* 44: 793–797.

Herson J. (2017). *Data and Safety Monitoring Committees in Clinical Trials*. Second edition. CRC Press, Taylor & Francis Group, New York.

Hwang IK, Shih WJ, and DeCani JS. (1990). Group sequential designs using a family of Type I error probability spending functions. *Statistics in Medicine* 9: 1439–1445.

ICH (International Conference on Harmonisation of Technical Requirements for Registration of Pharmaceuticals for Human Use). (1996). *Guideline for Industry: E3 Structure and Content of Clinical Study Reports*, http://www.fda.gov/downloads/drugs/guidancecomplianceregulatoryinformation/guidances/ucm073113.pdf (accessed on 4/20/2015).

ICH. (1998). *Guidance for Industry: E9 Statistical Principles for Clinical Trials*, http://www.fda.gov/downloads/drugs/guidancecomplianceregulatoryinformation/guidances/ucm073137.pdf (accessed on 2/17/2014).

Jennison C and Turnbull BW. (1997). Group-sequential analysis incorporating covariate information. *Journal of the American Statistical Association* 92: 1330–1341.

Kim KM and DeMets DL. (1987). Design and analysis of group sequential tests based on Type I error rate spending function. *Biometrika* 74: 149–154.

Kim KM, Boucher H, and Tsiatis AA. (1995). Design and analysis of group sequential Logrank tests in maximum duration versus information trials. *Biometrics* 51: 988–1000.

Lachin JM (1997). Group sequential monitoring of distribution-free analyses of repeated measures. *Statistics in Medicine* 16: 653–668.

Lan KKG and DeMets DL. (1983). Discrete sequential boundaries for clinical trials. *Biometrika* 70: 659–663.

Lan KKG and Wittes J. (1988). The B-value: a tool for monitoring data. *Biometrics* 44: 579–585.

Lan KKG and Zucker D. (1993). Sequential monitoring for clinical trials: the role of information and Brownian motion. *Statistics in Medicine* 12: 753–765.

Lan KKG, Reboussin DM, and DeMets DL. (1994). Information and information fractions for designing sequential monitoring of clinical trials. *Communications in Statistics (A)—Theory and Methods* 23: 403–420.

Lee JW and DeMets DL. (1991). Sequential comparison of changes with repeated measurements data. *Journal of American Statistical Association* 86: 757–762.

Llovet JM, Ricci S, Mazzaferro V, Hilgard P, Gane E, Blanc JF, de Oliveira AC et al. The SHARP Investigators Study Group. (2008). Sorafenib in advanced Hepatocellular Carcinoma. *New England Journal of Medicine* 359: 378–390.

Mok TSK, Wu YL, Kudaba I, Kowalski DM, et al. for the KEYNOTE-042 Investigators. (2019). Pembrolizumab versus chemotherapy for previously untreated, PD-L1-expressing, locally advanced or metastatic non-small-cell lung cancer (KEYNOTE-042): a randomised, open-label, controlled, phase 3 trial. *Lancet* 4;393(10183): 1819–1830.

Motzer RJ, Escudier B, Oudard S, et al. for the RECORD-1 Study Group. (2008). Efficacy of everolimus in advanced renal cell carcinoma: a double-blind, randomised, placebo-controlled phase III trial. *Lancet* 372: 449–456.

O'Brien PC and Fleming TR. (1979). A multiple testing procedure for clinical trials. *Biometrics* 35: 549–556.

Peto R, Pike MC, Armitage P, Breslow NE, Cox DR, Howard SV, Mantel N, et al. (1976). Design and analysis of randomized clinical trials requiring prolonged observation of each patient. *British Journal of Cancer* 35: 585–611.

Pocock SJ. (1977). Group sequential methods in the design and analysis of clinical trials. *Biometrika* 64: 191–199.

Proschan MA, Lan KKG, and Wittes JT. (2006). *Statistical Monitoring of Clinical Trials: A Unified Approach.* New York: Springer.

Reboussin DM, DeMets DL, Kim KM, and Lan KKG. (2000). Computations for group sequential boundaries using the Lan-DeMets spending function method. *Controlled Clinical Trials* 21: 190–207.

Ribas A, Kefford R, Marshall MA, et al. (2013). Phase III randomized clinical trial comparing tremelimumab with standard-of-care chemotherapy in patients with advanced melanoma. *Journal of Clinical Oncology* 31: 616–622.

Rudin CM, Awad MM, Navarro A, et al. for the KEYNOTE-604 Investigators. (2020). Pembrolizumab or placebo plus etoposide and platinum as first-line therapy for extensive-stage small-cell lung cancer: randomized, double-blind, phase III KEYNOTE-604 study. *Journal of Clinical Oncology* 38: 2369–2379.

Scandinavian Simvastatin Survival Study Group. (1993). Design and baseline results of the Scandinavian Simvastatin survival study of patients with stable Angina and/or previous myocardial infarction. *The American Journal of Cardiology* 71: 393–400.

Scharfstein DO, Tsiatis AA, and Robbins JM. (1997). Semiparametric efficiency and its implication on the design and analysis of group sequential studies. *Journal of the American Statistical Association* 92: 1342–1350.

Sellke T and Siegmund D. (1983). Sequential analysis of the proportional hazards model. *Biometrika* 70: 315–326.

Severe P, Juste MAJ, Ambroise A, et al. (2010). Early versus standard antiretroviral therapy for HIV-infected adults in Haiti. *The New England Journal of Medicine* 363: 257–65.

Shih WJ. (2000). Group sequential methods. In *Encyclopedia of Biopharmaceutical Statistics*, Chow SC (Ed.), New York: Marcel-Dekker.

Slud ER and Wei LJ. (1982). Two-sample repeated significance tests based on the modified Wilcoxon statistic. *Journal of the American Statistical Association* 77: 862–868.

Spurrier JD and Hewett JE. (1976). Two-stage Wilcoxon tests of hypotheses. *Journal of the American Statistical Association* 71: 982–987.

Tsiatis AA. (1981). The asymptotic joint distribution of the efficient scores test for the proportional hazards model calculated over time. *Biometrika* 68: 311–315.

Tsiatis AA. (1982). Repeated significance testing for a general class of statistics used in censored survival analysis. *Journal of the American Statistical Association* 77: 855–861.

Wei LJ, Su JQ, and Lachin JM. (1990). Interim analyses with repeated measurements in a sequential clinical trial. *Biometrika* 77: 359–364.

10

Monitoring the Maximum Information and Adaptive Sample Size Designs

We previously discussed the fixed-size design without interim analysis, as well as sequential designs with interim analyses in previous chapters. The alpha-spending function approach of the classical group sequential (GS) design is especially useful in providing a flexible tool for monitoring the safety and efficacy aspects of clinical trials. Particularly, this approach provides flexibility in the schedule and the number of interim analyses. The fundamental structure of the fixed-size design without interim analyses and the classical GS procedure with interim analyses relies on the maximum, fixed, and prespecified information in the study protocol. The information times (fractions) used for interim analyses are based on this fixed, prespecified, maximum information. What if the prespecified maximum information is incorrect? Can it be altered later if it is found to be inadequate? These questions are often asked. Recall that in Chapter 4 we discussed how sample size calculation, study power, and values for design parameters such as treatment effect, within-group variance, intra-class correlation for correlated observations, and compliance rate had to be assumed, ideally based on data derived from prior studies with very similar design conditions, especially for Phase III confirmatory studies. However, we often find that the prior studies, if any, usually involve different patient populations (defined by the inclusion and exclusion criteria and different disease staging technologies), medical practices (e.g., allowable concomitant medications), study durations, or treatment regimens. An intriguing idea, therefore, would be to see if these assumptions could be verified or updated with interim data from the ongoing study itself. For example, after checking the interim data, we find that an extension of the (initial) maximum information is necessary to ensure the study power. With this finding, we would then need to modify the original sample size and perhaps also the conventional fixed-size test or the classical sequential procedure. In performing all these modifications, we would then need to ensure that the type I error rate remained controlled. A recent development in this area is termed *adaptive designs* or *flexible designs*, which include the classical GS design discussed in Chapter 9. In this chapter, we first review some key points about adaptive designs in general. Then, we discuss three topics related to the adaptive/flexible designs: (i) sample size reestimation (SSR) with continuous or binary endpoints, (ii) monitoring trial duration for maximum information (for event-driven trials) or maximum duration (for

DOI: 10.1201/9781003176527-10

duration-driven trials) with survival endpoints, and (iii) modification of the maximum information in the classical GS to become adaptive GS. In SSR, we present methods involving either blinded data or unblinded data (i.e., with or without a comparative analysis on interim data). In monitoring trial duration, the method could involve only blinded data. For the modification of the maximum information in GS, we use unblinded interim data as well. Other topics of adaptive designs such as Phase II/III seamless (select-the-winner) design and various biomarker-guided designs including adaptive enrichment design are covered in Chapters 12 and 13, after studying methods for controlling the type I error rate due to multiple tests in Chapter 11. Overall, the recent development of adaptive designs offers trials great flexibility in making midcourse modifications of the maximum information or duration, but there could be some potential pitfalls. Examples are given to illustrate some vigilant points. We first give an overview on the adaptive design in the next section.

10.1 Adaptive Designs—Overview

Ever since the US FDA launched its Critical Path Initiative (CPI) in March 2004—the FDA's national strategy for transforming the way FDA-regulated medical products being developed, evaluated, and manufactured—innovative adaptive designs and methods have been the key for modernizing the field of clinical trials. The European Medicines Agency (EMEA) and Committee for Medicinal Products for Human Use (CHMP) also issued a similar paper on methodological issues in confirmatory clinical trials with flexible design and analysis plan in March 2006. Recently, the US FDA has updated its Guidance for Industry on adaptive designs for clinical trials in November 2019. There are several key points expressed in these documents.

- First, the terms are clarified by the regulatory agency in distinguishing adaptation methods by two types: adaptation with or without a comparative analysis of the interim data. It stated that *"A non-comparative analysis is an examination of accumulating trial data in which the treatment group assignments of subjects are not used in any manner in the analysis."* This corresponds to the term "blinded" analysis usually seen in the literature and in this book. Moreover, the guidance defines that *"A comparative analysis is an examination of accumulating trial data in which treatment groups are identified, either with the actual assigned treatments or with codes (e.g., labeled as A and B, without divulging which treatment is investigational)."* This corresponds to the term "unblinded" analysis usually used by trialists. It is important to recognize that an interim analysis can be comparative or non-comparative regardless of whether trial subjects, investigators, and other personnel such as the sponsor and data monitoring committee (DMC) have knowledge of individual treatment assignments or access to comparative results by treatment arm. For example, it is possible to include adaptations based on a non-comparative analysis even in open-label trials.

- Second, since adaptive designs all involve interim analysis, we need logistic procedures that ensure the interim data are of high quality and available in a timely manner so that adaptive decision making is based on up-to-date and reliable data. Preplanning adaptive design modifications usually require more effort at the design stage.

- Third, an adaptive design usually sets aims and hypotheses that are different from those without adaptation. We need to make sure the aims and corresponding hypotheses are clearly expressed in the protocol and analysis plan. Chapter 12 is devoted to addressing the hypotheses for various designs guided by predictive biomarkers, including the adaptive enrichment design.

- Fourth, and most critically, adaptive designs require specific analytical methods to avoid increasing the chance of erroneous conclusions and introducing bias in estimates. Particularly, the control of type I error rate is an overarching issue with adaptation. For this reason, we discuss multiplicity issue and methods of controlling the family-wise type I error rate in Chapter 11 before we cover more topics on adaptive designs.

10.2 Adaptive Sample Size Design: Sample Size Reestimation

Adaptive (or flexible) sample size design, also known as SSR, is one of the most popular forms of adaptive design for clinical trials. We first discuss SSR with non-comparative analysis (i.e., using blinded interim data) in Section 10.2.1, and then SSR with comparative interim analysis in Section 10.2.2. Because increasing the sample size of an ongoing trial involves many administrative and logistical matters and possibly delaying the trial, we usually perform SSR only once in the course of a study. The timing of when we perform an SSR also needs attention. We need enough data to make the interim analysis reliable. On the other hand, the later the interim analysis, the harder we find it to make administrative changes to the trial, such as amending the protocol, going through IRBs, selecting new medical centers, contracting new investigators, and enrolling more patients.

In the following, we consider a randomized parallel-arm clinical trial. Assume that the observations are normally distributed with means μ_X and μ_Y, respectively, for the two arms and a common variance σ^2. Follow the notation in Chapter 4, $\delta = \mu_X - \mu_Y$, and δ / σ is the standardized treatment effect. Suppose the original sample size is planned to be n_0 subjects per group, and the interim analysis for SSR is conducted with n_1 per group.

10.2.1 SSR with Non-Comparative Analysis

To protect the integrity of an ongoing trial, the concealment of the treatment group assignment is best kept intact. Our concern is on the assumed within-group variance. A simple method for SSR would be to check the total variance for trials using a continuous primary endpoint or to check the pooled event rate for trials using a binary primary endpoint, based on the blind interim data. If the total variance is found much higher or the pooled event rate is found much lower than the expected total variance or pooled event rate, respectively, compared to the original assumptions, then we increase the sample size to achieve the desired study power. Otherwise, the study continues with the original sample size. SSR using blind interim data without the possibility of downsizing will not change the type I error rate, because the variance and pooled event rate are the nuisance parameters (parameters that are separated from the treatment difference, delta). The power calculation in SSR still remains the treatment effect (delta) that the protocol authors assumed in the original alternative hypothesis.

More sophisticated methods for SSR are available. For example, we can use the EM (expectation-maximization) algorithm for solving a mixture of two normal distributions with a common variance (see Shih 1992; Gould and Shih 1992, 1998), which is based on the idea that the unavailable treatment group identification is "missing completely at random" (MCAR)—see Chapter 15 for the topic of missing data. However, most of the practitioners prefer the above simple methods (i.e., just using the total variance). If, however, concern remains that the total variance may be too large compared to the within-group variance used in the original sample size calculation, one may consider using a correction formula that involves assumed treatment difference, delta, as follows:

Let S_T^2 be the sample estimate of the total variance and S_W^2 be the (pooled) estimate of the within-group variance. We can show that

$$(2n_1 - 1)S_T^2 = n_1\hat{\delta}^2 / 2 + 2(n_1 - 1)S_W^2 \tag{10.1}$$

The proof may be done for a homework (Homework 10.1). Note that in the ANOVA setting the left-hand side of Equation 10.1 is the "corrected total of sum of squares," the second term of the right-hand side is the "within-group sum of squares," and the multipliers involving the per-group sample size n_1 are the corresponding degrees of freedom. Of course, because of the blinding, neither the estimate of the treatment effect, $\hat{\delta}$, nor the estimate of the within-group variance, S_W^2, are actually observed. Gould and Shih (1992, 1998) suggested the use of the original hypothesized δ_0 to replace $\hat{\delta}$

in Equation 10.1 and then obtained the following estimate of the pseudo-within-group variance:

$$S^2 = \left[(2n_1 - 1)S_T^2 - n_1 \hat{\delta}_0^2 / 2 \right] / 2(n_1 - 1) \tag{10.2}$$

An alternative correction strategy uses the mean squared error (MSE) of a regression model with some baseline (surrogate) covariate other than the (unavailable) treatment group. Of course, in either correction we never know whether the adjustment will be enough or inadequate, depending on the assumed delta, for the first way of correction, and on the correlation of the (surrogate) covariate with the response, for the second way of correction, relative to the true treatment effect.

Note that, as we have seen in Chapters 4 and 5, the MSE in ANCOVA is what we need for the within-group variance estimate in the sample size calculation. Therefore, the SSR discussed above actually targets the estimation of this MSE (but without the treatment group as a factor) in the ANCOVA model. Toward this end, we should use the residuals of the ANCOVA instead of the values of the response variable itself. For example, Shih and Long (1998) included the center effect as a covariate.

Proschan, Lan, and Wittes (2006) pointed out that based on Equation 10.1 the ratio of the total variance to the within-group variance can be expressed as

$$\frac{S_T^2}{S_W^2} = \frac{n_1 \hat{\delta}^2}{(2n_1 - 1)S_T^2} + \frac{2(n_1 - 1)}{2n_1 - 1} \approx 1 + \frac{1}{4}\left(\frac{\hat{\delta}}{S_W} \right)^2$$

The effect size $\dfrac{\hat{\delta}}{S_W}$ in a typical Phase III trial is around 0.2–0.5 (see Section 4.2). This gives us some idea of the range of the inflation when we use the total variance estimate instead of the (unobserved) within-group variance estimate. SSR without comparative analysis does not materially affect the type I error rate.

10.2.2 SSR with Comparative Analysis

When there is too much uncertainty around the treatment difference, or when a clinically meaningful effect is difficult to define, the treatment identification of each patient needs to be accessed to perform a comparative analysis for SSR. With a comparative interim analysis, the outcome information from the analysis influences the sample size of the second stage, and thus influences the sample size of the whole study with both stages combined. It is very important to limit the access to comparative interim results (see details in the FDA's guidance section VII).

In this section, we discuss four popular methods for SSR with comparative analysis. The first method uses the usual likelihood ratio test, score test, or Wald test, with an adjusted critical region (Li et al. 2002, Li, Shih and Wang

2005; Li, Shih and Wang 2016). Bowden and Mander (2014) termed it *LSW method*. The weighted method (Cui, Huang and Wang 1999), known as the *CHW weighted test*, adjusts the test statistic with given (fixed) weights rather than adjusting the critical region. The third method is the *dual test* introduced by Denne (2001). The fourth method is the *promising zone* approach by Chen et al. (2004). All four methods preserve the type I error rate and have included the estimation of treatment effect in the literature that we will leave to readers as homework readings.

We emphasize that, while the rule of the design is flexible, the structure of the decision process must be prespecified for the protocol to follow so that there is no ambiguity for the regulatory agencies to examine the validity of the statistical procedure.

10.2.2.1 The LSW Likelihood Method

Continuing the previous setup, a clinical trial is designed with an initial sample size of n_0 patients per group given in the protocol. We are interested in testing the null hypothesis $H_0: \delta = 0$ versus the one-sided alternative hypothesis $H_A: \delta > 0$. Different from the last section where we are concerned with the within-group variance, here we assume σ^2 can be consistently and stably estimated with the unblinded data, so that, for simplicity, we may let $\sigma^2 = 1$. Equivalently, we assume δ is the standardized treatment effect. At the first/interim stage when data from n_1 patients in each group are available, we calculate the sample means $\bar{X}_1$ and $\bar{Y}_1$ of the two groups. Let $\hat{\delta}_1 = \bar{X}_1 - \bar{Y}_1$ and

$$Z_1 = \frac{\hat{\delta}_1}{se(\hat{\delta}_1)} = \sqrt{\frac{n_1}{2}}\,\hat{\delta}_1.$$

It is common for a sequential design to consider possible early termination of a study for either futility or efficacy at the interim stage. For given constants h and k, we plan to (i) reject H_0 and terminate the trial if $z_1 > k$, (ii) accept H_0 and terminate the trial if $z_1 < h$, or (iii) continue the trial to the second (final) stage if $h \le z_1 \le k$. For the path (iii), the task is to determine an additional n_2 number of patients per group and a critical value c for the final test so that the overall type I error rate is preserved at the prescribed level α. In the literature, different forms of the final test and associated formula for n_2 and c have been discussed. Throughout the following, we write $n_2(z_1)$ and n_2 interchangeably; the former emphasizes the fact that n_2 depends on z_1 for flexible sample size designs.

Denote $\hat{\delta}_2 = \bar{X}_2 - \bar{Y}_2$ and $Z_2 = \dfrac{\hat{\delta}_2}{se(\hat{\delta}_2)}$ based on the second-stage samples. Z_2 is defined only if the study continues. At the end of the trial, the Wald test statistic is $Z(n) = \dfrac{n_1(\bar{X}_1 - \bar{Y}_1) + n_2(\bar{X}_2 - \bar{Y}_2)}{\sqrt{2(n_1 + n_2)}} = \dfrac{\sqrt{n_1}Z_1 + \sqrt{n_2(Z_1)}Z_2}{\sqrt{n_1 + n_2(Z_1)}}$ based on $n = n_1 + n_2$ patients per group. Of note, $Z(n)$ is a weighted combination of Z_1

and Z_2. We have seen this form of weighted combination in Appendix 8.3.1 before. However, this time, the second part of the weights involves $n_2(z_1)$ that depends on the first stage Z_1. We also have seen that we used conditional probability for the two-stage monitoring process in Chapter 8. We continue to use conditional probability here as follows.

The conditional probability for the final test to be significant is

$$CP_\delta(n_2, c \mid z_1) = \Pr(Z(n) > c \mid z_1, \delta)$$

$$= 1 - \Phi\left[\frac{c\sqrt{2(n_1 + n_2)} - z_1\sqrt{2n_1} - n_2\delta}{\sqrt{2n_2}}\right] \tag{10.3}$$

(Note: Eq. (10.3) is equivalent to Eq. (8.10) with $\sigma^2 = 1$; Homework 10.2.) The conditional probability (10.3) for given n_2 and c is conditioning on two quantities: the assumed treatment effect size δ for Stage 2 data and the observed $Z_1 = z_1$ from Stage 1 data. The treatment effect size can be based on several considerations and is up to the choice of the researcher, as alluded to in Section 8.2.1. When a design aims to provide a conditional power (CP) of $1 - \beta_1$ for detecting the current trend $\delta = \hat{\delta}_1 = \sqrt{\dfrac{2}{n_1}} z_1$ at the final stage given the interim result $h \le z_1 \le k$, Eq. (10.3) gives

$$CP_{\hat{\delta}_1}(n_2, c \mid z_1) = \Phi\left[\frac{z_1}{\sqrt{\dfrac{t}{T}\left(1 - \dfrac{t}{T}\right)}} - \frac{c}{\sqrt{1 - \dfrac{t}{T}}}\right] = 1 - \beta_1 \tag{10.4}$$

where $t = n_1/n_0$ is the information fraction in the scale of the original sample size n_0 and $T = \dfrac{n_1 + n_2}{n_0} = t + \dfrac{n_2}{n_0}$ is the sample size increase ratio relative to n_0.

Note that $\dfrac{t}{T} = \dfrac{n_1}{n_1 + n_2}$. We have seen a similar form to (10.4) in Section 8.2.1 (Eq. 8.12) as well.

Li et al. (2002) derived via Eq. (10.4) the following:

$$n_2(z_1) \ge \left[\left(\frac{c + z_{\beta_1}}{z_1}\right)^2 - 1\right]n_1$$

Or,

$$f = \frac{n_2(z_1)}{n_1} \ge \left(\frac{c + z_{\beta_1}}{z_1}\right)^2 - 1 \tag{10.5}$$

Furthermore, with practical considerations, we may set

$$n_2(z_1) \geq \max \left\{ \min \left(n_{2max}, \left[\left(\frac{c + z_{\beta_1}}{z_1} \right)^2 - 1 \right] n_1 \right), n_{2min} \right\}, \qquad (10.6)$$

where n_{2max} is the maximum resource-allowable and n_{2min} is the prespecified minimum sample sizes for the second stage. (Usually, $n_{2min} = n_0 - n_1$, indicating no decrease in sample size.) Of course, the cap of n_2 would limit the conditional power to not reaching the desired level of $1 - \beta_1$.

The critical value c may be solved by two ways. Both ways are to ensure the type I error rate is preserved at α. The first way given by Li et al. (2002) is to solve

$$1 - \Phi(h) - \alpha = \int_h^k \Phi \left[\frac{c\sqrt{n_1 + n_2(z_1)} - z_1\sqrt{n_1}}{\sqrt{n_2(z_1)}} \right] \phi(z_1) dz_1 \qquad (10.7)$$

for the given set of design parameters, β_1, h, k, n_{2max}, and n_{2min}. $\Phi(\cdot)$ is the cumulative distribution function, and $\phi(\cdot)$ is the density function of the standard normal, and $z_{\beta_1} = \Phi^{-1}(1 - \beta_1)$. However, as discussed in Section 8.2.2, futility is usually regarded as an internal business decision for the manufacturers; thus, health agencies often view the boundary h non-binding (not reinforceable) to the manufacturer. In this case, we replace h by $-\infty$ in Eq. (10.7) as an option. That is, set

$$1 - \alpha = \int_{-\infty}^k \Phi \left[\frac{c\sqrt{n_1 + n_2(z_1)} - z_1\sqrt{n_1}}{\sqrt{n_2(z_1)}} \right] \phi(z_1) dz_1 \qquad (10.8)$$

Note that Eq. (10.7) or (10.8) also involves $n_2(z_1)$, but only through the ratio to n_1. Appendix 10.1 provides an SAS code for solving c.

Another way to obtain the critical value c is not to integrate the conditional error rate over the density of the interim Z_1, but to recognize the following fact. Let the original critical value before conducting interim analysis be the conventional group sequential boundary c_g. That is, c_g satisfies the equation

$$\alpha = \Pr(Z_1 > k \mid \delta = 0) + \Pr(Z^0 > c_g, h \leq Z_1 \leq k \mid \delta = 0)$$

$$\leq \Pr(Z_1 > k \mid \delta = 0) + \Pr(Z^0 > c_g, -\infty < Z_1 \leq k \mid \delta = 0) \qquad (10.9)$$

where Z^0 is the Wald test statistic based on the planned sample size n_0. (Note: With $k > 4$ and no multiplicity adjustment, $c_g = 1.96$ for one-sided $\alpha = 0.025$. For $k \leq 4$, adjustment is needed as seen in Chapter 9. A numerical illustration is given in the sequel.) To preserve the type I error rate for $Z(n)$, the critical boundary c_g must be adjusted to c, so that

$$\Pr\big(Z(n) \geq c \,|\, z_1\big) = \Pr\big(Z(n_0) \geq c_g \,|\, z_1\big) \tag{10.10}$$

under the null hypothesis ($\delta = 0$). (That is, if the conditional error rate is the same, then the unconditional error rate must be the same, i.e., equal to α.) Following the same derivation process as in Eq. (10.3) with $\delta = 0$ for $Z(n)$ on the left-hand side and for $Z(n_0)$ on the right-hand side of Eq. (10.10), we obtain

$$\Phi\left[\frac{-c_g\sqrt{n_0} + z_1\sqrt{n_1}}{\sqrt{n_0 - n_1}}\right] = \Phi\left[\frac{-c\sqrt{(n_1+n_2)} + z_1\sqrt{n_1}}{\sqrt{n_2}}\right]$$

Solving for c produces the following explicit formula for the new critical value:

$$c = \sqrt{\frac{n_0}{n_1 + n_2}}\left\{\left(c_g - z_1\sqrt{\frac{n_1}{n_0}}\right)\sqrt{\frac{n_2}{n_0 - n_1}} + z_1\sqrt{\frac{n_1}{n_0}}\right\} \tag{10.11}$$

Equation (10.11) also involves n_2, but only through the ratio to n_0. Recall $t = n_1/n_0$ for Stage 1 and $T = \dfrac{n}{n_0} = \dfrac{n_1+n_2}{n_0} = t + \dfrac{n_2}{n_0}$ for Stage 2. Then, (10.11) is also expressed as

$$c = \frac{1}{\sqrt{T}}\left\{\frac{\sqrt{T-t}}{\sqrt{1-t}}\left(c_g - z_1\sqrt{t}\right) + z_1\sqrt{t}\right\} \tag{10.12}$$

Compared to the first approach, which integrated out z_1, (10.11) or (10.12) depends on the interim result z_1. This means that, with the second method, we cannot predetermine the critical value in advance in the statistical analysis plan.

Now, plug Eq. (10.11) into Eq. (10.5) or (10.6) to obtain the new sample size. Or, plug c directly to Eq. (10.4) and obtain:

$$T - t = \frac{n_2}{n_0} \geq \frac{t\big(z_{\beta_1}\sqrt{1-t} + c_g - z_1\sqrt{t}\big)^2}{z_1^2(1-t)} \tag{10.13}$$

Or,

$$\frac{n_2}{n_1} \geq \frac{\big(z_{\beta_1}\sqrt{1-t} + c_g - z_1\sqrt{t}\big)^2}{z_1^2(1-t)} \tag{10.14}$$

subject to the same n_{2max} and n_{2min} as in Eq. (10.6).

Discussion

Point 1: Note that for n_2, so long as it satisfies the inequality in formula (10.6) or (10.13), it does not really matter how the actual value is obtained. In practice, there are many other factors besides the interim result that could influence the sample size adjustment. n_2 can be obtained with internal or external information. Afterward, the actual sample size (say, $n_2^* > n_2$) may turn out to be different from n_2, but we expect that they would differ very little and that the minor difference should be due to administrative reasons only. At this point, just like the fixed-size design case, conditioning on the actual n^* for the final test is valid so long as the reason for the minor difference between them has nothing to do with the data itself. In Shih, Li, and Wang (2016), it was shown that so long as $n_2^* > n_2$, where n_2 provides a conditional power at least 50% under the current trend $\hat{\delta}_1$, then the overall type I error rate is still preserved for the LSW test $(Z(n), c)$.

Point 2: In the literature, it was said that the current trend $\hat{\delta}_1$, on which the conditional power is based, could be unreliable and some found that using it generally leads to large, expected sample sizes. For this issue, we advised that SSR should not be performed too soon so that n_1 of the interim analysis is not too small to provide a stable estimate of δ. (This advice applies to the SSR with non-comparative analysis in Section 10.2.1 for the within-group variance estimate as well.)

The level of conditional power should also be contemplated with different scenarios as $t = n_1/n_0$ varies. The effect of capping n_2 below $n_{2\max}$ on the conditional power $1-\beta_1$ should be considered as well. Shih, Li, and Wang (2016) suggested to consider the level of $1-\beta_1$ with $n_2 = n_0 - n_1$ (per group) with $z_1 = c_g$ at $t = n_1/n_0$, and then to set the target conditional power at this level. For example, if $c_g = 2$, we have $1-\beta_1 = \Phi\left(\dfrac{2\left(1-\sqrt{t}\right)}{\sqrt{t(1-t)}}\right)$. Thus, set $1-\beta_1 = 0.96$, 0.88, or 0.78 if the interim analysis (SSR) is performed at $t = 1/3$, $1/2$, or $2/3$, respectively. See Example 10.2 in In-Class Exercises below for illustration.

10.2.2.2 The CHW Weighted Test

The CHW weighted test statistic is $Z_W = \dfrac{\sqrt{n_1}\, Z_1 + \sqrt{(n_0 - n_1)}\, Z_2}{\sqrt{n_0}} = \sqrt{t}\, Z_1 + \sqrt{1-t}\, Z_2$. It uses the critical value c_g of the conventional group sequential design; see Eq. (10.9). Cui et al. (1999) showed that under the null hypothesis, $\Pr\left(Z_W \geq c_g\right) \leq \alpha$.

Discussion

Point 1: The critical value c_g for Z_W is readily obtainable from available software, in which the calculation uses the fact that the correlation between

Z^0 and Z_1 is the square root of the information time/fraction $t = n_1/n_0$ via the principle of partial sum process with independent increments in the group sequential setting (see Chapter 9). If there is no early stop planned, i.e., $-h = k = \infty$, then the critical value $c_g = z_\alpha$ as for the fixed sample size design. However, in the conventional group sequential design, where over-running or under-running of sample size may occur (see Example 9.4), the actual sample size (say n^*) should be used, i.e., the correlation should be $\sqrt{n_1/n^*}$, to determine the critical value for the final test. But for the CHW weighted test, the critical value c_g must be based on Eq. (10.9), i.e., assuming $n_0 = n^*$. Therefore, to say that the CHW weighted test uses the "same" critical value as in the conventional group sequential design, as some authors do, is not exactly accurate. Unlike the LSW method (previous section), where n_0 only appears in setting a minimum for n_2, the initial sample size n_0 plays a rather critical role in the CHW weighted test and hence needs to be carefully planned. Ironically, this n_0 is what we are not quite sure about when considering sample size flexible designs.

Point 2: The CHW weighted test comes from the interest of preserving the type I error rate. In Z_W the weights for the stage-wise Z_1 and Z_2 are only proportional to the planned sample size n_0, not to the reestimated sample size n. The fixed weights have been generalized, and the test has been extended to a p-value combination method; see Appendix 8.3.2.

Point 3: An advantage for the CHW weighted test is that it does not mandate a specific rule involving z_1 for calculating n_2. That is, it remains implicit (alias flexible) about how n_2 should be obtained. But any reasonable n_2 should be large enough to provide a certain level of power for the study.

10.2.2.3 The Dual Test

To control the type I error rate in the LSW method, the Wald test statistic Z uses the adjusted critical value c, while the CHW weighted statistic Z_W uses the naive critical value c_g. The dual test, suggested by Denne (2001), is a combination test of the above two by requiring $\min(Z, Z_W) \geq c_g$ to be statistically significant. By the construction, under H_0, $\Pr\left(\min\left(Z, Z_W\right) \geq c_g\right) \leq \Pr\left(Z_W \geq c_g\right) \leq \alpha$. Obviously, the dual test loses power compared to the weighted test in general.

10.2.2.4 Promising Zone Approach

Another recent development in this area is to further divide the continuation region with a sub-region called *promising zone*. When the interim result z_1 is "promising," measured by the conditional power or by the magnitude of z_1 itself, the sample size will be increased (i.e., $n_2 > n_0 - n_1$) and, without inflation of the type I error, the final test will be the naive test (Z, c_g).

To be specific, the CHW weighted test (Z_W, c_g) and the Wald test (Z, c) of the LSW method are linked in the following way: $Z = Z_W \ (= Z_1)$ in the early rejection and acceptance regions of the LSW method, where Z_2 does not exist. $Z = Z_W (= Z^0)$ in the region where the trial continues with the original sample size, i.e., $n = n_0$. Z and Z_W differ only in the region where we continue the trial with an increase in sample size, i.e., $n_2 > n_0 - n_1$. This sub-region in the continuation region is the so-called *promising zone*. Obviously, the focus is the construction of the promising zone. The promising zone needs to be prespecified in the protocol before the interim analysis. Chen et al. (2004) showed that increasing sample size when the interim result is "promising" (meaning conditional power at least 50% with the planned sample size n_0) will not inflate the type I error rate with the use of the naive test (Z, c_g). From Eq. (10.4), the conditional power (CP) under the current trend with the planned sample size n_0 is

$$CP_{\hat{\delta}_1}\left(n_0 - n_1, |z_1\right) = 1 - \Phi\left[c_g\sqrt{\frac{1}{1-t}} - z_1\sqrt{\frac{1}{t(1-t)}}\right] \qquad (10.15)$$

where $t = n_1/n_0$, the information time/fraction at the interim analysis gauged by the planned sample size. Note that for $CP_{\hat{\delta}_1}\left(n_0 - n_1, c_g|z_1\right) = 0.5$, $z_1 = \sqrt{t}\, c_g$. Hence, for Chen et al. (2004), their promising zone in the z-scale is $z_1 \geq \sqrt{t}\, c_g$, and the condition for n_2 is simply $n_2 > n_0 - n_1$.

Mehta and Pocock (2011) and Broberg (2013) extended the promising zone of Chen et al. to a region where conditional power is somewhat below 50%. Shih, Li, and Wang (2016) showed that the extension is somewhat narrow and accompanied with a rather complicated requirement for n_2.

In-Class Exercises

Example 10.1

For simplicity, let $c_g = z_\alpha = 1.96$ (i.e., $k = \infty$, no early stop for superiority, $\alpha = 0.025$) and $t = 1/2$. The upper bound of a promising zone is the "favorable zone" where the conditional power (CP) is sufficient with the original sample size (so the trial continues without an increase in the sample size). Let the CP=80% be considered sufficient for the favorable zone. Then from (10.15), $z_1 = 1.81$ is the upper bound. The promising zone of Chen et al. is from $z_1 = \sqrt{t}\, c_g = 1.38$ (50% CP) to 1.81 (80% CP).

Example 10.2

We illustrate the two-stage design with use of the LSW method. We also pay attention to the process of gathering design information during the study.

Assume that we plan to spend a type I error rate of $\alpha_1 = 0.005$ (out of the total $\alpha = 0.025$) at the first stage, then $k = 2.576$. (We need to commit this in the protocol). Suppose at $t = 1/2$ we perform the interim analysis with $n_1 = 200$ patients (per group) and find z_1 is less than 2.576. So, we are in the continuation region. Then, $\Pr(Z_1 < 2.576, Z > c_g) = \alpha - \Phi(-k) = 0.02$ gives $c_g = 2.003$. (This becomes known when the interim analysis at t is performed.) As a reference point for targeting the conditional power, if we have no cap in sample size, the maximum conditional power would be $CP_{\hat{\delta}_1}(n_0 - n_1, c_g | z_1 = 2.003) = 0.88$ from Eq. (10.15) for $t = 1/2$. At this point in time, n_{2max} should also become available, e.g., $f_{max} = \dfrac{n_{2max}}{n_1} = 3$ to indicate the limited resource.

Using the simple rule of Chen et al., the promising zone in the z-scale is $z_1 \geq \sqrt{t}\, c_g = 1.416$ (CP above 50%).

Consider the following scenario. Suppose that $z_1 = 1.20$, which corresponds to $CP_{\hat{\delta}_1}(n_0 - n_1, c_g | z_1 = 1.20) = 0.333$, indicating that the data are below the promising zone. In case one considers $CP = 0.33$ still somewhat hopeful and would like to continue the study with sample size adjustment, then LSW method can be used to do SSR as follows:

The LSW method with $k = 2.576$ and $1 - \beta_1 = 0.88$ (cf. the reference point), using the first approach, which integrates the distribution of z_1, from Eq. (10.5), $f = \dfrac{n_2}{n_1} = 6.32 > f_{max} = 3$. From Eqs. (10.6) and (10.8) the associated critical value is $c = 2.071$ and $n_2 = 600$ (per group) for $f_{max} = 3$. The critical value c is calculated by the SAS program in Appendix 10.1 when t and f_{max} are known at the time of conducting the interim analysis. It is independent of z_1. Using the second approach, which does need z_1, we obtain from Eq. (10.14) that $f = \dfrac{n_2}{n_1} = 5.47 > f_{max} = 3$. Thus, we may only increase n_2 up to 600 (per group), the same as in the first approach. Suppose we do carry out $n_2 = 600$, then $T = 2$, and the critical value is $c = 2.014$ obtained from Eq. (10.12), which agrees with the first method closely. The LSW design can still allow the trial to continue. With the sample size increase capped by $f_{max} = 3$, the highest achievable conditional power would be 0.628, compared to the 0.333 level without adjusting the sample size.

Summary

We first summarize what should be planned in a protocol for designing a flexible sample size Phase III trial. We pay attention to preserving the type I error and avoiding potential bias. We distinguish between planning and monitoring. In planning, we need to be explicit about what must be committed throughout the study and what may be implicit and subject to modification during monitoring. We also distinguish requiring a specific value given to the design parameter from requiring a formula for which the parameter value may be realized when information is available. The more we permit a design parameter to be implicit or given by a formula instead of a committed value at the planning stage, the more flexibility we have for conducting a valid and adequately powered trial.

Toward this end, for a two-stage sequential design, the protocol needs to specify an α spending, $\alpha_1 = 1 - \Phi(k)$ at the interim stage with information fraction $t = n_1/n_0$, gauged by the planned sample size n_0 that is determined with a certain power level. The α_1 or equivalently, the early rejection region $z_1 > k$, must be explicit so that the overall α level may be preserved without ambiguity. This α_1 or k is the only design quantity besides n_0 that needs to be explicitly fixed in the protocol. Notice that $t = n_1/n_0$ is a formula for planning; we project n_1 in the protocol, but its exact value becomes known only at the time when we conduct the interim analysis. At that point in time, the critical value c_g is then determined by Formula (10.9).

The early acceptance (i.e., futility) region, on the other hand, needs not be explicit in the protocol since, as commented previously, it is regarded as non-binding and should not be used to "buy back some alpha." However, when considering sample size for the second stage, there will be a maximum resource-allowable sample size, n_{2max} for consideration, but that is also a business matter and needs not be decided in the protocol. If the reestimated sample size exceeds the maximum allowable sample size, we have two options. We either continue the study with the maximum allowable sample size and let the power be compromised to a certain extent, or stop the study and declare futility. For the LSW method or Chen et al.'s promising zone approach, n_{2max} needs not be decided in the protocol, but for Mehta and Pocock's promising zone (2011), n_{2max} is needed to determine the lower bound of the promising zone.

For the LSW method, we also need to specify the conditional power. The critical value c for the Wald test statistic is determined for the given set of design parameters: $\alpha, \beta_1, k, n_{2max}$, and $n_{2min} (= n_0 - n_1)$. Again, among these, the values of α, k, and n_0 are necessarily explicit in the protocol, and n_1 is projected but only realized when doing the interim analysis; at that time, n_{2max} and β_1 should be known to consider the sample size of the next stage, $n_2(z_1)$.

10.3 Monitoring Trial Duration for Studies with Survival Endpoints

Clinical trials with survival endpoints usually require a long duration in order to enroll enough patients and incur enough events. When we specify maximum information (i.e., the total number of events) in the protocol for a desirable study power, the length of the trial then becomes random. Although we specify the projected length of the study at the beginning of the trial, we believe it prudent, and in fact a common practice, for the sponsor of such a resource-demanding trial to reestimate the end time of the trial based on interim data during the trial's progress. Below is an example to illustrate this point.

Example 10.3

A trial is designed to require 120 primary events with a plan to enroll 230 patients. Eighteen months after randomizing the first patient, an interim analysis with blinded data reveals a total of 111 enrolled subjects and shows the following information: total patient exposure time of 65 patient-years, 16 primary events out of the 111 enrolled subjects, and 10 subjects who dropped out early (lost to follow-up) without a primary event before withdrawal.

Using simple or crude estimates, we calculate the rate of subject recruitment at about $111/18=6$ patients per month, the event rate at $16/65=0.25$ events per patient-year, and the patient early withdrawal rate at $10/65=0.15$ withdraws per patient-year. The question we then pose is: If the trial continued at the same enrollment rate, withdrawal rate, and event rate, how long would it take for the study to reach the full 120 events?

We first derive the general solution and then come back to this specific example.

Let T_j be the potential event time and U_j the censoring time of subject j. The variable T_j will be observed whenever $T_j < U_j$. Let $X_j = \min(T_j, U_j)$, and $\delta_j = I_{\{T_j \leq U_j\}}$, where I_A is the indicator function for event A. The data are the set $\{X_j, \delta_j, j=1, \ldots, n\}$, and the counting process as a function of time t is $N_j(t) = I_{\{X_j \leq t, \delta_j=1\}}$. Then, we derive

$$E[N_j(t)] = Pr(X_j \leq t, \delta_j = 1) = Pr(T_j \leq t, T_j \leq U_j)$$

$$= Pr(\text{subject } j \text{ will have event by time } t, \text{ from time } 0)$$
$$(\text{i.e., observation period is } t)$$

$$= E_T[Pr(T_j \leq t, T_j \leq U_j | T_j)]$$

Assuming T and U are independent, we find that

$$E[N_j(t)] = \int_0^t H(s)f(s)ds \tag{10.16}$$

where $H(s)=Pr(U>s)$ and $f(\cdot)$ is the density of T.

The above censoring mechanism U may be a competing risk to the primary event, including dropout (i.e., loss to follow-up), or administrative censoring due to staggered entry and data review at time t. The origin of time $(t=0)$ is the study start (first patient randomization) day.

For example, suppose that the primary event and censoring are independent with exponential distributions: $H(s)=Pr(U>s)=e^{-\eta s}$, $f(s)=\lambda e^{-\lambda s}$. Then following Equation 10.16, Pr(subject j will have event by time t)

$$= \int_0^t H(s)f(s)ds = \int_0^t e^{-\eta s}\lambda e^{-\lambda s}ds = \lambda \int_0^t e^{-(\eta+\lambda)s}ds$$

$$(10.17)$$

$$= \frac{\lambda}{(\eta+\lambda)}\int_0^t (\eta+\lambda)e^{-(\eta+\lambda)s}ds = \frac{\lambda}{(\eta+\lambda)}\left[1-e^{-(\eta+\lambda)t}\right]$$

We saw this formula previously in Chapter 4 for sample size calculation and continue to use this convenient exponential model to monitor the study progress.

Let n be the total number of subjects planned to be enrolled in the study and n_1 be the number of subjects enrolled at the interim analysis time t_1 ($n=230$, $n_1=111$, $t_1=18$ months in the above example). Suppose that, when we reviewed the data at time t_1, we found d_1 events and r dropouts. Hence, (n_1-d_1-r) subjects remain to be followed up until the final analysis time, t_2. We call these n_1-d_1-r patients Cohort Q_a.

For Cohort Q_a,

Pr(subject j in these (n_1-d_1-r) will have an event by time t_2, *from time* t_1)

$$\int_{t_1}^{t_2} H(s)f(s)ds = \frac{\lambda}{(\eta+\lambda)}\left[1-e^{-(\eta+\lambda)(t_2-t_1)}\right]$$

$$(10.18)$$

$$\left(\text{observation period is } t_2 - t_1\right)$$

The expected number of events by time t_2 in the patients of Cohort Q_a then is

$$E_a = (n_1 - d_1 - r)\frac{\lambda}{(\eta+\lambda)}\left[1-e^{-(\eta+\lambda)(t_2-t_1)}\right]$$

$$(10.19)$$

Furthermore, when we review the data at time t_1, another $n_2=n-n_1$ future subjects are to be enrolled between the time interval (t_1, t_R) and followed up until t_2 (the final analysis time). We call these n_2 subjects Cohort Q_b.

For Cohort Q_b, we need to include the patient entry time distribution into Equation 10.16. Let y_j be subject j's entry time. Y has the density function g(y) for $t_1 \le y \le t_R$. Let T_j be the potential event time and U_j be the censoring time of subject j; both are relative to the entry time y_j, and all are mutually independent. At calendar/real time t (relative to the study start time 0), the patient's study duration is $t-y_j$. We count subject j as having an event at time t only when the event happens within his or her study duration, $T_j \le (t-y_j)$, *and* happens before he/she drops out, $T_j \le U_j$; that is, the variable T_j will be observed whenever $T_j \le \min((t-y_j), U_j)$. Let $X_j(t)=\min(T_j, U_j, t-y_j)$, and $\delta_j = I_{\{T_j \le \min(t-y_j, U_j)\}}$, the data are the set $\{X_j, \delta_j, j=1, ..., n\}$ as before, and the counting process as a function of time t is $N_j(t)=I_{\{X_j \le t, \delta_j = 1\}}$.

For Cohort Q_b, the observation period length is t_2-t_1; the cumulative event rate at time $t_2 \geq t_R$ is

$$E[N_j(t_2)] = Pr(X_j \leq t_2,\ \delta_j = 1)$$

$$= Pr(\text{subject } j \text{ will have event by time } t_2,\ \textit{from time } t_1)$$

$$= E_y\left[Pr(T_j \leq t_2,\ T_j \leq U_j,\ T_j \leq (t_2-y_j)|y_j)\right]$$

$$= E_y\left[Pr(T_j \leq U_j,\ T_j \leq (t_2-y_j)|y_j)\right]$$

Y, T, and U are mutually independent, and from Equation 10.16,

$$= \int_{t_1}^{t_R}\left[\int_0^{t_2-y} H(s)f(s)ds\right]g(y)dy \qquad (10.20)$$

For example, with the exponential model as before, $H(s)=Pr(U>s)=e^{-\eta s}$, $f(s)=\lambda e^{-\lambda s}$, and with uniform entry pattern between $t_1 \leq y \leq t_R$, $g(y)=1/(t_R-t_1)$. Equation 10.20 indicates that

Pr (subject j in Cohort Q_b will have event by time t_2, *from time t_1*)

$$= \int_{t_1}^{t_R}\left[\int_0^{t_2-y} H(s)f(s)ds\right]g(y)dy$$

$$= \frac{1}{t_R-t_1}\int_{t_1}^{t_R}\left[\int_0^{t_2-y} H(s)f(s)ds\right]dy$$

$$= \frac{1}{t_R-t_1}\int_{t_1}^{t_R}\frac{\lambda}{(\eta+\lambda)}\left[1-e^{-(\eta+\lambda)(t_2-y)}\right]dy$$

$$= \frac{\lambda}{(\eta+\lambda)}\left[1-\left(\frac{1}{(\eta+\lambda)(t_R-t_1)}\right)^{\left(e^{-(\eta+\lambda)(t_2-t_R)}-e^{-(\eta+\lambda)(t_2-t_1)}\right)}\right]$$

The expected number of events by time t_2 in the patients of Cohort Q_b is

$$E_b = (n-n_1)\frac{\lambda}{(\eta+\lambda)}\left[1-\left(\frac{1}{(\eta+\lambda)(t_R-t_1)}\right)^{\left(e^{-(\eta+\lambda)(t_2-t_R)}-e^{-(\eta+\lambda)(t_2-t_1)}\right)}\right] \qquad (10.21)$$

Therefore, the additional total number of events expected at time t_2 is $d_2 = E_a + E_b$, the sum of Equations 10.19 and 10.21.

Given a fixed total information (event-driven trials) $E_T = d_1 + d_2$, we can solve for t_2 to answer the question: How long will it take for the study to reach the full number of required events?

On the other hand, for a maximum-duration trial (t_2 is fixed) to reach a certain number of events determined by power, we can solve for the required number of patients, n.

For either question, the parameters η and λ are plugged in by their estimates from the interim data. For Example 10.3, which is an event-driven trial, the required total number of events to reach is $120 = d_1 + d_2$. At the interim analysis, we have $n_1 = 111$, $n - n_1 = 230 - 111 = 119$, $d_1 = 16$, $r = 10$, $\lambda = 16/(65*12)$, $\eta = 10/(65*12)$, $t_1 = 18$ (months). Assuming the trial continues with the same uniform enrollment rate ($111/18 \approx 6$ patients per month), then $t_R = 18 + (119/6) \approx 38$ months. If we assume a more conservative uniform enrollment rate of 5 patients per month, then $t_R = 18 + (119/5) \approx 42$ months.

Therefore, we plug in the above information from the interim data in the following equation and solve for t_2:

$$120 - d_1 = (n_1 - d_1 - r)\frac{\lambda}{(\eta+\lambda)}\left[1 - e^{-(\eta+\lambda)(t_2-t_1)}\right]$$

$$+ (n - n_1)\frac{\lambda}{(\eta+\lambda)}\left[1 - \left(\frac{1}{(\eta+\lambda)(t_R-t_1)}\right)^{\left(e^{-(\eta+\lambda)(t_2-t_R)} - e^{-(\eta+\lambda)(t_2-t_1)}\right)}\right] \quad (10.22)$$

Using the R function in Appendix 10.2, we obtain $t_2 = 79$ months. This information is useful in managing the trial. For example, if the end time or sample size required is considered too long or too large, then effort at increasing the accrual rate and decreasing withdrawals should be strategized, or the trial might be judged to be futile (Homework 10.4–10.6).

10.4 Modification of the Classical GS Alpha-Spending Function Procedure

The previous sections discussed monitoring the maximum information or trial duration while keeping the trial blinded. This section discusses the situation using the classical GS procedure with unblinded interim analyses of the treatment effect. As we discussed in Chapter 9, we design the classical GS procedures with a fixed maximum total information. The expected total information may, however, be reduced with chances of early termination of the trial as a result of interim analyses. The alpha-spending function approach gives us the advantage of a flexible schedule and frequency of interim analyses, with the information times calculated by the fixed maximum total information as specified in the study protocol. In the FDA's *Guidance for Industry: Adaptive Design Clinical Trials for Drugs and Biologics* (CDER and CBER 2019), it was emphasized that trials with GS designs should clearly specify, in the protocol, how the alpha is to be spent during the trial. However, we also illustrated in Chapter 9 that the alpha-spending function may be altered when the observed maximum total information turns out to be different from the originally designed maximum total information. Therefore, in practice, we strive to keep the actual and designed maximum total information as close as possible in order to minimize the alteration. Regardless, only when the trial continues to its final analysis without early termination will we know the actual final total information. When this occurs, the final critical value should be updated with the actual information times of all interim analyses.

When the prespecified maximum information is uncertain and a reestimation based on an interim stage data is desired, Gould and Shih (1998) suggested performing a blinded SSR before the first GS (unblinded) interim analysis, and then using the reestimated maximum total information to reschedule the (classical) GS analyses.

Recently, *adaptive GS* (as opposed to classical GS) methods have developed as a popular topic, in which not only the frequency and schedule of the interim analyses may change, but the maximum total information may also increase in the middle of the trial. This section and the next only discuss the case where the changes are because of administrative reasons or external information (such as the COVID-19 pandemic interruption of accrual and visits), and not because of a comparative analysis of the interim data from the current trial. However, we must remain cautious that, unless there is a good reason to alter the plan designed in the protocol, the adaptive GS may not be a good idea, as illustrated in the following examples.

Example 10.4

A trial was planned with one interim analysis using an overall two-sided $\alpha=0.05$ and the linear spending function: $\alpha(t)=\alpha t$. Thus, $\alpha(1/2)=\alpha/2=0.025$, which leads to $|c_1|=2.2414$, and $\alpha(1)=\alpha=0.05$, $|c_2|=2.1251$. However, suppose that after $t_1=1/2$, the investigator, for administrative reasons, would like to add another interim analysis at $t_2=3/4$, with the same maximum information. We explore the available two options:

Option 1: Follow the classical GS procedure, keep the same $\alpha(t)=\alpha t$, and add $t_2=3/4$. Then, $|c_1|=2.2414$, $|c_2|=2.2885$, $|c_3|=2.2296$. All of these values can be calculated by the Lan-DeMets program and remain within the realm of the flexible alpha-spending function method. However, we emphasize that an observer will rightly make an issue of the change and ask whether the additional interim look at $t_2=3/4$ is "t_1-data-driven." Operationally, we must justify and convince others that the additional look at $t_2 = 3/4$ resulted from an administrative reason and was not driven by the unblinded t_1-data. Along this precautionary line, keeping the DMC independent from the sponsor and keeping the sponsor blinded to the efficacy data remains vital in avoiding data-driven changes in the monitoring process.

Note that $|c_1| = 2.2414$ remains unchanged (already occurred); the new $|c_2| = 2.2885 > |c_1|$ and also > the old $|c_2|$ (2.1251). Hence, unless there is a justifiable administrative reason, adding another look at $t_2 = 3/4$ is not always logical. Furthermore, the more interim analyses we perform, the more we suffer loss of power.

Option 2: Changing to a new spending function. A skeptic would express even more suspicion if the trial switched to another spending function after the first look. For example, if we switch to spending the rest of the 0.025 type I error via the Pocock-type boundary, then the new critical values are $|c_1| = 2.2414$, $|c_2| = 2.2551$, $|c_3| = 2.2551$. (The first value is fixed because it has already occurred. The second and third values are the same, as characterized by the Pocock-type boundary. A program can be found in Appendix 10.3 for the above calculation.) Suppose $Z_1 = 2.22$, then the regulatory agency would also rightly feel suspicious, because the Z_1 appears so close to $|c_1| = 2.2414$. On the other hand, switching to the OBF-type boundary after t_1 would also seem foolish, because the new critical values then would be $|c_1| = 2.2414$, $|c_2| = 2.4900$, $|c_3| = 2.1564$. (Again, the first value is fixed since it has already occurred. The second and third values have the relationship of $|c_2|\sqrt{3/4} = |c_3|$, as characterized by the OBF-type boundary.) We also note that the boundary jumps higher at t_2.

For both options, alpha = 0.05 remains preserved. We thus conclude that changing the frequency and/or the schedule of a planned interim analysis must be performed carefully. Even without changing the fixed maximum information, using a technically correct flexible alpha-spending function method, and preserving the type I error, the boundaries can look obscured, as demonstrated in Example 10.4. Flexibility can also cause loss of efficiency, as seen with a larger critical value for the additional interim analysis.

10.5 Adaptive GS Procedure—Change Not Dependent on Unblinded Interim Data

In Section 10.2.2, we discussed SSR with comparative analysis using the conditional power based on unblinded treatment effect at the interim analysis, where we studied how to adjust either the critical value of the final test (LSW likelihood method) or the final test statistic (CHW weighted test). Basically, SSR is a two-stage procedure. With more stages in the group sequential setting, Example 10.4 illustrated a situation where the maximum sample size remained unchanged, but an extra interim analysis was added after the first stage. Let us now examine a situation where the maximum total information is increased midstream of a group sequential trial. The key questions for finding the boundaries to preserve the overall α are: How large is the total information increased, and how will we spend the rest of the alpha sensibly? Here, we assume that the increase in the total information and the new schedule of the interim analyses are not driven by the unblinded interim efficacy data. We thus always ask up front, what is the purpose or cause of the change? Although the adaptive GS procedure is flexible, change without a justifiable reason derails the spirit of the design or method flexibility. Although efficiency is not the only or most important consideration in clinical trials, we should bear in mind that design or method for flexibility can cause loss of efficiency. Again, we discuss with examples.

We first work on a one-sided test ($\alpha=0.025$) with three planned analyses (two interim and one final analysis) based on the total information N, with boundary (c_1, c_2, c_3) given by

$$\alpha = \Pr\left(Z_1 > c_1 \text{ or } Z_2 > c_2 \text{ or } Z_3 > c_3 \mid H_0\right).$$

Suppose $c_1 = z_{\alpha_1}$ with a prespecified spending function that spends the type I error rate of α_1 for the first interim analysis at t_1. After the first interim analysis, the total information N is changed to N* ($>$N) and the new interim information at the second interim analysis is n_2^*. With this new total information, the new information times are $t_i^* = \dfrac{n_i^*}{N^*}$, for i=1, 2, 3, as shown in Table 10.1. Note that the old schedule ($t_1, t_2, 1$) becomes irrelevant for calculating the new boundary.

The new critical values are obtained by

$$\alpha - \alpha_1 = \Pr(Z_1 < z_{\alpha_1}, Z_2 > c_2 \text{ or } Z_3 > c_3 \mid H_0)$$

$$= \Pr(Z_1 < z_{\alpha_1}, Z_2^* > c_2^* \text{ or } Z_3^* > c_3^* \mid H_0) \quad (10.23)$$

TABLE 10.1

With Two Interim Analyses and One Final Analysis Planned Based on Total Information N

Original Schedule		Revised Schedule	
n_1	t_1	$n_1^* = n_1$	$t_1^* = \dfrac{n_1}{N^*}$
n_2	t_2	n_2^*	$t_2^* = \dfrac{n_2^*}{N^*}$
N	1 (old schedule no longer relevant)	$n_3^* = N^*$	$t_3^* = 1$

Note: After the first interim analysis, the total information N is changed to N* ($>$N).

We then solve the above equation for $\left(c_2^*,\ c_3^*\right)$ by numerical integration of the centered multivariate normal distribution with the following covariances/correlations:

$$\text{Cov}\left(Z_1,\ Z_2^*\right) = \text{Corr}\left(Z_1,\ Z_2^*\right) = \sqrt{n_1 / n_2^*} = \sqrt{t_1^* / t_2^*}$$

$$\text{Cov}\left(Z_1,\ Z_3^*\right) = \text{Corr}\left(Z_1,\ Z_3^*\right) = \sqrt{n_1 / N^*} = \sqrt{t_1^*}$$

$$\text{Cov}\left(Z_2^*,\ Z_3^*\right) = \text{Corr}\left(Z_2^*,\ Z_3^*\right) = \sqrt{n_2^* / N^*} = \sqrt{t_2^*}$$

and a specified relationship between c_2^* and c_3^*. For example, we may specify $c_2^* = c_3^*$ for the (z-value flat) Pocock-type boundary, $c_3^* = c_2^*\sqrt{\dfrac{n_2^*}{n_3^*}}$ for the (B-value flat) OBF-type boundary, or a general $c_3^* = f \times c_2^*$ for any $f \le 1$.

Example 10.5

Consider an initial plan that defines three analyses with equal time intervals, $t_1 = 1/3$, $t_2 = 2/3$, and $t_3 = 1$. The OBF-type boundary with corresponding critical values is ($c_1 = 3.71$, $c_2 = 2.51$, $c_3 = 1.99$). This implies that the alpha at the first interim analysis is $\alpha_1 = 0.00021$ (two-sided). Suppose that after $n_1 = 20$ patients, the sample sizes are revised to the following: $n_2 = 40$ becomes $n_2^* = 70$, $n_3 = N = 60$ becomes $n_3^* = N^* = 100$. This implies that the new schedule for analyses is $t_1^* = 0.2$, $t_2^* = 0.7$, and $t_3^* = 1$. If we continue to use the OBF-type boundary, then the revised critical values are calculated as ($c_1 = 3.71$, $c_2^* = 2.401$, $c_3^* = 2.009$). If we switch to using the Pocock-type boundary, then the revised critical values are ($c_1 = 3.71$, $c_2^* = 2.1397$, $c_3^* = 2.1397$).

The calculation cannot be performed using the Lan-DeMets program from Chapter 9, because their program is for the classical GS design with the alpha-spending function approach, not for the adaptive design as just described. Appendix 10.3 contains the R program used for the above calculation.

Example 10.6

Continue with the same setting of Example 10.5, but instead of modifying the schedule after the first interim analysis, we modify it after the second interim analysis: After $n_1 = 20$ and $n_2 = 40$, $n_3 = N = 60$ is revised to $n_3^* = N^* = 100$. This revision implies that the new schedule for analyses is $t_1^* = 0.2$, $t_2^* = 0.4$, and $t_3^* = 1.0$. If we continue to use the OBF-type boundary, then we calculate the revised critical values as ($c_1 = 3.71$, $c_2^* = 2.51$, $c_3^* = 2.0289$). Because the first two interim analyses have already occurred, the only change is their information times, not the critical values. Of course, the final critical value is also altered due to the change of the correlation structure.

In summary, increasing the sample size at an interim stage changes the information fraction/time. It also changes the critical values for later analyses in order to preserve the overall type I error rate. The final critical value will most likely be larger than the original design specified in the protocol. In Examples 10.5 and 10.6, the number of analyses remained unchanged. We thus generalize the adaptation to also changing the number of analyses with the increase in the total maximum information. That is, after j-th interim analysis, N changes to N* (>N), and K analyses change to K* analyses.

Example 10.7

Let us again look at the same scenario of having a one-sided test ($\alpha = 0.025$) with three planned analyses (two interim and one final) based on the total information N, with boundary (c_1, c_2, c_3) given by

$$\alpha = P\left(Z_1 > c_1 \text{ or } Z_2 > c_2 \text{ or } Z_3 > c_3 \mid H_0\right).$$

Suppose after the second interim analysis, N increases to N*, and K=3 increases to K*=5, as shown in Table 10.2.

Similar to Equation 10.23, we obtain critical values of the new boundary by solving

$$\alpha - \alpha_1 - \alpha_2 = P\left(Z_1 < z_{\alpha_1}, Z_2 < z_{\alpha_2}, Z_3 > c_3 \mid H_0\right)$$

$$= P\left(Z_1 < z_{\alpha_1}, Z_2 < z_{\alpha_2}, Z_3^* > c_3^* \text{ or } Z_4^* > c_4^* \text{ or } Z_5^* > c_5^* \mid H_0\right) \quad (10.24)$$

TABLE 10.2

With Two Interim Analyses and One Final Analysis Planned Based on Total Information N

Original Schedule		Revised Schedule	
n_1	t_1	$n_1^* = n_1$	$t_1^* = \dfrac{n_1}{N^*}$
n_2	t_2	$n_2^* = n_2$	$t_2^* = \dfrac{n_2}{N^*}$
N	1 (old schedule no longer relevant)	n_3^*	$t_3^* = \dfrac{n_3^*}{N^*}$
		n_4^*	$t_4^* = \dfrac{n_4^*}{N^*}$
		$n_5^* = N^*$	$t_5^* = 1$

Note: After the second interim analysis, the total information N is changed to N* (>N) and the total number of analyses K=3 is changed to K*=5.

With the notation $Z_i^* = Z_i$, $n_i^* = n_i$ for $i=1, 2$, we solve the above equation for $\left(c_3^*, c_4^*, c_5^*\right)$ by numerical integration of the centered multivariate normal distribution with the following covariances/correlations:

$$\text{Cov}\left(Z_i^*, Z_j^*\right) = \text{Corr}\left(Z_i^*, Z_j^*\right) = \sqrt{n_i^*/n_j^*} = \sqrt{t_i^*/t_j^*} \ \ i, j = 1, \ldots, 5$$

and a specified relationship among c_3^*, c_4^*, and c_5^*. Similar to the previous setting, we may specify $c_5^* = c_4^* = c_3^*$ for the (z-value flat) Pocock-type boundary, $c_j^* = c_3^* \sqrt{\dfrac{n_3^*}{n_j^*}} \, (j = 4, 5)$ for the (B-value flat) OBF-type boundary, or a general constraint $c_j^* = f_j \times c_3^*$ for any $f_5 \le f_4 \le 1$.

Example 10.7 (Continued)

Consider again the initial plan to have three equally spaced analyses at $t_1 = 1/3$, $t_2 = 2/3$, and $t_3 = 1$. The OBF-type boundary with corresponding critical values is then $(c_1 = 3.71, c_2 = 2.51, c_3 = 1.99)$. This implies that $\alpha_1 + \alpha_2 = 0.0121$ (two-sided). Suppose that after $n_1 = 20$ and $n_2 = 40$ patients, we revise the sample sizes and frequency of analyses to the following: $n_3 = N = 60$ becomes $n_3^* = 100$, $n_4^* = 120$, and $n_5^* = N^* = 150$. This further implies the new schedule for analyses as $t_1^* = 2/15$, $t_2^* = 4/15$, $t_3^* = 10/15$, $t_4^* = 12/15$, and $t_5^* = 1$. If we continue to use the OBF-type boundary, then we calculate the revised critical values as $(c_1 = 3.71, c_2 = 2.51, c_3^* = 2.592, c_4^* = 2.366, c_5^* = 2.116)$. If we switch to using the Pocock-type boundary, then we find the revised critical values as $(c_1 = 3.71, c_2 = 2.51, c_3^* = 2.274, c_4^* = 2.274, c_5^* = 2.274)$. We further note a jump in the OBF-type boundary in the new schedule at t_3^*. We have seen this kind of jump previously (Option 2 of Example 10.4 in this chapter; Practice 9.4 in Chapter 9).

Final Note: As we noted earlier, discussion of adaptive designs, including adaptive GS procedures, the change of the total maximum information may or may not depend on the unblinded interim effect size (i.e., with or without comparative analysis). The FDA's *Guidance for Industry: Adaptive Design Clinical Trials for Drugs and Biologics* (CDER and CBER 2019) specifically differentiates these two kinds of adaptations. In either case, we should always pay particular attention to the following issues: controlling the study-wide type I error rate, statistical bias in estimates of treatment effect associated with the study design adaptations, potential for increased type II error rate (i.e., loss of power), role of trial simulation in adaptive design planning and evaluation, and the role of a prospective statistical analysis plan.

Appendix 10.1

The SAS code for calculating (n_2, c) according to Eqs. (10.6) and (10.7) as in Li et al. (2002) and Shih et al. (2016) with default $h = -\infty$.

```
***Program for the calculation of critical values of LRT ;
***Last update: Oct 14, 2012;

option mprint symbolgen ps=58 nocenter;
%let prgnm=LRTCriticalValue;


*******************specify the function for n2/n1
***************************;
%macro n2_lrt;
      aa=(c_lrt+zbeta)*(c_lrt+zbeta)/(z*z)-1 ;
      n2_lrt=max( min(&n2max, aa*&n1), &n2min);
%mend n2_lrt ;


%macro C_lrt(n1=, n2min=, n2max=, h=, k=,   cp=, alpha=, inc=);

**** CP is conditional power ******;
****  inc is the increment used in integrations ****;
%if &inc= %then %let inc=0.0001;    ***set the default inc= 0.0001;
%if &h= %then %let h=-3.5;          ***set the default h= -3.5;

data alpha ;
      alpha=&alpha;
      zbeta=probit(&cp) ;
      h=max(-3.5, &h);
      k= min(4, &k) ;
        c1=1.0;
        c2=3.;
        c_lrt =2;
        do i=1 to 12;
            sum1=0;
            do z=&h to &k by &inc;
              %n2_lrt ;
              sum1=sum1+ probnorm((c_lrt*sqrt(&n1+n2_lrt)-
              z*sqrt(&n1))/sqrt(n2_lrt)) *
                    PDF('NORMAL', z);
            end;
            cnvg = sum1*&inc+&alpha-(1-probnorm(&h));
            if cnvg >0 then c2=c_lrt ;
            else if cnvg < 0 then c1=c_lrt ;
            c_lrt=0.5*(c1+c2);
```

```
        end;
        output;
        call symput('c_lrt',put(c_lrt,5.3));
run;

title "Generated by &prgnm..sas";
title2 "n1=&n1, n2min=&n2min, n2max=&n2max, alpha=&alpha,
h=&h, and k=&k";
footnote 'cnvg should be close to zero when the numerical
approximation procedure converges';
proc print noobs;
var  C_lrt   C1 C2      cnvg ;
run;


%mend c_lrt;

%c_lrt(n1=100, n2min=20, n2max=200, h=,   k=2.5,      cp=0.90,
alpha=0.025, inc=0.0001);
%*c_lrt(n1=100, n2min=20, n2max=200, h=0.675,   k=2.5,
cp=0.90, alpha=0.025, inc=0.0001);
```

Appendix 10.2

The R function to solve for t_2 in Equation 10.22.

```
# Monitoring time to study end at an interim analysis of an
    event-driven trial
# Input: n1 = number of patients at the interim analysis
    (first cohort)
# t1 = time of the interim analysis
# n2 = number of patients yet to enroll after the time of
    interim analysis (second cohort)
# lambda = estimated event rate
# nta = estimated loss-to-follow-up rate
# d1 = number of events occurred at the interim analysis in
    the first cohort
# d2 = number of additional events yet to occur after the
    interim analysis
# loss = number of patients lost-to-followup before observing
    event in the first cohort
# tr = enroll period of time from t1 for the second cohort

bisect <- function(n1 = 111,n2 = 119, lambda = 16/(65*12),nta =
    10/(65*12),t1 = 18, d1 = 16, d2 = 104, loss = 10, tr = 42,
    e = 0.001) {
a = tr
b = 5*tr
for(i in 1:100) {
    f = function(x) {
```

```
    lam_nta = lambda+nta
    Qa = (n1-d1-loss)*(lambda/lam_nta)*
            (1-exp(0-lam_nta*(x-t1)))
    Qb = (n2*lambda/lam_nta)*(1-(exp(0-lam_nta*(x-tr))-
            exp(0-lam_nta*(x-t1)))/(lam_nta*(tr-t1)))
    d2-Qa-Qb
    }
    if (f (a) *f (b) < 0 & abs (f (a) -f (b) ) >e) {
        c = (a+b)/2
        if (f(c)*f(a)<0) b = c
        else a = c
        }
        g = cbind(i,c, a, b)
        }
        g
}
# Run the example
bisect()
```

Appendix 10.3

The R program for adaptive GS procedure—change does not depend on
unblinded interim data.

```
# Written by Yong Lin at the Biostatistics Department Rutgers
    School of Public Health
# See example runs and lecture notes for input notation
# Need to Load package mvtnorm first
Library(mvtnorm)
c.values.adapt <- function(n.new, fi.new = rep(1,length(n.
    new)), n.old, C.old, alpha = 0.05, side = 1) {
    set.seed(501)
    j <- length(n.old)
    k <- length(n.new)
    n <- c(n.old, n.new+n.old[j])
    cor.mat <- n%o% (1/n)
    cor.mat[lower.tri(cor.mat)] <- 1/cor.mat[lower.tri(cor.mat) ]
    cor.mat <- sqrt(cor.mat)

if(side = =1) {
    fun <- function(ci, fv) sapply(ci, function(x) abs(1-
      pmvnorm(upper = c(C.old, x*fv),corr = cor.mat,
          algorithm = GenzBretz(abseps = 1e-12))-alpha))
    fun2 <- function(ci, fv) sapply(ci, function(x)
      1-pmvnorm(upper = c(C.old, x*fv),corr = cor.mat,
          algorithm = GenzBretz(abseps = 1e-12))-alpha)
}
else if (side = =2) {
    fun <- function(ci, fv) sapply(ci, function(x)abs(1-
```

```
      pmvnorm(lower = -c(C.old, x*fv),upper = c(C.old, x*fv),
            corr = cor.mat,algorithm = GenzBretz(abseps =
                          1e-12))-alpha))
      fun2 <- function(ci, fv) sapply(ci, function(x)1-
        pmvnorm(lower = -c(C.old, x*fv),upper = c(C.old, x*fv),
          corr = cor.mat,algorithm = GenzBretz(abseps =
                          1e-12))-alpha)
  }

  c.val <- optimize(f = fun,interval = c(0,10),fv = fi.new,tol =
      1e-9)$minimum
  c.val2 <- uniroot(f = fun2,interval = c(0,10),fv = fi.new,tol
      = 1e-9)
  Ci<- c.val*fi.new
  names(C.old) <- paste('C',1:j,'.old',sep = '')
  names (Ci) <- paste('C',1:k,'.new',sep = '')
  ti <- n/n[j+k]

  if(j = =i) alpha.left <- alpha - (1-pnorm(C.old))
  else alpha.left <- alpha - (1-pmvnorm(upper = C.old, corr =
      cor.mat[1:j,1:j]))
    return(list(C = c.val,C2 = c.val2, cut_value = c(C.old,Ci),
      corr = cor.mat, information_time = ti, alpha =
      c(alpha,alpha.left)))
  }
# Chapter10-Example 10.4-option2
    # switch to Pocock type
c.values.adapt(n.new = c (30-20,4 0-20),fi.new = 0(1,1), n.old =
    c(20), C.old = 0(2.2414), side = 2)
    # switch to OBF type
c.values.adapt(n.new = c(30-20,40-20),fi.new =
    c(1,sqrt(30/40)),n.old = c(20), C.old = c(2.2414),
    side = 2)
# Chapter10-Example 10.5
# switch to OBF type
c.values.adapt(n.new = c (70-20,100-20),fi.new =
    c(1,sqrt(70/100)),n.old = c(20),C.old = c(3.71), side = 2)
# Chapter10-Example 10.6
    c.values.adapt(n.new = c(100-40),fi.new = c(1),n.old =
    c (20,40), C.old = 0(3.71,2.51), side = 2)
# Chapter10-Example 10.7
    c.values.adapt(n.new = c(100-4 0,120-4 0,150-40),fi.new =
    c(1,sqrt(100/120),sqrt(100/150)),n.old = c(20,40),C.old =
    c(3.71,2.51), side = 2)
```

HOMEWORK 10.1

Prove Equation 10.1.

HOMEWORK 10.2

Show that Eq. (10.3) is equivalent to Equation (8.10) by setting $1.96 = c$, $t = \dfrac{N_1}{N}$, $N_1 = 2n_1$, $N - N_1 = 2n_2$, $\sigma = 1$.

HOMEWORK 10.3

Follow Example 10.2, and obtain the final critical value if $f_{max} = \dfrac{n_{2max}}{n_1} = 2$ and $t = 0.4$.

HOMEWORK 10.4

Refer to Example 10.3. Vary the patient early withdrawal rate to different levels: 10/65, 9/65, 8/65, ..., 1/65, and 0 (per patient-year). Comment on its effect on the solution of t_2.

HOMEWORK 10.5

In Equation 10.20, use the exponential model as before, $H(s) = Pr(U > s) = e^{-\eta s}$, $f(s) = \lambda e^{-\lambda s}$. However, instead of the uniform entry pattern, use the (general) truncated exponential model:

$$g(\gamma, y) = \frac{\gamma e^{-\gamma y}}{1 - e^{-\gamma(t_R - t_1)}}, \qquad \gamma \neq 0$$

$$= 1/(t_R - t_1) \qquad \gamma = 0 \ (\text{the uniform entry case})$$

for $t_1 \leq y \leq t_R$.
Show that, for $\gamma \neq 0$,
$Pr(\text{subject } j \text{ in Cohort } Q_b \text{ will have event by time } t_2, \text{ from time } t_1)$

$$= \int_{t_1}^{t_R} \left[\int_0^{t_2 - y} H(s)f(s)ds \right] g(y)dy$$

$$= \frac{\lambda}{(\eta + \lambda)} \left[e^{-\gamma t_1} - \frac{\gamma}{(\eta + \lambda - \gamma)\left[1 - e^{-\gamma(t_R - t_1)}\right]} \left[e^{-(\eta + \lambda)(t_2 - t_R) - \gamma t_R} - e^{-(\eta + \lambda)(t_2 - t_1) - \gamma t_1} \right] \right]$$

HOMEWORK 10.6

Refer to the formula $d_2 = E_a + E_b$, where d_2 is the additional total number of events expected by time t_2; E_a and E_b are given by Equations 10.19 and 10.21, respectively. Assume the same exponential models for the primary event and loss to follow-up and uniform enrollment as in Equation 10.22. For a maximum-duration trial (t_2 is fixed) to reach a certain number of events (d_1 and d_2) determined by power, write an R program (similar to the one in Appendix 10.2) to solve for the required number of subjects, n.

HOMEWORK 10.7

Use the R program c.values.adapt in Appendix 10.3 to perform the following adaptive GS design:

A trial was designed with a maximum total sample size of 120 subjects with six equally spaced analyses planned (five interim and one final) using the Pocock-type boundary: (2.453758, 2.453758, 2.453758, 2.453758, 2.453758, 2.453758) to control two-sided alpha=0.05.

a. After the third interim analysis, the investigator wishes to change the plan and would like to conduct four additional analyses with the following revised sample sizes: 80, 100, 130, 150 (instead of the original three at 80, 100, 120) and continue to use the Pocock-type boundary. Assume the change occurred due to some administrative reason. Find and discuss the new boundary.

b. Suppose that, after the second interim analysis, the investigator wishes to change the plan and would like to conduct only two additional analyses with the sample sizes set at 80 and 100 (instead of the original four at 60, 80, 100, and 120). Continue to use the Pocock-type boundary. Assume the change occurred due to some administrative reason. Find and discuss the new boundary.

(This exercise explores how flexible the adaptive GS procedure can be by using the R program c.values.adapt. We do not suggest that anyone should conduct a study in such a fashion without a justifiable, administrative reason.)

References

Bowden J. and Mander A. (2014). A review and re-interpretation of a group-sequential approach to sample size re-estimation in two-stage trials. *Pharmaceutical Statistics* 13: 163–172.

Broberg P. (2013). Sample size re-assessment leading to a raised sample size does not inflate type I error rate under mild conditions. *BMC Medical Research Methodology* 13:94

CDER and CBER (US Department of Health and Human Services, Food and Drug Administration, Center for Drug Evaluation and Research and Center for Biologics Evaluation and Research). (2019). *Guidance for Industry: Adaptive Design Clinical Trials for Drugs and Biologics*, November 2019. *https://www.fda.gov/regulatory-information/search-fda-guidance-documents/adaptive-design-clinical-trials-drugs-and-biologics-guidance-industry/* (accessed on March 1, 2021).

Chen YH, DeMets DL, Lan KKG. (2004). Increasing the sample size when the unblinded interim result is promising. *Statistics in Medicine* 23: 1023–1038.

Cui L, Hung HM, Wang SJ. (1999). Modification of sample size in group sequential clinical trials. *Biometrics* 55: 853–857.

Denne JS. (2001). Sample size recalculation using conditional power. *Statistics in Medicine* 20: 2645–2660.

EMEA (European Medicines Agency) CHMP (Committee for Medicinal Products for Human Use). Refection paper on methodological issues in confirmatory clinical trials with flexible design and analysis plan. London, 23 March 2006 Doc. Ref. CHMP/EWP/2459/02. http://www.emea.eu.int

Li G, Shih WJ, Xie T and Lu J. (2002). A sample size adjustment procedure for clinical trials based on conditional power. *Biostatistics* 3(2): 277–287.

Li G, Shih WJ, Wang Y. (2005). Two-stage adaptive design for clinical trials with survival data. *Journal of Biopharmaceutical Statistics* 15: 707–718.

Gould AL and Shih WJ. (1992). Sample size reestimation without unblinding for normally distributed outcomes with unknown variance. *Communications in Statistics (A)* 21: 2833–2853.

Gould AL and Shih WJ. (1998). Modifying the design of ongoing trials without unblinding. *Statistics in Medicine* 17: 89–100.

Mehta CR and Pocock SJ. (2011). Adaptive increase in sample size when interim results are promising: A practical guide with examples. *Statistics in Medicine* 30: 3267–3284.

Proschan MA, Lan KKG, and Wittes JT. (2006). *Statistical Monitoring of Clinical Trials: A Unified Approach*. New York: Springer.

Shih WJ. (1992). Sample size reestimation in clinical trials. In *Biopharmaceutical Sequential Statistical Applications*; Peace, KE (Ed.), New York: Marcel Dekker, 285–301.

Shih WJ and Long J. (1998). Blinded sample size re-estimation with unequal variances and center effects in clinical trials. *Communications in Statistics, Theory & Method* 27: 395–408.

Shih WJ, Li G, Wang Y. (2016). Methods for flexible sample-size design in clinical trials: Likelihood, weighted, dual test, and promising zone approaches. *Contemporary Clinical Trials* 47: 40–48.

Wang Y, Li G, Shih WJ. (2010). Estimation and confidence intervals for two-stage sample-size-flexible design with LSW likelihood approach. *Statistics in BioSciences* 2: 180–190.

11

Multiplicity Issues and Methods for Controlling the Type I Error Rate

Multiplicity refers to situations in a trial in which multiple statistical tests or analyses create multiple ways to "win" for treatment efficacy or safety. Multiplicity arises in clinical trials such as multiple endpoints, multiple treatment arms, multiple subgroups, multiple time points, multiple analyses, composite endpoints and their components, and combinations of the above. In fact, we have seen some of these topics in previous chapters, such as the group sequential procedure, which belongs to the category of multiple analyses at multiple times. We have learned how to control the overall type I error rate by the Lan-DeMets alpha-spending function approach (see Chapter 9). We have also used the simplest Bonferroni method to adjust for multiple testing of hypotheses when calculating the power and sample size (see Chapter 4). The increasing interest in this topic reflects apparent trends in clinical drug development, where much emphasis is placed on increasing efficiency of clinical drug development through sophisticated adaptive designs and comprehensive characterization of the efficacy and safety profiles of new treatments. Modern clinical trials use complex sets of objectives and hypotheses, particularly involving multiple endpoints evaluated at several dose levels or in several patient populations, with interim analyses, which gives rise to increasingly more complex multiplicity problems. An example can be found in the pembrolizumab KEYNOTE-048 trial (Medical Director Merck Sharp & Dohme Corp 2019), where 12 primary objectives/hypotheses were formed from a combination treatment groups, endpoints, and patient populations. In this chapter, before we discuss more adaptive designs in the next few chapters, we learn the fundamental concept of controlling the rate of false-positive inferences (known formally as the familywise error rate, or FWER), which is the requirement in confirmatory clinical trials with multiple objectives. Several commonly used methods are discussed and illustrated with examples taken from the literature of recent clinical trials.

11.1 General Notation and Familywise Error Rate

The following notation will be used throughout this chapter. Consider a general multiplicity problem in a confirmatory clinical trial with several objectives, for example, several endpoints or dose–control comparisons.

Let m denote the number of objectives expressed by scientific hypotheses. The null hypotheses related to the objectives are denoted by $H_1, ..., H_m$. Each null hypothesis is defined by such treatment differences corresponding to lack of expected treatment effect. As in some of the previous chapters, let θ_i denote the true value of the treatment difference for the i-th objective ($i = 1, ..., m$). For example, in a trial with m endpoints, θ_i represents the true treatment effect difference for the i-th endpoint between the test group and the control group. As we have seen in Chapter 4, for continuous endpoints, mean changes from baseline are usually the measure of a group treatment effect. For binary endpoints, the measure is the probability of an event. In oncology trials, log-hazard ratios of, say PFS (progression-free survival time) and OS (overall survival time), are often seen for comparing treatment effects between test and control groups, and then $m = 2$. In the next section, as we discuss several commonly used methods, the (unadjusted) p-values $p_1, ..., p_m$ for testing the corresponding null hypotheses $H_1, ..., H_m$ will be used. Let $p_{(1)} \leq ... \leq p_{(m)}$ denote the ordered p-values, and the associated ordered null hypotheses are $H_{(1)}, ..., H_{(m)}$. Finally, a one-sided setting is assumed throughout this chapter, and the overall one-sided error rate is set to be $\alpha = 0.025$.

The intersection of hypotheses $H_0 = \bigcap_{i=1}^{m} H_i$ (i.e., H_1 and H_2 and ... and H_m) is the so-called *global hypothesis*. Under this global hypothesis, all the m null hypotheses in this family are true. Rejecting this global hypothesis simply says "rejecting H_1 or H_2, ..., or H_m". In other words, it means "rejecting some (at least one) of the m (null) hypotheses." This is rather non-specific. We usually are also interested in knowing which individual hypothesis (member) of the family of m null hypotheses is being rejected. (Rejecting the null hypothesis j, for example, means "winning" the endpoint, or subgroup, or dose group j.) Global tests (i.e., tests for the global hypothesis) are usually used in early-stage development. The later phase confirmatory trials also require more specific conclusions on individual hypotheses. We shall focus on confirmatory trials in this chapter.

A global test procedure is said to control the FWER *weakly* if it ensures that the probability of rejecting at least one (null) hypothesis when all (null) hypotheses are true is no greater than α. In notation, it is written as

$$\Pr(\text{rejecting any } H_i \mid H_0) \leq \alpha.$$

where "rejecting any H_i" is equivalent to "rejecting H_0". In the one-way analysis of variance (ANOVA, see Chapter 5), where there are several treatment groups in comparison, the general F-test is such a global test. We usually would follow the F-test to perform "contrasts" for specific pairwise comparisons. The Bonferroni test, which splits the overall α level evenly among the individual tests for each member hypothesis, that is, a specific hypothesis H_i is rejected when $p_i < \alpha/m$, is also such a test. This is because

$$\Pr(\text{rejecting any } H_i \mid H_0) = P_{H_0}\left\{ \bigcup_{i=1}^{m}\left(p_i < \frac{\alpha}{m} \right) \right\}$$

$$\leq \sum_{i=1}^{m} P_{H_0}\left\{ p_i < \frac{\alpha}{m} \right\} = m \times \frac{\alpha}{m} = \alpha \tag{11.1}$$

Notice that in the above second to the last equality, we have used a well-known property that the p-value has a uniform (0, 1) distribution under the null hypothesis (see Appendix 11.1).

Actually, the Bonferroni test guarantees the following stronger property. Let $H = \{H_1, \ldots, H_m\}$, and let H' be a subset of H. Let $\mathcal{H}$ denote the family of all the 2^m-1 subsets of H. Then, like the global hypothesis H_0 defined before for H, denote by $\mathcal{H}_0$ the intersection of all the subsets H' in $\mathcal{H}$. The probability of rejecting the hypothesis $\mathcal{H}_0$ when it is true is not greater than α. This property is referred to as *strong* control of the FWER and can be expressed as

$$\Pr(\text{rejecting } \mathcal{H}_0 \mid \mathcal{H}_0) \leq \alpha, \tag{11.2}$$

where "rejecting $\mathcal{H}_0$" is equivalent to "rejecting any subset H' of H". Since H is also a subset of itself, in addition to all the individual hypotheses and others, the above criterion is stronger than the "weak control." Further, the above criterion is equivalent to

$$\max\{\Pr(\text{rejecting } H' \mid H')\} \leq \alpha, \tag{11.3}$$

where the maximum is over all H' in $\mathcal{H}_0$.

Example 11.1

We have $(\theta_1, \theta_2, \theta_3)$ as unknown treatment effect values (test vs. control) for three endpoints in a superiority trial. The individual (null) hypotheses are: $H_1 : \theta_1 = 0$, $H_2 : \theta_2 = 0$, and $H_3 : \theta_3 = 0$. $H = \{H_1, H_2, H_3\}$. The global hypothesis of H is $H_0 : \theta_1 = \theta_2 = \theta_3 = 0$. There are $2^3-1 = 7$ possible subsets of H, corresponding to null hypotheses configurations as follows: (0, 0, 0), $(\theta_1, 0, 0)$, $(0, \theta_2, 0)$, $(0, 0, \theta_3)$, $(\theta_1, \theta_2, 0)$, $(\theta_1, 0, \theta_3)$, and $(0, \theta_2, \theta_3)$, where (0, 0, 0) is H (or written as $H_1 \cap H_2 \cap H_3$), $(\theta_1, 0, 0)$ is $\{H_2, H_3\}$ (or written as $H_2 \cap H_3$), $(0, \theta_2, \theta_3)$ is H_1, etc. They compose $\mathcal{H}$ and the hypothesis $\mathcal{H}_0$: intersection of all these 7 subsets. Rejecting $\mathcal{H}_0$ means to reject any of these 7 subsets.

The International Conference on Harmonization (ICH) guidelines as well as the guidance documents released by the European Medicines Agency (EMA) and the US Food and Drug Administration (FDA) all require in confirmatory clinical trials with multiple objectives that the test procedures being used should control FWER strongly.

11.2 Multiple Endpoints and Efficacy Win Criteria

All confirmatory clinical trials involve more than one endpoint. Some are designated as primary and co-primary, some are designated as secondary endpoints, etc. Carefully triaging endpoints to primary and secondary is a very important consideration, but not sufficient in the trial design. When there are multiple primary endpoints, the trial should specify a "win scenario" for the set of primary endpoints that determines whether the trial has met its efficacy objectives. Examples of efficacy win criteria may be as follows: (1) All specified primary endpoints need to show clinically meaningful and statistically significant treatment efficacy; (2) at least one of the specified primary endpoints needs to show clinically meaningful and statistically significant treatment efficacy; and (3) a prespecified subset of primary endpoints need to show clinically meaningful and statistically significant treatment efficacy. For criterion (1), there is no concern of type I error rate inflation, hence no multiplicity issue. However, we need to make sure the design has adequate statistical power for each endpoint. For criterion (2), simply rejecting the global hypothesis only controls the FWER weakly, as discussed in the last section. We need to identify which primary endpoint did win. The control of FWER in the strong sense becomes necessary for criterion (2). Criterion (3) implies there is a hierarchical order existing among the endpoints, so the test procedure should take it into consideration as well.

11. 3 Commonly Used Methods

We introduce commonly used methods that strongly control the FWER in this section. We start from the simple ones to gradually more sophisticated procedures for complex situations. As we can see, all these procedures pay attention to the individual hypothesis.

11.3.1 Bonferroni Method

The Bonferroni method is the commonly used for sample size calculation when there are multiple (m) objectives to share the same overall α. It is the simplest and most conservative procedure. Simply split the overall α evenly to each objective. The objective-associated hypothesis H_i is rejected when $p_i < \alpha/m$. It is easy to see that the Bonferroni procedure preserves the FWER strongly. First, for each individual H_i, $\Pr(H_i \mid H_i) = P_{H_i}(p_i < \alpha/m) = \dfrac{\alpha}{m} < \alpha$. Second, for any intersection of H_i's, $\Pr(\text{intersection of } H_i\text{'s}|H_i\text{'s}) \leq \Pr(\text{an individual } H_i|H_i\text{'s}) = \dfrac{\alpha}{m} < \alpha$ Therefore, (11.2) or (11.3) is satisfied.

11.3.2 Holm's Method

Holm (1979) gave the following improved Bonferroni procedure based on ordered p-values.

Step 1. If $p_{(1)} < \alpha/m$, reject $H_{(1)}$ and go to Step 2; otherwise, stop.

Step 2. If $p_{(2)} < \alpha/(m-1)$, reject $H_{(2)}$ and go to Step 3; otherwise, stop.

...

Step m. If $p_{(m)} < \alpha$, reject $H_{(m)}$ and stop.

The above is known as a "step-down" procedure since it starts with the most significant (smallest p-value) to the least significant objective.

Example 11.2

There are three endpoints, m=3, in a trial. $H_{(1)}$ is rejected when $p_{(1)} < \alpha/3$. $H_{(2)}$ is rejected when $p_{(1)} < \dfrac{\alpha}{3}$ and $p_{(2)} < \dfrac{\alpha}{2}$. $H_{(3)}$ is rejected when $p_{(1)} < \dfrac{\alpha}{3}$, $p_{(2)} < \dfrac{\alpha}{2}$, and $p_{(3)} < \alpha$. Thus, all individual hypotheses, regardless of its order in the significance level, are controlled by α. Any intersection hypothesis will have its level less than that of an individual hypothesis involved in the intersection and thus is also controlled by α.

11.3.3 Hochberg's Method

Hochberg (1988) gave the following improved Bonferroni procedure based on ordered p-values.

Step 1. If $p_{(m)} < \alpha$, reject $H_{(i)}$ for all i=1, ..., m and stop; otherwise, go to Step 2.

Step 2. If $p_{(m-1)} < \alpha/2$, reject $H_{(i)}$ for i=1, ..., m-1 and stop; otherwise, go to Step 3.

...

Step m. If $p_{(1)} < \alpha/m$, reject $H_{(1)}$ and stop.

The above is known as a "step-up" procedure since it starts with the least significant (largest p-value) to the most significant objective.

Example 11.3

There are three endpoints, m=3, in a trial. We win all three endpoints (i.e., reject all hypotheses) if $p_{(3)} < \alpha$. We win only two endpoints that correspond to $p_{(1)} < p_{(2)} < \dfrac{\alpha}{2}$ when $p_{(3)} > \alpha$. We win only one endpoint that corresponds $p_{(1)} < \dfrac{\alpha}{3}$ when $p_{(2)} > \dfrac{\alpha}{2}$ and $p_{(3)} > \alpha$.

Comment: Holm's method is based on the Bonferroni inequality (11.1) and is valid regardless of the joint distribution of the test statistics (i.e., it is nonparametric). Hochberg's method is more powerful than Holm's method, but the test statistics need to be independent or have a distribution with multivariate total positivity of order two or a scale mixture thereof for its validity (Sarkar 1998).

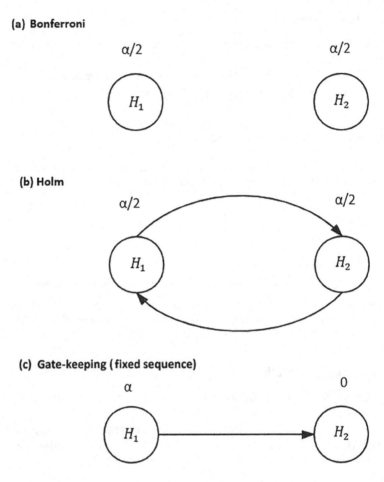

(a) Bonferroni

(b) Holm

(c) Gate-keeping (fixed sequence)

FIGURE 11.1
Bonferroni, Holm, and gate-keeper methods.

Therefore, Holm's method is usually preferred. Since Holm's method is based on the Bonferroni inequality, it is sometimes also called the Holm–Bonferroni procedure. Figure 11.1 depicts how Holm's method works for $m = 2$ in relation to the Bonferroni method and gate-keeper method, which is one of the several generalizations of the Holm–Bonferroni procedure introduced in the next section.

11.3.4 Generalization of Holm's Method

The generalization of the Holm–Bonferroni procedure is particularly useful in dealing with complex multiplicity situations. However, it is easier to follow by considering only two endpoints (or two populations) first. We started with the familiar Bonferroni method, which is known to be conservative by splitting the whole α by half to each endpoint. An improvement in gaining power and still strongly controlling the FWER is Holm's step-down method: First, allocate α/2 to each endpoint. Then, when winning on one endpoint at α/2, test the other endpoint at α. In other words, when we reject one hypothesis (at α/2 level), the α/2 is added to the next endpoint so that the next endpoint is tested at α/2+α/2=α level. Power gain is easily seen here. See Figure 11.1(a) and (b). Further generalization has two important parts: (1) Allocate the alpha unevenly when there is an initial (*a priori*) *weighing* consideration on the endpoints, say one endpoint gets wα and the other one gets (1-w)α, where 0≤w ≤1, and (2) assign connection chain (also with weight) for each endpoint to propagate the initially allocated alpha to test another endpoint when winning one endpoint. For there are connection chains between endpoints, this procedure is also known as *chain procedure*.

The "initially allocated alpha" in the chain procedure is also called "local alpha." The special case of w=0 or 1 of this chain procedure becomes the so-called *gate-keeping (fixed sequence) procedure*, where the endpoint given w=1 is the "gate-keeper" and the connection (weight) chain from the gate-keeper to the next is a one-way direction. See Figure 11.1(c). The "gate-keeper" is tested first at the whole α level. Only when it wins will the next endpoint in line be tested, also at the whole α level, etc. Obviously, the order of the endpoints becomes crucial in this testing strategy and requires careful consideration by both clinical meaning and statistical power of the endpoints. The pembrolizumab KEYNOTE-048 trial with 12 primary hypotheses, which we mentioned earlier, is a good example that illustrates the use of the gate-keeper procedure.

When there are m>2 endpoints, let $\alpha_i = w_i\alpha$ be the initial local alpha assigned to endpoint $i, i = 1, \ldots, m$, such that the sum of them is the total α. The chain procedure is best handled with graphs as shown by Maurer and Bretz (2013) and Dmitrienko, D'Agostino, and Huque (2013), which has become very popular for complex multiplicity situations. In the graphical chain procedure, the circles (as seen in Figure 11.1) represent the null hypotheses, and the weight w_i is displayed aside each hypothesis circle defining the initial alpha level used in the corresponding significance test prior to any alpha propagation. The rules of alpha propagation are defined by a set of (directed) connecting chain weights (g_{ij}) from H_i to H_j. The connection weights are chosen such that $g_{ii} = 0, g_{i1} + g_{i2} + \ldots + g_{im} \leq 1$, for every $i = 1, \ldots, m$. These chain weights specify the fractions of the error rate available after rejecting H_i that are transferred to other hypotheses. They are labeled by "Transition Matrix" in the R package "gMCP" GUI (see Appendix 11.2) and are conditional probabilities, which is better explained in the following illustrative Example 11.4 for m=3.

Example 11.4:

In Figure 11.2, we consider a trial with objectives regarding the hypotheses of three endpoints. The initial local alpha allocated to H_1 and H_2 are positive weights $w_1 = 0.25$ and $w_2 = 0.75$, respectively. A zero weight is assigned to H_3. Thus, for an overall one-sided $\alpha = 0.025$, we test H_1 at $\alpha_1 = 0.00625$ and H_2 at $\alpha_2 = 0.01875$, and do not test H_3 at the first step. (This is a situation where H_1 and H_2 could be hypotheses for two primary endpoints with unequal importance or priority, and H_3 could be for the secondary endpoint.) The alpha propagation rule defined by the weight of the (directed) connection weights from H_1 to H_2 is $g_{12} = 0.9$, and to H_3 is $g_{13} = 0.1$. They specify the fractions of the error rate available after rejecting H_1 that are transferred to H_2 ($0.9 \times \alpha_1$) and H_3 ($0.1 \times \alpha_1$), respectively. Notice that the rejection of H_1 opens a possibility to test H_3 and increases the chance of rejecting H_2.

Similarly, the weights of the outgoing connections for H_2 are given by $g_{21} = 0.8$ (from H_2 to H_1) and $g_{23} = 0.2$ (from H_2 to H_3). Notice that the rejection of H_2 increases the chance of rejecting H_1 and opens a possibility to test H_3 (by a greater extent than the case of rejecting H_1 seen above since $\alpha_2 > \alpha_1$ and $g_{23} > g_{13}$).

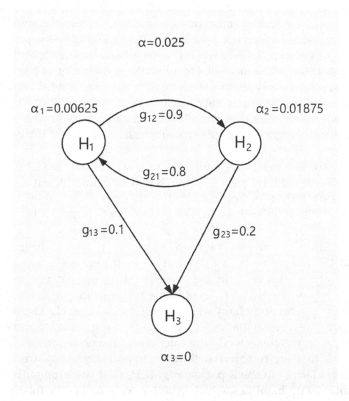

FIGURE 11.2
Three endpoints with different initial local alphas and chain weights (Example 11.4).

It is easy to see the meaning of g_{ij} as conditional probabilities of rejecting H_j given H_i has been rejected under $\{H_i, H_j\}$ by looking at H_1 and H_2 first in the following. Let A denote "rejecting H_1" and B denote "rejecting H_2". We use the following basic principle: $\Pr(A)=\Pr(A \mid B)\Pr(B)+\Pr(A \mid B^c)\Pr(B^c)$, where B^c denotes "not B" (or "complementary set of B"). Then, $\Pr(\text{rejecting } H_1)=\Pr(\text{rejecting } H_1 \mid \text{rejecting } H_2)\Pr(\text{rejecting } H_2)+\Pr(\text{rejecting } H_1 \mid \text{not rejecting } H_2)\Pr(\text{not rejecting } H_2)$. Under $\{H_1, H_2\}$, $\Pr(\text{rejecting } H_1) = g_{21}\alpha_2 + \alpha_1(1-\alpha_2) \le \alpha_1 + \alpha_2 = 0.00625 + 0.01875 = 0.025$. By the same way, $\Pr(\text{rejecting } H_2) = g_{12}\alpha_1 + \alpha_2(1-\alpha_1) \le \alpha_1 + \alpha_2 = 0.025$. As for H_3, it can only be tested after either H_1 or H_2 is rejected. Thus, under $\{H_1, H_2, H_3\}$, $\Pr(\text{rejecting } H_3)=\Pr(\text{rejecting } H_3 \mid \text{rejecting } H_1)\Pr(\text{rejecting } H_1)+\Pr(\text{rejecting } H_3 \mid \text{rejecting } H_2)\Pr(\text{rejecting } H_2) = g_{13}\alpha_1 + g_{23}\alpha_2 \le \alpha_1 + \alpha_2 = 0.025$.

Notice that in general, every individual hypothesis H_i is tested at

$$(w_i\alpha)\prod_{j\ne i}^{m}(1-w_j\alpha)+\sum_{j\ne i}^{m} g_{ji}(w_j\alpha) \le \alpha\left(w_i + \sum_{j\ne i} w_j\right)=\alpha.$$ The allocation

of the local alphas $\alpha_i = w_i\alpha$ and the strategy of placing the connecting weights g_{ij} are important design considerations for trials with multiple hypotheses. The graphical chain procedure is obviously a very helpful tool for the clarity of the design. After the initial setup in the design, we also need to do the test when data arrive. The testing then involves a dynamic updating of the initial graph. We continue the discussion in the next section.

11.3.5 Updating Algorithm of the Graphical Chain Procedure

Let us recap the two key components of the graphical chain procedure:

- $\alpha_i = w_i\alpha$ are the initial local alpha assigned to endpoint $i, i = 1, \ldots, m$, such that the sum of them is the total α.
- The rules of alpha propagation are defined by a set of (directed) connecting chain weights (g_{ij}) from H_i to H_j, which specify the fractions of the error rate available after rejecting H_i that are transferred to H_j. They are chosen such that $g_{ii} = 0, g_{i1} + g_{i2} + \ldots + g_{im} \le 1$, for every $i = 1, \ldots, m$.

The updating algorithm when testing occurs is summarized in the following: Set $J=\{1, \ldots, m\}$.

1. Select a "winning" H_j (i.e., its associated $p_j \le \alpha_j$) and continue. If no such hypothesis exists, then stop. The algorithm does not depend on the rejection sequence.

2. Update the graph's local alphas and the connecting chain weights:

   a. $J \to J \setminus \{j\}$ (that is, eliminate H_j from the graph)

   b. $\alpha_k \to \begin{cases} \alpha_k + \alpha_j g_{jk} & \text{for } k \text{ in } J \\ 0, & \text{otherwise} \end{cases}$

$$
\text{c.} \quad g_{kl} \rightarrow
\begin{cases}
\dfrac{g_{kl} + g_{kj}g_{jl}}{1 - g_{kj}g_{jk}} & \text{for } k, l \text{ in } \mathbf{J}, k \neq l, g_{kj}g_{jk} < 1 \\[2ex]
0, & \text{otherwise}
\end{cases}
$$

3. Go to Step 1.

Example 11.5:

We continue the example in Figure 11.2. Suppose we observed $(p_1, p_2, p_3) = (0.009, 0.016, 0.020)$ for (H_1, H_2, H_3). Compared to the local $(\alpha_1, \alpha_2, \alpha_3) = (0.00625, 0.01875, 0)$, we reject H_2, so the graph now only has H_1 and H_3 left. For H_1, we update its local alpha to $\alpha_1 + \alpha_2 g_{21} = 0.00625 + 0.01875*0.8 = 0.02125$. We also update the local level of H_3 to $\alpha_3 + \alpha_2 g_{23} = 0 + 0.01875*0.2 = 0.00375$. The chain from H_1 to H_3 becomes $\dfrac{g_{13} + g_{12}g_{23}}{1 - g_{12}g_{21}} = \dfrac{0.1 + 0.9*0.2}{1 - 0.9*0.8} = 1$.

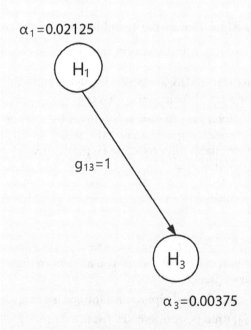

$\alpha = 0.025$

$\alpha_1 = 0.02125$

H_1

$g_{13} = 1$

H_3

$\alpha_3 = 0.00375$

FIGURE 11.3
Updating Figure 11.2 with observed p-values (Example 11.5).

The chain from H_3 to H_1 becomes $\frac{g_{31} + g_{32}g_{21}}{1 - g_{32}g_{23}} = \frac{0 + 0^*0.8}{1 - 0^*0.2} = 0$. The updated graph is shown in Figure 11.3.

Then, we compare $(p_1, p_3) = (0.009, 0.020)$ for (H_1, H_3) to the updated $(\alpha_1, \alpha_3) = (0.02125, 0.00375)$. We reject H_1. Finally, propagate all α_1 to H_3 (since the updated $g_{13} = 1$) and have $\alpha_1 + \alpha_3 = 0.02125 + 0.00375 = 0.025$. We also reject H_3 since $0.020 < 0.025$. Notice that, since $p_{(1)} = 0.009 > 0.025/3$, no hypothesis could be rejected by Holm's procedure.

11.4 Graphical Chain Procedure for Two Families of Null Hypotheses

The multiplicity problems discussed in Section 11.3 were defined as problems with a single source of multiplicity or a single family of null hypotheses, such as multiple endpoints in Section 11.2. A more complex setting is multiplicity problems with several sources of multiplicity or several families of null hypotheses. In Section 11.5, we will consider multiple analyses in the group sequential setting for multiple endpoints. In this section, we consider the situation where one family is multiple endpoints and another family is multiple treatment or dose groups. For example, we have high and low doses versus a common control, for which there is no preference which dose may win. For the endpoints, however, often one is primary and the other is secondary. We, of course, would prefer winning on the primary as priority to winning on the secondary endpoint. However, there may be a chance that high dose may win on the secondary endpoint while the low dose may win on the primary endpoint. How do we deal with this consideration? Figure 11.4 is a design strategy depicted by the graphical chain procedure (Dmitrienko et al. 2003) for such a situation.

The parallel (H_1, H_2) on the first row represent hypotheses of the primary endpoint for high-dose (left) and low-dose (right) groups versus the control, respectively. This is called the primary family of hypotheses. Similarly, (H_3, H_4) are the family for the secondary endpoint on the second row. As shown, the design is to start testing for the primary endpoint for high and low doses with their local alpha levels α_1 and $\alpha_2 = (1 - \alpha_1)$, respectively. There is no testing for the secondary endpoint until the primary endpoint is tested and rejected (won). If one of the dose groups wins on the primary endpoint, then a proportion (π) of the local alpha will be passed to the other dose group and $(1-\pi)$ to the testing for the secondary endpoint of the respective dose. What is interesting is that, if the high dose wins on both primary and secondary endpoints, the whole α_1 will be passed to the low dose for testing the primary endpoint at the total α. So, the low dose will have a second chance for testing the hypotheses (H_2, H_4) if it did not win at the first run. Likewise, if the low dose wins on both the endpoints, the whole α_2 will be passed to the high dose for testing the primary endpoint at the level of the total α. So,

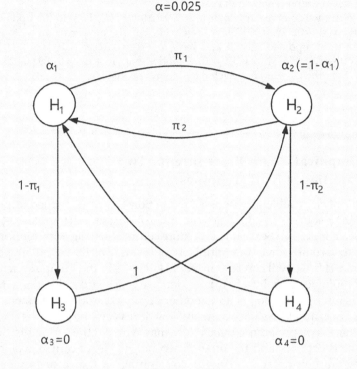

FIGURE 11.4
Graphical chain procedure for two Families of null hypotheses.

the high dose will have a second chance for testing the hypotheses (H_1, H_3) if it did not win at the first run. Calculations follow the formula given in Section 11.3.5 and Example 11.5 (Homework 11.2). Again, at the design stage, how to allocate the initial local alphas and the chain weights (π_1, π_2) as conditional probabilities depends on the assumptions about effect sizes in each treatment group and correlation between endpoints and further clinical and regulatory considerations. The graphical view of the chain procedure helps facilitate the discussions among research team members.

11.5 Monitoring Multiple Endpoints in Group Sequential Trials

We use A and B to illustrate the two primary endpoints monitored in a group sequential trial (see Chapter 9). We first split α between the two endpoints, $\alpha_A = w\alpha$ and $\alpha_B = (1 - w)\alpha$. Let c_j (d_j) be the group sequential boundaries for endpoint A (B) derived from some prespecified alpha-spending function at significance level α_A (α_B), $j=1, \ldots, J$. The two endpoints may have different error spending functions and different numbers of analyses. The trial is terminated early only when both endpoints win. The first (naive) method is to monitor the endpoints according to these group sequential boundaries independently without alpha propagation. This is called *group sequential Bonferroni* (GSB).

Ye et al. (2013) proposed another two methods that utilize the alpha propagation. In addition to c_j and d_j, let c'_j and d'_j be the revised boundaries at significance level α for endpoints A and B, respectively. Notice that, since $\alpha_A \leq \alpha$, we see that $c_j \geq c'_j$ for all j. Similarly, since $\alpha_B \leq \alpha$, $d_j \geq d'_j$ for all j. The second procedure is as follows: We monitor endpoint A using the level α_A group sequential boundary c_j and endpoint B using the level α_B boundary d_j. If either of the two endpoints crosses its boundary, then the other endpoint is tested using the full level α boundary. For example, if endpoint A crossed its level α_A boundary c_{j^*} at some look j^*, then endpoint A wins, and its α_A propagates to endpoint B so that endpoint B is tested using $\alpha_A + \alpha_B = \alpha$, with the full level α boundary d'_j for $j \geq j^*$. In short, endpoint B is tested with boundaries $(d_1, \ldots, d_{j^*-1}, d'_{j^*}, \ldots, d'_J)$. This method is called *group sequential Holm variable* (GSHv). Since $d_j \geq d'_j$ for $j=1, \ldots, j^*-1$ (the first portion), the overall significance level would be $\leq$ that of $(d'_j, j=1, \ldots, J)$, which is α. But, since $d'_j \leq d_j$ for $j=j^*,\ldots, J$ (the second portion), the overall significance level would be $\geq$ that of $(d_j, j=1, \ldots, J)$, which is α_B. Hence, GSHv is more powerful than GSB.

Alternatively, Ye et al. (2013) also suggested to retain boundaries unchanged at the interim analyses except at the final analysis J. In notation, after endpoint A wins, one may continue using the predefined interim boundaries, i.e., "fix" $d'_j = d_j$ for $j < J$. In summary, endpoint B is tested with boundaries $(d_1, \ldots, d_{J-1}, D_J)$, where D_J is fitted so that the overall level is α. This method is called *group sequential Holm fixed* (GSHf). The calculation of D_J can be done using Lan-DeMets spending function program available at the University of Wisconsin website (see Chapter 9).

Example 11.6:

Suppose a trial with two co-primary endpoints A and B with one-sided $\alpha_A = 0.006$ and $\alpha_B = 0.019$ allocated to A and B, respectively, such that $\alpha = \alpha_A + \alpha_B = 0.025$. The endpoints are tested in a group sequential design with at most two analyses for A and three analyses for B. IA1 and IA2 are scheduled on a calendar time that maps to the information fraction (0.86, 1.0) for endpoint A and to (0.60, 0.76) for endpoint B. Note that IA2 is the final analysis for endpoint A. Of course, if the trial continues, the final analysis for endpoint B is scheduled on a calendar time and its information fraction would be 1.0. For illustration of GSB, GSHv, and GSHf, we assume the information fractions are carried out as planned in this case.

Assume both endpoints use OBF-type boundaries (see Chapter 9). For $\alpha_A = 0.006$, $(c_1, c_2) = (2.7427, 2.5686)$, and for $\alpha_B = 0.019$, $(d_1, d_2, d_3) =$

TABLE 11.1

GSB, GSHv, and GSHf Group Sequential Boundaries with Two
Endpoints when Analyses are Performed on the Information Time
Planned as per the Protocol

	IA1	IA2	FA
$\alpha_A = 0.006$	$t_1 = 0.86$	$t_2 = 1.0$	
	$c_1 = 2.7427$	$c_2 = 2.5686$	
$\alpha_A = 0.025$	$c'_1 = 2.1532$	$c'_2 = 2.0419$	
$\alpha_B = 0.019$	$t_1 = 0.60$	$t_2 = 0.76$	$t_3 = 1.0$
(GSB)	$d_1 = 2.8121$	$d_2 = 2.4901$	$d_3 = 2.1271$
$\alpha_B = 0.025$	$d'_1 = 2.6686$	$d'_2 = 2.3660$	$d'_3 = 2.0188$
GSHv	$d_1 = 2.8121$	$d'_2 = 2.3660$	$d'_3 = 2.0188$
(d_1, d'_2, d'_3)			
alpha attained = 0.0246			
GSHf	$d_1 = 2.8121$	$d_2 = 2.4901$	$D_3 = 1.9901$
(d_1, d_2, D_3)			
alpha attained = 0.025			

(2.8121, 2.4901, 2.1271). For $\alpha = 0.025$, $(c'_1, c'_2) = (2.1532, 2.0419)$ and $(d'_1, d'_2, d'_3) = (2.6686, 2.3660, 2.0188)$.

Suppose, at IA1, none of the endpoints crossed their boundaries at their local levels. At IA2, only endpoint A crosses the boundary $c_2 = 2.5686$. We reject the null hypothesis regarding A and continue to test the hypothesis regarding endpoint B at the full level $\alpha = \alpha_A + \alpha_B = 0.025$ ($j^* = 2$). For endpoint B, the GSB boundaries are $(d_1, d_2, d_3) = (2.8121, 2.4901, 2.1271)$. The GSHv boundaries are $(d_1, d'_2, d'_3) = (2.8121, 2.3660, 2.0188)$, completely different values after alpha allocation. Notice that, since elementwise $(d'_2, d'_3) < (d_2, d_3)$, GSHv is easier to cross, and hence more powerful than GSB. Also notice that $d_1 = 2.8121 > d'_1 = 2.6686$, so GSHv loses some power as the overall alpha is attained at $0.0246 < 0.025$. For GSHf, the boundaries are $(d_1, d_2, D_3) = (2.8121, 2.4901, 1.9901)$, where D_3 is obtained by iterative fitting so that the overall level is $\alpha = 0.025$. The calculation is done using the Lan-DeMets spending function program available at the University of Wisconsin website (see Chapter 9), with "Compute Probability" and "User Input" options for "Determine Bounds." Compared to GSHv, GSHf is easier to cross with $D_3 = 1.9901 < 2.0188 = d'_3$ since it attains the full $\alpha = 0.025$ at the final analysis. Table 11.1 summarizes the results.

The above numerical illustration mimics the planned group sequential schema of KEYNOTE-604 trial. It assumes the time fractions stay the same as planned or the total information remains the same as prespecified in the protocol (for maximum information trials) throughout the trial. For maximum-duration trials, the total information may exceed the design's projection (over-running) as we have discussed in Chapter 9 (Appendix 9.3), also as actually happened in the KEYNOTE-604 trial (Homework 11.4).

As seen, the GSHv does not exploit the full potential of power gain, unless the propagation takes place at the first stage. On the other hand, the power gain associated with the GSHf is realized only if the trial continues to the final stage. Xi and Tamhane (2015) proposed an extension method by specifying a stage r at which the boundary is modified, $1 \le r \le J$, regardless of when either hypothesis is actually rejected and the significance level assigned to it is propagated to the other hypothesis. This general procedure is termed GSP(r), where GSHf is denoted by GSP(J). Following our description of the GSHv procedure before, the GSP(r) is explained as follows. For example, if endpoint A crossed its level α_A boundary c_{j^*} at some look j^*, then endpoint A wins, and its α_A propagates to endpoint B so that endpoint B is tested using $\alpha_A + \alpha_B = \alpha$, with the full level α boundary d'_j starting at the stage r regardless of j^*. In brief, endpoint B is tested with the new boundary $(d_1, \ldots, d_{r-1}, d''_r, \ldots, d''_J)$. The new boundary is calculated such that under the null hypothesis of endpoint B (unrejected),

$$1 - \alpha = \Pr\left(Z_1 \le d_1, \ldots, Z_{r-1} \le d_{r-1}, Z_r \le d''_r, \ldots, Z_J \le d''_J \mid H_{0B}\right) \quad (11.4)$$

The solution of (11.4) is obtained by the multivariate normal numerical integration method as we presented in Section 10.5, where $d_1, \ldots, d_{r-1}$ were known from the J-stage group sequential α_B level. The rest $d''_r, \ldots, d''_J$ follows the restriction: $d''_r = d''_{r+1} \ldots = d''_J = d''$ if the Pocock form boundary is initially used; $d''_r \sqrt{t_r} = d''_{r+1} \sqrt{t_{r+1}} \ldots = d''_J$ if the OBF form boundary is initially used.

It is tempting to choose r adaptively according to when the rejection of a hypothesis (A or B endpoint) occurs instead of prespecifying it. However, Xi and Tamhane (2015) showed that the adaptive GSP does not strongly control the FWER in general. Choosing r=1 has certain practical benefits although it may not be optimal. In fact, the optimality may not easily be defined in this case since there are many different considerations that dictate the choice of r.

Appendix 11.1

a. We first note a property of the uniform U[0, 1] distribution: If X has a uniform distribution U[0, 1], then 1-X also has a uniform U[0, 1] distribution.
   Proof: $\Pr(1 - X \le a) = \Pr(X \ge 1 - a) = 1 - (1 - a) = a$, for all $0 \le a \le 1$.

b. Let $F_T(t)$ denote the cumulative distribution function of the test statistic T. For practical purposes, assume its inverse F_T^{-1} exists[*]. Then, $F_T(t)$ has a uniform U[0,1] distribution.

---

[*] Note: In most of the practical cases, when sample size is large enough, such is the case for confirmatory clinical trials, F_T^{-1} exists.

Proof: Let $U(t) = F_T(t) \equiv \Pr(T \le t)$. Notice that U ranges between 0 and 1. The following equation shows the distribution of U: $\Pr(U(T) \le a) = \Pr(F_T(T) \le a) = \Pr(T \le F_T^{-1}(a)) = F_T(F_T^{-1}(a)) = a$, for all $0 \le a \le 1$.

c. Let $F_T(t)$ denote the cumulative distribution function of the test statistic T under the null hypothesis. By its definition, the p-value is the tail probability of T: $p = P_{H_0}(T > t) = 1 - F_T(t)$. Therefore, from (a) and (b), the p-value is uniformly distributed on [0,1] under the null hypothesis.

Appendix 11.2

a. An R package is available for the graphical chain procedure. Follow the steps:

- Install package: gMCP
- Load package: gMCP
- ?gMCP (to study the package)
- graphGUI() (to use the graphical display)
- Use one of the Example graphs, then modify the Transition Matrix
- Can save it (File: Save Graph to R); give a name (Load Graph from R)
- Export Graph to PNG Image → and then open it or use it in PowerPoint
- In the right lower panel, input the observed p-values
- Hit the triangle on the top of the left panel (start testing)
- File → Save Word Docx Report or Save LaTex Report.

b. The following is an SAS IML program to run an example of Section 11.4.

```
/* This program is adopted from ASA Webinar held on March 5, 2015, given
by Frank Bretz and Dong Xi */

/*
h: indicator whether a hypothesis is rejected (= 1) or not (= 0)
(1 x n vector)
a: initial significance level allocation (1 x n vector)
g: weights for the edges (n x n matrix)
p: observed p-values (1 x n vector)
*/

proc IML;
start mcp(h, a, g, p);
   n=ncol(h);
```

```
    mata=a;
    crit=0;
    do until (crit=1);
        test=(p<a);
        if (any(test)) then do;
            rej=min(loc(test#(1:n)));
            h[rej]=1;
            g1=J(n,n,0);
            do i=1 to n;
              a[i]=a[i]+a[rej]*g[rej,i];
              if g[i,rej]*g[rej,i]<1 then do j=1 to n;
                  g1[i,j]=(g[i,j]+g[i,rej]*g[rej,j])/
(1-g[i,rej]*g[rej,i]);
                end;
                g1[i,i]=0;
              end;
              g=g1; g[rej,]=0; g[,rej]=0;
              a[rej]=0;
              mata=mata//a;
          end;
          else crit=1;
  end;
  print h;
  print (round(mata, 0.0001));
  print (round(g, 0.01));
  Finish;
  /* Example */

  h={0 0 0 0 };
  a={0.0125 0.0125 0 0 };
  g={0 0.5 0.5 0 ,
      0.5 0 0 0.5 ,
      0 1 0 0 ,
      1 0 0 0 };
  p={0.01 0.02 0.07 0.001};

  run mcp(h, a, g, p);
  quit;
```

HOMEWORK 11.1

A trial has two independent endpoints, and we test each endpoint at level 0.05.

1. Explain why the FWER for rejecting the global hypothesis is: $FWER = 1 - (0.95)^2 = 0.0975$.

2. To control the FWER (weakly) at 0.05 for the global hypothesis, what should be the local level of the test for each endpoint?

HOMEWORK 11.2

Work out the graphic chain approach step by step in Figure 11.4 for $\alpha=0.025$, $\alpha_1=\alpha/3$, $(\pi_1, \pi_2)=(0.5, 0.5)$. Suppose that the observed p-values are $p_1=0.01$, $p_2=0.02$, $p_3=0.005$, and $p_4=0.0075$, respectively, for (H_1, H_2, H_3, H_4). Find out the rejected hypotheses. Also use the SAS program in Appendix 11.2(b) to verify your answer.

HOMEWORK 11.3

Use the R package gMCP GUI (see Appendix 11.2) to test the hypotheses using the observed p-values with the following design. Two hypotheses (H_1, H_2) from the primary family are initially assigned the local level $\alpha/2$ each, whereas (H_2, H_4) from the secondary family of endpoints are assigned the local level 0. If H_1 and/or H_2 is rejected, the local level $a/2$ is split into half and passed to H_3 and H_4 with weights 0.5. If H_3 (H_4) is rejected in the subsequence at its local significance level, then this level is passed to H_4 (H_3) with weight 1. Let $\alpha=0.025$ (one-sided), and suppose that we observe $p_1=0.01$, $p_2=0.02$, $p_3=0.005$, and $p_4=0.0075$. Make the chain graphs, work out the steps, and find out the rejected hypotheses. Compare the design and outcome with that in Homework 11.2.

HOMEWORK 11.4

1. Continue Example 11.6 to fill in Table 11.1 with GSP(r) with $r=1, 2, 3$.

2. Read the following paper: Rudin CM, Awad MM, Navarro A, et al. *Pembrolizumab or placebo plus etoposide and platinum as first-line therapy for extensive-stage small-cell lung cancer: Randomized, double-blind, phase III KEYNOTE-604 study.* DOI: 10.1200/JCO.20.00793. Journal of Clinical Oncology 38, no. 21 p. 2369–2379. Also read the protocol that is included in the appendix of the paper for the group sequential testing for the primary endpoints (OS and PFS) according to the graphic chain design. Find the protocol-estimated (planned) information time versus the actual (true) information time for each analysis. Reconstruct Table 11.1 for GSB, GSHv, and GSHf group sequential boundaries with the two endpoints using the actual information time when analyses were performed.

References

Bretz F, Maurer W, Brannath W, and Posch M. (2009). A graphical approach to sequentially rejective multiple test procedures. *Statistics in Medicine* 28:586–604.

Dmitrienko A, D'Agostino RB, and Huque MF. (2013). Key multiplicity issues in clinical drug development. *Statistics in Medicine* 32: 1079–1111.

Hochberg Y. (1988). A shaper Bonferroni procedure for multiple tests of significance. *Biometrika* 75: 800–802.

Holm S. (1979). A simple sequentially rejective multiple test procedure. *Scandinavian Journal of Statistics* 6: 65–70.

Maurer W and Bretz F. (2013). Multiple testing in group sequential trials using graphical approaches. *Statistics in Biopharmaceutical Research* 5: 311–320.

Medical Director Merck Sharp & Dohme Corp (2019). A Study of Pembrolizumab (MK-3475) for First Line Treatment of Recurrent or Metastatic Squamous Cell Cancer of the Head and Neck (KEYNOTE-048). https://clinicaltrials.gov/ct2/show/NCT02358031

Millen B and Dmitrienko A. (2011). Chain procedures: a class of flexible closed testing procedures with clinical trial applications. *Statistics in Biopharmaceutical Research* 3: 14–30.

Rudin CM, Awad MM, Navarro A, et al. (2020). Pembrolizumab or placebo plus etoposide and platinum as first-line therapy for extensive-stage small-cell lung cancer: randomized, double-blind, phase III KEYNOTE-604 study. *Journal of Clinical Oncology* 38(21): 2369–2379.

Sarkar S. (1998). Some probability inequalities for ordered MTP2 random variables: a proof of the Simes conjecture. *Annals of Statistics* 26: 494–504.

Xi D and Tamhane AC. (2015). Allocating recycled significance levels in group sequential procedures for multiple endpoints. *Biometrical Journal* 57(1): 90–107.

Ye Y, Li A, Liu L, and Yao B. (2013). A group sequential Holm procedure with multiple primary endpoints. *Statistics in Medicine* 32: 1112–24.

12

Clinical Trials with Predictive Biomarkers

In the booklet entitled *Cancer Biomarkers* by the Institute of Medicine of the US National Academies, a biomarker is defined as "any characteristic that can be objectively measured and evaluated as an indicator of normal biological processes, pathogenic processes, or pharmacological response to a therapeutic intervention." For our purpose, we can think of a biomarker as a demographic, genetic, or pathophysiologic characteristic that is thought to be related to the drug's mechanism of action. The medical use of biomarkers includes screening, diagnosis, monitoring, and treatment of diseases. In this chapter, we focus on the areas where biomarkers are developed for enhancing the effectiveness and safety of patient care by allowing physicians to tailor treatment for individual patients—an approach known as personalized medicine, or precision medicine, according to the US FDA's initiative on personalized medicine (FDA, 2013). Particularly, we discuss how the recent trend of precision medicine in utilizing predictive biomarkers has impacted on study design and analysis of modern clinical trials. There have increasingly been discussions and proposals of various trial designs and comparisons among them in the literature. In the following sections, we review several kinds of designs commonly used in oncology and other clinical trials involving one dichotomized biomarker or a combination of biomarkers. We emphasize on distinguishing what hypotheses each design is able to test for, including a special design strategy known as *adaptive enrichment design* that aims to increase the chance of successful development of treatment by utilizing biomarkers. The first part assumes perfect marker assay and classification rules for simplicity. The second part expands to the more realistic situation where misclassification is present.

12.1 General Notion

In the following sections, we will discuss "targeted and untargeted designs," "stratified designs," "precision medicine designs," and "adaptive enrichment designs." We pay attention to the salient features of these designs and delineate what clinical hypotheses could be of interest and tested by the respective design. We consider the case of two treatment groups, test (T) versus control or standard of care (C), in the context of mean difference of a continuous endpoint. One can generalize to binary and survival endpoints as well. Let μ_{ij} denote the true mean response of treatment group i (i = T or C) for patients in marker cohort j (j = 0 being marker-negative or j = 1 being marker-positive). For the sake of clarity in presenting the hypotheses that each design is able to test, we first consider the ideal situation of perfect sensitivity and specificity of a biomarker assay, then followed by the more realistic situation of imperfect sensitivity and specificity in Section 12.5.

We focus on the fundamental aims and clinical hypotheses of interest in each design (see Chapter 1, Sections 1.2.3 and 1.2.4). The test procedures for these hypotheses and comparisons of their statistical efficiencies can be found in Shih and Lin (2018) and Lin, Shih, and Lu (2019).

12.2 Designs and Hypotheses in the Absence of Classification Errors

Targeted and Untargeted Designs

In a *targeted design*, only marker-positive patients, who are predicted to be responsive, are randomized to the treatment groups. In contrast, an *untargeted design* is an all-comers design, which is the traditional randomized trial without the biomarker information. Simon and Maitournam (2004) and Maitournam and Simon (2005) reported that targeted designs are more efficient (for requiring fewer subjects) than untargeted or all-comers designs. However, it is obvious that the treatment effect in a targeted design is limited to the marker-positive cohort only, while for the untargeted design, the treatment effect refers to the overall unselected population. Expressed in notation, the null hypothesis is

$$H_{0a}: \mu_{T\#} = \mu_{C\#}$$

for untargeted designs, where

$$\mu_{T\#} = p\mu_{T1} + (1-p)\mu_{T0} \tag{12.1}$$

$$\mu_{C\#} = p\mu_{C1} + (1-p)\mu_{C0} \tag{12.2}$$

and p is the prevalence rate of marker-positives.

Since there is no biomarker information available for patients in the untargeted design, the treatment group means are a mixture of means of the two (unidentified) marker cohorts. H_{0a} is interpreted as the hypothesis of *treatment's group effects* or *treatment utility*, as opposed to the absolute treatment effect (see H_{0T} below).

For targeted designs, the null hypothesis is

$$H_{0+}: \mu_{T1} = \mu_{C1}.$$

The two hypotheses H_{0a} and H_{0+} are not compatible unless there is no treatment effect for the marker-negatives (i.e., $\mu_{T0} = \mu_{C0}$). The premise for a targeted design is that the investigator has strong preliminary data (such as a retrospective study) indicating that marker-positive patients may benefit from the test treatment and is interested in focusing on this cohort only. See the example of pembrolizumab in non-small cell lung cancer when the enrichment design is discussed in Section 12.4.

For the untargeted design, the biomarker is not recognized as being predictive and patients are not "typed" by the biomarker. We caution that statistical (power) efficiency comparison must be based on testing the same hypothesis. (Recall design efficiency was discussed in Chapter 3.) Another concept of design strategy is to maximize the expected number of "responders" for the trial for the prefixed sample size. Targeted designs perhaps aim on optimizing ethics rather than efficiency in terms of sample size; see discussion in Appendix 3.3.

Marker-Stratified Designs

With untargeted designs, as seen above, treatment groups may not be balanced with respect to the biomarker-defined cohorts, despite randomization. A *marker-stratified design* (Figure 12.1), which also includes all eligible patients, but recognizing the predictive value of the biomarker, randomizes treatments within each marker stratum so that treatment groups are more likely balanced with respect to the marker status. (See Chapter 2 for stratified randomization.) Therefore, in addition to the hypotheses H_{0a} and H_{0+}, a marker-stratified design also allows testing for the treatment effect in the biomarker-negative cohort (H_{0-}), the absolute treatment effect (H_{0T}), the biomarker effect (H_{0B}), as well as the marker-by-treatment interaction effect (H_{0I}). That is, we may test

$$H_{0-}: \mu_{T0} = \mu_{C0}$$

$$H_{0T}: \mu_{T0} + \mu_{T1} = \mu_{C0} + \mu_{C1}$$

$$H_{0B}: \mu_{T0} + \mu_{C0} = \mu_{T1} + \mu_{C1}$$

$$H_{0I}: \mu_{T0} - \mu_{C0} = \mu_{T1} - \mu_{C1}$$

Hypothesis H_{0B} relates to the prognostic effect of the biomarker across treatment groups. Contrasting H_{0a} with H_{0T}, the latter does not factor in the marker prevalence rate and thus is termed absolute (or marginal) treatment effect.

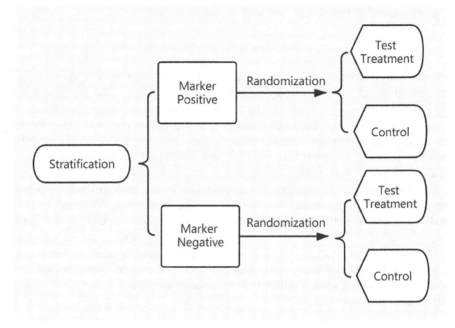

FIGURE 12.1
Marker-stratified design: treatment are randomized within each marker stratum.

The untargeted design can only test H_{0a} and is not able to test H_{0T}. It is debatable which hypothesis, H_{0a} (with marker-positive prevalence) or H_{0T} (without marker-positive prevalence), is more clinically relevant.

The interaction hypothesis H_{0I} is of particular interest to Sargent et al. (2005) and Mandrekar and Sargent (2009, 2010) so that this design was called marker-by-treatment interaction design in their papers. It checks whether and how the biomarker status modifies the treatment effect. If the interaction effect is significant, then a closer examination is needed to find out whether the modification is directional (*qualitative interaction*) or in magnitude (*quantitative interaction*). In this case, hypotheses H_{0+} and H_{0-} specifically regarding the marker-positive and marker-negative cohorts, respectively, would be of interest, while the absolute treatment effect hypothesis H_{0T} would not be.

However, we think that the composite hypothesis

$$H_{0C}: H_{0+} \text{ and } H_{0-}$$

and the individual component hypotheses H_{0+} and H_{0-} are more meaningful than the interaction hypothesis H_{0I} because they answer the clinical questions more directly regarding the treatment effect in each marker-defined stratum. (Note: In Chapter 11, H_{0C} was called the global hypothesis, and the multiple test procedures studied there are useful for testing the individual hypotheses.)

Precision Medicine Designs

Precision medicine designs randomize patients into two arms (Figure 12.2). The first arm is a marker-dependent arm, and the second arm is a marker-independent arm. For the marker-independent arm, patients are further randomized to treatment group T or C without biomarker information. For the marker-dependent arm, marker-positive patients all receive the test treatment T and marker-negative patients all receive the control treatment C (standard of care, SOC). This kind of designs is also called *marker-based strategy design* in Mandrekar and Sargent (2009, 2010) and Young, Laird, and Zhou (2010).

The marker-independent arm is just like that in untargeted designs; hence, the pooled treatment means $\mu_{T\#}$ and $\mu_{C\#}$ are estimable directly in this arm. The marker-dependent arm provides information to estimate μ_{T1} and μ_{C0}. With known or an estimate of the prevalence rate p of the marker-positive patients and by relationship (12.1), μ_{T0} will be estimated. Similarly, μ_{C1} can be estimated via relationship (12.2).

Having all μ_{ij}, $i = T$ or C, $j = 0$ or 1 estimable, the hypotheses of marker-specific treatment effects, H_{0+} and H_{0-}, the treatment and marker (main) effects, H_{0T} and H_{0B}, the treatment-by-marker interaction effect, H_{0I}, and the composite H_{0C} can all be tested.

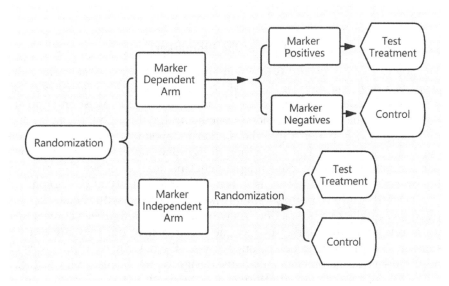

FIGURE 12.2
Precision medicine design.

12.3 Comparison between Stratified Design and Precision Medicine Design

12.3.1 Stratified Design is More Efficient

From Section 12.2, we see that all the hypotheses H_{0a} to H_{0C} are testable in both stratified designs and precision medicine designs. Shih and Lin (2018) calculated the relative efficiency between the stratified design and the precision medicine design in full detail with respect to testing the same hypotheses and concluded that the stratified design has greater efficiency than the precision medicine design in terms of sample size and power. The reason for better efficiency of the stratified design is conceivable because the precision medicine design includes patients treated with the same treatment on both marker-independent and marker-dependent arms. This overlap increases as the prevalence of marker-defined cohorts increases, leading to greater efficiency loss for the precision medicine design.

Obviously, the stratified design is simpler in structure and all the effects are estimated directly from the marker–treatment components. In contrast, the precision medicine design has a double-randomization structure and the treatment-by-marker interaction and the marker (main) effects are estimated indirectly, as shown in Section 12.2. Thus, intuitively, the precision medicine design would require a larger overall sample size. However, the precision medicine design has the merit that it provides direct information on clinical utility of the biomarker, which may be provided, but is not so apparent, from the stratified design; see the next section.

12.3.2 Test the Clinical Utility of the Biomarker

The question of clinical utility of a biomarker is *"whether the use of the biomarker supports a treatment decision that produces a better outcome for the patient than if the marker results were not available"* (Hayes, 2016). This question is potentially answerable by the precision medicine design through the first layer of randomization of patients into the marker-independent versus the marker-dependent arms, which the stratified design does not have. Thus, the comparison between the marker-independent and marker-dependent arms in the precision medicine design is to test the clinical utility of the biomarker. The clinical utility hypothesis should not be confused with the marker-by-treatment qualitative interaction. As we shall see, a biomarker's clinical utility is related to the marker-by-treatment interaction, but they are not the same in general. To map one-to-one between them, we need another design requirement for the precision medicine design, as we discuss in the sequel.

The assessment of clinical utility especially needs external information of the sensitivity and specificity of the biomarker assay and classification rule. If the sensitivity and specificity are low, there will be no clinical utility of the biomarker. In discussions of the designs so far, we have not factored in the sensitivity and specificity of the biomarker assay and classification rule. That is, we have assumed perfect sensitivity and specificity for classification so far, for the sake of simplicity and clarity as we focus on the hypotheses that each design is able to test. We will add the consideration of assay and classification errors in Section 12.5.

To explore the clinical utility of the biomarker, let μ^{DP} be the mean of the marker-dependent arm and μ^{IN} be the mean of the marker-independent arm. The null hypothesis of clinical utility of the biomarker is expressed as

$$H_U: \mu^{DP} = \mu^{IN}$$

Assuming perfect sensitivity and specificity of the biomarker assay and classification,

$$\mu^{DP} = p\mu_{T1} + (1-p)\mu_{C0} \qquad (12.3)$$

Furthermore, let r be the randomization proportion to the test treatment group T in the marker-independent arm, then

$$\mu^{IN} = r\mu_{T\#} + (1-r)\mu_{C\#} \qquad (12.4)$$

$$= r\left[p\mu_{T1} + (1-p)\mu_{T0}\right] + (1-r)\left[p\mu_{C1} + (1-p)\mu_{C0}\right]$$

from Eqs. (12.1) and (12.2).

We define the marker's clinical utility as a function of r and p by

$$MU_{(r,p)} = \mu^{DP} - \mu^{IN}$$

$$= (1-r)p(\mu_{T1} - \mu_{C1}) - r(1-p)(\mu_{T0} - \mu_{C0}) \qquad (12.5)$$

We see that, when there is no treatment effect, i.e., $\mu_{T1} = \mu_{C1}$ and $\mu_{T0} = \mu_{C0}$, there is no marker utility, $MU_{(r,p)} = 0$. But even when there is treatment effect, as along as $(\mu_{T1} - \mu_{C1})/(\mu_{T0} - \mu_{C0}) = r(1-p)/(1-r)p$, $MU_{(r,p)} = 0$.

When the clinical utility $MU_{(r,p)} \neq 0$, it depends on the randomization ratio r, which expresses the option of treatment decision if the marker results are not available. For example, when $r = 0$, patients are always treated with the control/SOC,

$$MU_{(0,p)} = p(\mu_{T1} - \mu_{C1})$$

When $r = 1/2$, patients have a half–half chance to receive either the test treatment or the control,

$$MU_{(1/2,p)} = \left[p(\mu_{T1} - \mu_{C1}) - (1-p)(\mu_{T0} - \mu_{C0})\right]/2.$$

The clinical utility expressed by (12.5) in general, as a function of r and p, is not the same as the marker-by-treatment interaction. To see this, let $w = (\mu_{T1} - \mu_{C1}) - (\mu_{T0} - \mu_{C0})$ be the marker-by-treatment interaction effect. For equal randomization, $r = 1/2$, $MU_{(1/2,p)} = [(1-p)w + (2p-1)(\mu_{T1} - \mu_{C1})]/2$. So, even with no interaction effect, $MU_{(1/2,p)} = (p - 1/2)(\mu_{T1} - \mu_{C1}) \neq 0$ unless the prevalence rate of the marker-positives $p = 1/2$.

To link a one-to-one relationship between clinical utility and the marker-by-treatment interaction effect, we need to choose $r = p$ in the design. Add this requirement to the design, and then

$$MU_{(p, p)} = \mu^{DP} - \mu^{IN} = (1-p)p[(\mu_{T1} - \mu_{C1}) - (\mu_{T0} - \mu_{C0})] = (1-p)pw$$

In this case, $MU_{(p, p)} = 0$ if and only if $w = 0$. However, it is difficult, if not impossible, to set $r = p$ exactly in practice.

We see that the marker-stratified design can also address (12.5), which is not directly obvious from the stratified design itself. Nevertheless, we may compare the statistical efficiency in testing the same hypothesis H_U (as well as the interaction hypothesis H_{0I}) between the stratified design and the precision medicine design. Shih and Lin (2018) found that the stratified design is also more efficient than the precision medicine design in testing the utility hypothesis (Homework 12.1.a). We therefore recommend the stratified design be used in practice.

12.4 Adaptive Enrichment Designs

In 2012, the US FDA issued a draft guidance on enrichment design to pave its 2013 initiative on personalized medicine (FDA 2012, 2013). One purpose of enrichment designs is for better treatment response potential for a selected marker-positive cohort. An example is the trastuzumab benefit on HER2+ breast cancer patients (Smith et al. 2007). However, sometimes the enrichment design is easily confused with the targeted design. To avoid confusion, the *adaptive enrichment design* is referred by Wang et al. (2007) as a two-stage adaptive design with an interim analysis for possible enrichment of the patient population at the second stage. The targeted design is suitable when there is already evidence that the treatment may have beneficial effect only on the marker-positive subset, but not on the maker-negative subset. In contrast, the sequential two-stage enrichment design is suitable for the situation where such evidence is lacking. For example, it is interesting to notice that the landmark pembrolizumab (Merck's immune checkpoint inhibitor) KEYNOTE-010 trial, which included all TPS≥1% NSCLC patients to receive test treatment as the second-line therapy, showed significant treatment benefit of pembrolizumab over the SOC control group for the PD-L1 strongly positive subset, but not in the overall cohort (Herbst et al., 2016). With this evidence as background, the next trial KEYNOTE-024 using pembrolizumab to treat NSCLC patients as their first-line therapy used a targeted design, enrolled only the PD-L1 strongly positive cohort (TPS$\geq$50%), and was a successful study to win the US FDA's fast-track approval (Reck et al., 2016).

Specifically, for an adaptive enrichment deign the trial follows the following scheme: The first stage is a stratified design with both marker-defined cohorts. If the global (composite) hypothesis H_{0G} (H_{0a} and H_{0+}) is rejected (see below), we stop the trial and claim that treatment is effective either for the overall (unselected) patient population or for the marker-positive patients. The test for the individual hypothesis H_{0a} and H_{0+} would shed more light on the conclusion. However, if H_{0G} is not rejected, the trial will then continue to accrue more patients in Stage 2 with two different scenarios, 2a or 2b, depending on the futility assessment for the marker-negative patients (Figure 12.3). A futility analysis is performed with the Stage 1 data for the marker-negative patients. If the marker-negative cohort is shown futile, then the second stage will accrue only the marker-positive patients, thus enriching the design. The chance of dropping the marker-negative and enriching the design with marker-positive patients depends on the futility criterion set for the marker-negative cohort. In case of enriching, the duration of the accrual will be longer, depending on the prevalence rate of the marker-positive cohort.

Notice that even though the first stage (and the scenario 2a) is a stratified design, the hypothesis of interest for an enrichment design is not the marker-by-treatment interaction, but the composite hypothesis of H_{0a} (for the "overall" treatment utility) and H_{0+} (for the marker-positive subgroup treatment effect):

$$H_{0G}: H_{0a} \text{ and } H_{0+}$$

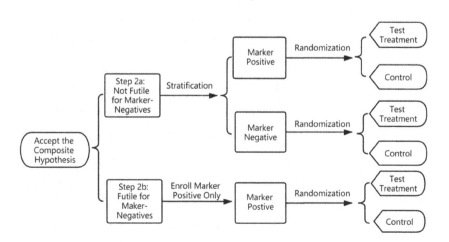

FIGURE 12.3
The second stage of the adaptive enrichment design.

and its components. If the marker-negative cohort is deemed futile, then the hypothesis of interest for the second stage will be just H_{0+}, as a targeted design. H_{0+} will be tested by using all the marker-positive patients from both stages. Otherwise, the hypothesis of interest will continue to be the composite H_{0G} and its components, tested by using all patients from both stages.

The main concern in performing the testing procedures for the adaptive enrichment design is on how to allocate the alpha levels in the interim and final analyses between multiple hypotheses so that the overall type I error rate is controlled. Lin, Shih, and Lu (2019) discussed the testing procedure in much more detail (Homework 12.1.b).

Table 12.1 is a summary of the various designs and the relevant hypotheses we have discussed above, assuming that the biomarker assay and classification rule are perfect.

TABLE 12.1

Summary of Designs and Hypotheses (Absence of Classification Error)

Design	Hypothesis (null) to test	Note
Untargeted design	$H_{0a}: \mu_{T\#} = \mu_{C\#}$	Test treatment group effects for the overall unselected population
Targeted design	$H_{0+}: \mu_{T1} = \mu_{C1}$	Test treatment effects for the biomarker-positive sub-population
Stratified design (Alias: marker-by-treatment interaction design)	$H_{0a}: \mu_{T\#} = \mu_{C\#}$ $H_{0+}: \mu_{T1} = \mu_{C1}$ $H_{0-}: \mu_{T0} = \mu_{C0}$	Test treatment effects for the biomarker-negative sub-population
	$H_{0T}: \mu_{T0} + \mu_{T1} = \mu_{C0} + \mu_{C1}$	Test the marginal absolute treatment effects for unselected population
	$H_{0B}: \mu_{T0} + \mu_{C0} = \mu_{T1} + \mu_{C1}$	Test the marginal biomarker effect across treatment groups
	$H_{0I}: \mu_{T0} - \mu_{C0} = \mu_{T1} - \mu_{C1}$	Test the biomarker-by-treatment interaction
	$H_{0C}: H_{0+}$ and H_{0-}	Composite hypotheses of treatment effects in both marker-positive and marker-negative sub-populations
	$H_U: (1-r)p(\mu_{T1} - \mu_{C1})$ $= r(1-p)(\mu_{T0} - \mu_{C0})$	See below

(*Continued*)

TABLE 12.1 (*Continued*)

Summary of Designs and Hypotheses (Absence of Classification Error)

Design	Hypothesis (null) to test	Note
Precision medicine design (Alias: marker-based strategy design)	$H_{0a}, H_{0+}, H_{0-}, H_{0T}, H_{0B}, H_{0I}, H_{0C}$ $H_U: \mu^{DP} = \mu^{IN}$ Or equivalently: $(1-r)p(\mu_{T1} - \mu_{C1})$ $= r(1-p)(\mu_{T0} - \mu_{C0})$	Test the marker's clinical utility in supporting a treatment decision to produce a better outcome
Adaptive enrichment design (Alias: two-stage sequential enrichment design)	$H_{0G}: H_{0a}$ and H_{0+} at the first stage H_{0+} or H_{0G} at the second stage, depending on the interim analysis	Composite hypotheses of treatment effects in the overall population and in the marker-positive sub-population

12.5 Designs and Hypotheses in the Presence of Misclassification

Unlike other stratification factors such as gender, age, or disease stage, biomarker assays and classification rules with the choice of cut-offs are prone to be imperfect. The assay and classification accuracy are measured by sensitivity (λ_{sen}) and specificity (λ_{spec}). We discuss the hypotheses in the previous sections when sensitivity and specificity are considered. We assume p, λ_{sen}, and λ_{sen} parameters are known in the following discussions on trial designs and relevant hypotheses in parallel to Section 12.2. (Note: In Chapter 8, Section 8.1.3 defines positive predictive value (PPV) in relation to disease prevalence and sensitivity of a diagnostic device.)

Targeted Designs and Untargeted Designs

For untargeted designs, since no markers are involved, H_{0a} remains the same, where formulas (12.1) and (12.2) apply with no change. For the targeted design, patients are marker-appeared-positives. Together with the prevalence rate p, by Bayes theorem (see Section 8.1.3), the positive predictive value (PPV) is

$$\theta = \frac{p\lambda_{sen}}{p\lambda_{sen} + (1-p)(1-\lambda_{spec})}$$

The mean response now becomes

$$\mu_{T*} = \theta\mu_{T1} + (1-\theta)\mu_{T0} \tag{12.6}$$

for the test group, and

$$\mu_{C*} = \theta\mu_{C1} + (1-\theta)\mu_{C0} \qquad (12.7)$$

for the control group.

Thus, to test the hypothesis H_{0+} by the targeted design in the presence of classification error, we need to perform some algebra (Homework 12.2). Otherwise, the direct comparison of the two treatment groups is to test

$$H'_{0+}: \mu_{T*} = \mu_{C*}$$

which is comparing the mean responses between the two treatment groups on marker-appeared-positive patients. The "targeted" is approaching the "untargeted" when sensitivity and specificity approach ½ (i.e., ineffective marker assay). In that case, θ approaches p, μ_{i*} approaches $\mu_{i\#}$ for i = T and C, and H'_{0+} approaches H_{0a}.

Marker-Stratified Designs

For the marker-stratified design, in addition to (12.6) and (12.7), there are marker-appeared-negative patients, for which we need to consider the negative predictive value (NPV):

$$\eta = \frac{(1-p)\lambda_{spec}}{p(1-\lambda_{sen}) + (1-p)\,\lambda_{spec}}$$

The mean responses for the test group and the control group in this cohort become

$$\mu_{T\emptyset} = (1-\eta)\mu_{T1} + \eta\mu_{T0} \qquad (12.8)$$

and

$$\mu_{C\emptyset} = (1-\eta)\mu_{C1} + \eta\mu_{C0} \qquad (12.9)$$

respectively.

From Equations (12.6)–(12.9), we can obtain the following conversions (Homework 12.3):

$$\mu_{T1} = \frac{-\eta}{1-\theta-\eta}\mu_{T*} + \frac{1-\theta}{1-\theta-\eta}\mu_{T\emptyset} \qquad (12.10)$$

$$\mu_{T0} = \frac{1-\eta}{1-\theta-\eta}\mu_{T*} + \frac{-\theta}{1-\theta-\eta}\mu_{T\emptyset} \qquad (12.11)$$

$$\mu_{C1} = \frac{-\eta}{1-\theta-\eta}\mu_{C*} + \frac{1-\theta}{1-\theta-\eta}\mu_{C\varnothing} \qquad (12.12)$$

$$\mu_{C0} = \frac{1-\eta}{1-\theta-\eta}\mu_{C*} + \frac{-\theta}{1-\theta-\eta}\mu_{C\varnothing} \qquad (12.13)$$

Having all μ_{ij}, i = T or C, j = 0 or 1 estimable, the hypotheses of marker-specific treatment effects, H_{0+} and H_{0-}, the treatment and marker (main) effects, H_{0T} and H_{0B}, the treatment-by-marker interaction effect, H_{0I}, and the composite hypothesis H_{0C} can all be tested. The efficiency loss due to classification errors is another matter; see discussion in Shih and Lin (2018). Note that

$$(\mu_{T1} - \mu_{C1}) - (\mu_{T0} - \mu_{C0}) = \frac{-1}{1-\theta-\eta}\left[(\mu_{T*} - \mu_{C*}) - (\mu_{T\varnothing} - \mu_{C\varnothing})\right].$$

Therefore, the marker-by-treatment interaction hypothesis may be tested directly by the observed mean responses without going through the conversions.

Precision Medicine Designs

The marker-independent arm is the untargeted design; no marker is involved. Thus, the treatment utility hypothesis H_{0a} remains the same, where formulas (12.1) and (12.2) apply with no change. The marker-dependent arm allows estimates of (12.6) and (12.9). From (12.1), (12.2), (12.6), and (12.9), we can obtain the following conversions (Homework 12.4):

$$\mu_{T1} = \frac{1-p}{\theta-p}\mu_{T*} - \frac{1-\theta}{\theta-p}\mu_{T\#} \qquad (12.14)$$

$$\mu_{T0} = \frac{-p}{\theta-p}\mu_{T*} + \frac{\theta}{\theta-p}\mu_{T\#} \qquad (12.15)$$

$$\mu_{C1} = \frac{1-p}{1-p-\eta}\mu_{C\varnothing} - \frac{\eta}{1-p-\eta}\mu_{C\#} \qquad (12.16)$$

$$\mu_{C0} = \frac{-p}{1-p-\eta}\mu_{C\varnothing} + \frac{1-\eta}{1-p-\eta}\mu_{C\#} \qquad (12.17)$$

Having all μ_{ij}, i = T or C, j = 0 or 1 estimable, the hypotheses H_{0+} to H_{0C} can all be tested.

We now examine how the marker utility hypothesis H_U alters in the presence of misclassification.

Let $q = p\lambda_{sen} + (1-p)(1- \lambda_{spec})$, then $1-q = p(1-\lambda_{sen}) + (1-p)\lambda_{spec}$. The mean of the marker-dependent arm becomes

$$\mu_m^{DP} = q\mu_{T*} + (1-q)\mu_{C\varnothing}$$

$$= q[\theta\mu_{T1} + (1-\theta)\mu_{T0}] + (1-q)[(1-\eta)\mu_{C1} + \eta\mu_{C0}]$$

$$= p\lambda_{sen}\mu_{T1} + (1-p)(1- \lambda_{spec})\mu_{T0} + p(1-\lambda_{sen})\mu_{C1} + (1-p)\lambda_{spec}\mu_{C0} \qquad (12.18)$$

where μ_{T*} is from (12.6) and $\mu_{C\varnothing}$ is from (12.9).

The mean of the marker-independent arm is still the same as (12.4):

$$\mu^{IN} = r\mu_{T\#} + (1-r)\mu_{C\#}$$

$$= r[p\mu_{T1} + (1-p)\mu_{T0}] + (1-r)[p\mu_{C1} + (1-p)\mu_{C0}]$$

The marker utility becomes, as a function of r, sensitivity, and specificity:

$$MU_{(r, p)}(\lambda_{sen}, \lambda_{spec}) = \mu_m^{DP} - \mu^{IN}$$

$$= p(\lambda_{sen} - r)(\mu_{T1} - \mu_{C1}) + (1-p)(1- \lambda_{spec} - r)(\mu_{T0} - \mu_{C0}) \qquad (12.19)$$

Note that (12.19) becomes (12.5) when $\lambda_{sen} = \lambda_{spec} = 1$. Corresponding to H_U, the marker utility hypothesis becomes

$$H_U': \mu_m^{DP} = \mu^{IN}.$$

Again, we see that, when there is no treatment effect, i.e., $\mu_{T1} = \mu_{C1}$ and $\mu_{T0} = \mu_{C0}$, there is no marker utility, $MU_{(r, p)} = 0$. When there is only treatment effect in the marker-positives and no effect in the marker-negatives, $MU_{(r, p)}(\lambda_{sen}, \lambda_{spec}) = p(\lambda_{sen} - r)(\mu_{T1} - \mu_{C1})$. But even when there is treatment effect on both cohorts, as along as $(\mu_{T1} - \mu_{C1})/(\mu_{T0} - \mu_{C0}) = (r-1+ \lambda_{spec})(1-p)/(\lambda_{sen} -r)p$, $MU_{(r, p)}(\mu_{sen}, \mu_{spec}) = 0$. The ratio $(\mu_{T1} - \mu_{C1})/(\mu_{T0} - \mu_{C0})$ may also be interpreted as a measure of marker-by-treatment interaction, as long as $\mu_{T0} - \mu_{C0} \neq 0$. Hence, when a marker-by-treatment interaction is expressed at a specific level shown above, $MU_{(r, p)}(\lambda_{sen}, \lambda_{spec}) = 0$. On the other hand, even when there is no marker-by-treatment interaction,

$$MU_{(r, p)}(\lambda_{sen}, \lambda_{spec}) = [p(\lambda_{sen} - r) + (1-p)(1- \lambda_{spec} - r)](\mu_{T1} - \mu_{C1})$$

generally is not zero.

Compared to (12.5), (12.19) shows that the marker utility is diluted by classification errors. When $\lambda_{sen} = \lambda_{spec} = 1/2$ (i.e., useless assay),

$$MU_{(r,p)}\left(\lambda_{sen} = \lambda_{spec} = 0.5\right) = \left(\frac{1}{2} - r\right)\left[p(\mu_{T1} - \mu_{C1}) + (1-p)(\mu_{T0} - \mu_{C0})\right]$$

which is 0 when $r = 1/2$ (equal randomization design).

When clinical utility $MU_{(r,p)}\left(\lambda_{sen}, \lambda_{spec}\right) \neq 0$, it depends on the randomization ratio r, which expresses the option of treatment decision if the marker results are not available. For example, when $r = 0$, patients are always treated with the control/SOC, and then

$$MU_{(0,p)}\left(\lambda_{sen}, \lambda_{spec}\right) = p\lambda_{sen}(\mu_{T1} - \mu_{C1}) + (1-p)(1 - \lambda_{spec})(\mu_{T0} - \mu_{C0}) \qquad (12.20)$$

Compared to the case of perfect assay, $MU_{(0,p)}(1,1) = p(\mu_{T1} - \mu_{C1})$, we see the trade-off between the misclassification errors and the treatment effect on the marker-negative patients.

Notice that the stratified design, with the same randomization ratio r, can also address (12.19). Shih and Lin (2018) found that the marker-stratified design has much greater statistical efficiency in testing the marker utility hypothesis H'_U than the precision medicine design. Hence, the precision medicine design is no longer recommended.

Adaptive Enrichment Designs

The adaptive enrichment design now is really enriching the marker-appeared-positive subjects. At the first stage, where the stratified design is placed, the composite (global) hypothesis will still be H_{0G}, with components H_{0a} and H_{0+}. The futility rule still depends on the inference on $\mu_{T0} - \mu_{C0}$, from Equations (13) and (15). However, the second stage, when enriching by accruing marker-appeared-positive without marker-appeared-negative subjects, is a targeted design, which can only contribute to Equations (12.6) and (12.7). In order to test H_{0+} we not only combine the marker-appeared-positives from both stages (for μ_{T*} and μ_{C*}), but also need to borrow the marker-appeared-negative stratum (for $\mu_{T\varnothing}$ and $\mu_{C\varnothing}$) to form Equations (12.10) and (12.12). The power and sample size calculations for the global hypothesis, overall cohort, and marker-positive cohort, impacted by classification's sensitivity and specificity, are addressed in Lin, Shih, and Lu (2019), where the enrichment design is shown to be more efficient than the marker-stratified design (one stage without enrichment consideration) in testing both the global hypothesis H_{0G} and the hypothesis of the treatment effect on the marker-positive cohort H_{0+}. The two-stage enrichment design enhances the power for testing the more hopeful marker-positive subset and the global hypothesis with a smaller sample size by reducing the power for the less hopeful overall cohort.

HOMEWORK 12.1

a. Read Shih and Lin's (2018) "Relative efficiency of precision medicine designs for clinical trials with predictive biomarkers" (*Statist Med*. 54(3): 411–424) to study the test procedures for all the hypotheses and comparisons of their efficiencies in testing the same hypotheses.

b. Read Lin, Shih, and Lu's (2019) "Two-stage enrichment trial design with adjustment for misclassification in predictive biomarkers" (*Statist. Med.* 38: 5445–5469) to identify the hypotheses and to study the test procedures of the two-stage enrichment design.

HOMEWORK 12.2

Derive (12.6) and (12.7), and comment on how the hypothesis H_{0+} on the marker-positive cohort may be tested.

HOMEWORK 12.3

Obtain Equations (12.10)–(12.13) from Equations (12.6)–(12.9).

HOMEWORK 12.4

Obtain Equations (12.14)–(12.17) from Equations (12.1), (12.2), (12.6), and (12.9).

HOMEWORK 12.5

a. Read Herbst, Baas, Kim, et al.'s (2016) "Pembrolizumab versus docetaxel for previously treated, PD-L1-positive, advanced non-small-cell lung cancer (KEYNOTE-010): a randomised controlled trial" (*The Lancet*. 387(10027): 1540–1550). What were the primary and secondary aims and hypotheses? What was the biomarker used in this study?

b. Read Reck, Rodriguez-Abreu, Robinson AG, et al.'s (2016) "Pembrolizumab versus chemotherapy for PD-L1-positive non-small-cell lung cancer" (*New England J Med.* 375: 1823–1833). What was the trial design? What were the primary and secondary aims and hypotheses? What was the biomarker-defined cohort?

References

Hayes DF. (2016). A bad tumor marker test is as bad a bad drug: The case for more consistent regulation of cancer diagnostics. *ASC Connection* Dec 22, 2016. http://connection.asco.org/blogs. (Last access: 12/30/2020).

Herbst RS, Baas P, Kim DW, et al. (2016). Pembrolizumab versus docetaxel for previously treated, PD-L1-positive, advanced non-small-cell lung cancer (KEYNOTE-010): a randomised controlled trial. *The Lancet* 387(10027):1540–1550.

Lin Y, Shih WJ and Lu SE. (2019). Two-stage enrichment trial design with adjustment for misclassification in predictive biomarkers. *Statistics in Medicine* 38:5445–5469.

Maitournam A and Simon R. (2005). On the efficiency of targeted clinical trials. *Statistics in Medicine* 24:329–339.

Mandrekar SJ, Sargent DJ. (2009). Clinical trial designs for predictive biomarker validation: one size does not fit all. *Journal of Biopharmaceutical Statistics* 19:530–542.

Mandrekar SJ, Sargent DJ. (2009). Clinical trial designs for predictive biomarker validation: theoretical considerations and practical challenges. *Journal of Clinical Oncology* 27:4027–34.

Mandrekar SJ, Sargent DJ. (2010). Predictive biomarker validation in practice: lessons from real trials. *Clinical Trials* 7:567–573.

Moses HL, Carbone D, Hartwell L, et al. (2007). *Cancer Biomarkers – The promises and challenges of improving detection and treatment.* Committee on Developing Biomarker-based Tools for Cancer Screening, Diagnosis, and Treatment. Washington, DC: The National Academies Press.

Reck M, Rodriguez-Abreu D, Robinson AG, et al. (2016). Pembrolizumab versus chemotherapy for PD-L1-positive non-small-cell lung cancer. *New England Journal of Medicine* 375:1823–1833.

Sargent DJ, Conley BA, Allegra C, Collette L. Clinical trial designs for predictive marker validation in cancer treatment trials. *Journal of Clinical Oncology* 2005; 23: 2020–27.

Shih WJ, Lin Y. (2017). On study designs and hypotheses for clinical trials with predictive biomarkers. *Contemporary Clinical Trials* 62:140–145.

Shih WJ, Lin Y. (2018). Relative efficiency of precision medicine designs for clinical trials with predictive biomarkers. *Statistics in Medicine* 54(3):411–424.

Simon R and Maitournam A. (2004). Evaluating the efficiency of targeted designs for randomized clinical trials. *Clinical Cancer Research* 10:6759–6763.

Smith I, Procter M, Gelber RD, Guillaume S, Feyereislova A, Dowsett M, et al. (2007). 2-year follow-up of trastuzumab after adjuvant chemotherapy in HER2-positive breast cancer: a randomised controlled trial. *Lancet* 369:29–36.

US Food and Drug Administration. (2012). Guidance for industry. *Enrichment strategies for clinical trials to support approval of human drugs and biological products.* Silver Spring, MD: US Food and Drug Administration.

US Food and Drug Administration. (2013). *Paving the way for personalized medicine: FDA's role in a new era of medical product development.* Silver Spring, MD: US Food and Drug Administration.

Wang SJ, Hung HMJ, O'Neill RT. (2009). Adaptive patient enrichment designs in therapeutic trials. *Biometrical Journal* 51:358–374.

Wang SJ, O'Neill RT, Hung HMJ. (2007). Approaches to evaluation of treatment effect in randomized clinical trials with genomic subset. *Pharmaceutical Statistics* 6:227–44.

Young KY, Laird A, Zhou XH. (2010). The efficiency of clinical trial designs for predictive biomarker validation. *Clinical Trials* 7:557–566.

13

Seamless Phase II/III: Select-the-Winner Design

Previously, we overviewed the conventional drug development steps (Section 1.4.3), in which the evaluations of dose, safety, pharmacokinetic (PK) and pharmacodynamic (PD) activity, and comparative benefit are performed in a sequence of phases using trial designs and endpoints specifically devised for each phase. The discrete development programs have intrinsic inefficiencies and pause between phases of research while investigators interpret results, design, and initiate the next study. Following the US FDA's Critical Path Initiative launched in 2004, the 21st Century Cures Act was signed into law in 2016. The Cures Act specifically calls on FDA to assist sponsors in incorporating complex adaptive and other novel trial designs into proposed clinical protocols and applications for new drugs and biological products to facilitate more efficient product development. One of the key innovations in drug development is to seek consolidation of the phases and to rapidly expand accrual with "seamless" trial designs.

Some of the seamless (Phase I/IIA) designs has been used in early-phase exploratory dose-ranging trials. An adaptive dose-ranging trial might begin with several doses and incorporate interim analyses based on comparative data to select doses for continued evaluation, with the goal of providing improved characterization of the dose–response relationship relative to a non-adaptive design and allowing selection of an optimal dose or doses for evaluation in future confirmatory trials. Bretz et al. (2005) combined multiple comparison procedure and modeling (MCP-Mod) for analyzing dose finding trials, which includes a PoC (proof-of-concept) assessment and a dose-selection step. Tao et al. (2015) extended MCP-Mod to finding MTD (maximum tolerated dose) and MED (minimum effective dose) with joint models. In oncology, the seamless Phase I/II usually is performed by single-arm dose escalation or de-escalation instead of several doses in parallel. Sometimes it is called Phase I/IIA, or Phase I with Phase II expansion. The Phase I part is for dose-finding with safety and tolerability as objectives and the Phase II expansion is for preliminary efficacy assessment on perhaps certain specific tumor sites.

Lin and Shih (2001) studied statistical properties of the traditional algorithm-based designs for Phase I cancer clinical trials, which included the so-called "3+3" designs in the general class of "A+B" designs. Shih and Lin (2006) further advanced the study to the modified "A+B" designs. The

DOI: 10.1201/9781003176527-13

Bayesian designs such as "mTPI" (Ji et al. 2010) and "BOIN" (Liu and Yuan 2015) have also gained popularity among practitioners recently.

We often find that, after the Phase I/IIA study, there may still be two or three doses left for testing in Phase IIB studies. In the pivotal Phase III trial, at most 2 doses are feasible in terms of sample size and other operational factors. The seamless Phase II/III design that we will discuss in this chapter is to further connect the selection of a dose (the "winner") portion to the Phase III portion, where confirmation of efficacy of the selected dose can be considered based on data combined from the entire trial. Such an adaptive design could in principle allow interim modifications to additional aspects of the design such as endpoint selection, the number of additional patients that will be enrolled, and/or the randomization ratio for treatment arms carried forward. As for trials intended to provide substantial evidence of effectiveness, statistical hypothesis testing methods should account for the adaptive selection of a best dose or doses from the multiple doses evaluated in the trial, as well as any additional adaptive modifications, such as the potential to stop the trial early or to modify future sample sizes. Some trials only operationally connect the Phase II dose selection part to the Phase III confirmatory testing of the selected dose by having the same study centers, investigators and laboratories using one trial protocol to save operation efforts and time (not sample size) in the trial process. For example, the Phase II dose selection is based on an endpoint as its primary objective and the Phase III is based on a different endpoint as its primary objective. See Merck's (2021) INSIGNIA-PAH trial (NCT04732221) for an example. In this case, separate statistical inferences are performed and data are not combined from the Phase II and Phase III parts of the same protocol. This kind of design is known as *operationally seamless design* to distinguish it from what we consider in the following, which is *inferentially seamless design*. Incidentally, most Phase I/II designs are operationally seamless. An example is given by Bardia et al. (2019).

In this chapter, we consider a design with two doses (say high and low) and a control group with a planned interim analysis. The inferior dose group will not be expanded after the interim analysis, and only the winning dose and the control groups will be expanded to the end of the study. (But the inferior dose group might still be followed up.) The interim evaluation may be based on a different but correlated (surrogate) endpoint than the primary endpoint for the final analysis when the primary endpoint needs more time to measure or observe. The correlation between the two endpoints plays an important role in this situation. Seamless trials require rigorous, prespecified, statistical analysis plans, and sample sizes commensurate with the objectives and endpoints under study. This is especially interesting since, as we shall discuss in Chapter 15, the strategy of handling intercurrent events may well be different for an early-phase trial versus a late-phase trial, while this phase II/III seamless design is a combination of both. We consider the continuous endpoints in this chapter and leave the readers to consult Fang et al. (2013) for the case of more complicated survival endpoints.

13.1 Trial Setting, Hypothesis, and Test Statistic

13.1.1 Trial Setting and Hypothesis

Consider a two-stage winner design with two dose groups of an experimental treatment and one control group. The randomization is 1:1:1; equal sample size n_1 per group for the first stage. One interim selection is planned to select a more effective ("winner") treatment dose at information time $\tau = n_1/n$, where n is the final sample size combining both stages for the winning dose (and the control group) as the "winner" treatment dose is continued with the control group for testing the hypothesis in the final analysis. Hence, the total sample size of the trial is $N = 2n + n_1$.

Let $\{X_i^{(j)} \mid i = 1, \ldots, n_1\}$ denote the interim continuous measurements that are assumed to be independently, identically distributed with $N(v_j^X, \sigma_X^2)$, where j=0 represents the control arm and j=1, 2 denote the two dose arms of the experimental treatment (j=1 for low dose and j=2 for high dose). Likewise, let $\{Y_i^{(j)} \mid i = 1, \ldots, n\}$, j=0, 1, 2, denote the final continuous measurements that are independently, identically distributed with $N(\mu_j^Y, \sigma_Y^2)$. The continuous variable X used at the interim analysis could be the same as or a surrogate of the continuous variable Y used at the final analysis. Assume that the variances σ_X^2 and σ_Y^2 are known, and $X_i^{(j)}$ and $Y_i^{(j)}$ are correlated with a correlation ρ, i.e., $\mathrm{corr}(X_i^{(j)}, Y_i^{(j)}) = \rho$, for $1 \le i \le n_1$ and j =0, 1, 2. Notice that when the endpoints at the interim and final analyses are the same, $X_i^{(j)} = Y_i^{(j)}$ and hence $\rho = 1$.

Let $\delta_j = \mu_j^Y - \mu_0^Y$ be the unknown treatment effect of dose j of the experimental treatment versus the control at the final analysis for j =1 or 2. We consider the following noninferiority (NI) hypotheses:

$$H_{01} : \delta_1 \le -\Delta, \text{ verses } H_{A1} : \delta_1 > -\Delta$$

$$H_{02} : \delta_2 \le -\Delta, \text{ verses } H_{A2} : \delta_2 > -\Delta$$

$$H_0 = H_{01} \cap H_{02} : \delta_1 \le -\Delta \text{ and } \delta_2 \le -\Delta, \text{ verses } H_A : \delta_1 > -\Delta \text{ or } \delta_2 > -\Delta \quad (13.1)$$

where $\Delta \; (\ge 0)$ is the prespecified NI margin which can be interpreted as the largest clinically and statistically acceptable difference in means. If $\Delta = 0$, then (13.1) becomes superiority hypothesis. Notice that, in the case of $\Delta = 0$, the null hypothesis in (13.1) is more appropriate than $H'_0 : \delta_1 = 0$ and $\delta_2 = 0$ as expressed in Shun et al. (2008) for one-sided hypothesis. The familywise type I error rate (FWER) is controlled by the application of the closed testing procedure (Marcus, Peritz, and Gabriel 1976). That is, in this case, the two doses with comparisons to the common control and the corresponding hypotheses H_{01} and H_{02} are to be tested, and the overall type I error rate is

0.025 (one-sided noninferiority) by the following: H_{01} can be rejected at alpha level of 0.025 if and only if both $H_0 = H_{01} \cap H_{02}$ and H_{01} are rejected using valid tests with level 0.025; H_{02} can be rejected at level 0.025 if and only if $H_0 = H_{01} \cap H_{02}$ and H_{02} are rejected using valid tests with level 0.025. Hence, we start to work on testing $H_0 = H_{01} \cap H_{02}$ first in the following sections since it applies to both doses. Notice that H_0 is a global or composite hypothesis (see Chapter 10). The alternative hypothesis H_A states that either dose 1 or dose 2 of the experimental treatment is NI to the control. (See Figure 4.3 in Chapter 4.) To control strongly the FWER, we will also test the individual hypothesis for each dose at the same alpha level after we finish testing (and rejecting) H_0.

13.1.2 Test Statistic for the Global Hypothesis

Let the interim sample means be $\overline{X}_{n_1}^{(j)} = \left(\dfrac{1}{n_1}\right)\sum_{i=1}^{n_1} X_i^{(j)}$, $j = 0$, 1, 2, and $V_{n_1} = \sqrt{\dfrac{n_1}{2\sigma_X^2}}\left(\overline{X}_{n_1}^{(1)} - \overline{X}_{n_1}^{(2)}\right)$. Let the final sample means be $\overline{Y}_n^{(j)} = \left(\dfrac{1}{n}\right)\sum_{i=1}^{n} Y_i^{(j)}$, for $j = 0$, 1, 2, and $Z_n^{(i)} = \sqrt{\dfrac{n}{2\sigma_Y^2}}(\overline{Y}_n^{(i)} - \overline{Y}_n^{(0)})$ for $i = 1$ or 2. The selection rule at the interim look is as follows: Select treatment dose 1 (low dose) when $\overline{X}_{n_1}^{(1)} - \overline{X}_{n_1}^{(2)} > c$, or equivalently, $V_{n_1} > c'$ where $c' = c\sqrt{\dfrac{n_1}{2\sigma_X^2}}$; otherwise, select treatment dose 2, where $c > 0$ is a constant that dictates a minimum amount of difference for low dose to be considered better than the high dose to demonstrate its preference. It may be reasonable clinically to relate c to Δ. Remember, however, the NI margin is to compare with the control in the primary endpoint, while c is to compare the two doses in the surrogate endpoint. This is a generalization of Wang et al. (2017) where c=0. Notice that no statistical test is involved in the selection rule and that the design is to select only one dose arm of the experimental treatment to expand with the control group after the first stage. For the unselected dose, there are two scenarios depending on the disease and the primary endpoint. One scenario is called "complete follow-up," where patients in the unselected dose group are still followed up for the primary endpoint (such as survival) even though no new additional patients will be enrolled in the second stage. The other scenario is called "discontinued follow-up," where the patients treated with the unselected dose are simply discontinued from the trial and no further data are collected (such as the multiple sclerosis case; see Friede et al. 2011). We will discuss further this point later when considering the test for individual dose hypotheses.

We define the final test statistic as

$$W = Z_n^{(1)} + \Delta' \text{ if } V_{n_1} > c'; \text{ otherwise, } W = Z_n^{(2)} + \Delta' \qquad (13.2)$$

where $\Delta' = \Delta\sqrt{\dfrac{n}{2\sigma_Y^2}}$ and $c' = c\sqrt{\dfrac{n_1}{2\sigma_X^2}}$.

V_{n_1} follows a normal distribution with mean λ and variance 1, where

$$\lambda = \sqrt{\dfrac{n_1}{2\sigma_X^2}}\left(v_1^X - v_2^X\right) \equiv \sqrt{\dfrac{n_1}{2\sigma_X^2}}v_{12}. \qquad (13.3)$$

The probability of selecting dose 1 and continuing to test its efficacy against the control group is $p = \Pr(V_{n_1} > c') = \Phi(\lambda - c') \equiv \Phi(\lambda')$; $q = 1 - p$ is the probability of selecting dose 2. The null global hypothesis $H_0 = H_{01} \cap H_{02}$ is rejected when the value of W is large, say $W > w_\alpha$. To determine the critical value w_α, and to estimate power at δ_j, we need to know the distribution of W. The distribution of W involves the correlation between the interim endpoint and final analysis endpoint as follows:

$$F_W(w) = \Pr(W \le w) = \Pr\left(W \le w,\ V_{n_1} > c'\right) + \Pr\left(W \le w,\ V_{n_1} < c'\right)$$

$$= \Pr\left(Z_n^{(1)} + \Delta' \le w,\ V_{n_1} > c'\right) + \Pr\left(Z_n^{(2)} + \Delta' \le w,\ V_{n_1} < c'\right)$$

$$= \Pr\left(Z_n^{(1)} - \delta_1' \le w - \Delta' - \delta_1',\ V_{n_1} - \lambda > c' - \lambda\right)$$

$$+ \Pr\left(Z_n^{(2)} - \delta_2' \le w - \Delta' - \delta_2',\ V_{n_1} - \lambda < c' - \lambda\right)$$

$$\equiv \Pr\left(T_n^{(1)} \le w - \Delta' - \delta_1',\ S_{n_1} > c' - \lambda\right)$$

$$+ \Pr\left(T_n^{(2)} \le w - \Delta' - \delta_2',\ S_{n_1} < c' - \lambda\right) \qquad (13.4)$$

where $\delta_i' = \sqrt{\dfrac{n}{2\sigma_Y^2}}\delta_i$, $T_n^{(i)} = Z_n^{(i)} - \delta_i'$, and $S_{n_1} = V_{n_1} - \lambda$. The joint distribution of $(T_n^{(i)}, S_{n_1})$ is bivariate standard normal with covariance (correlation) $\eta = \mathrm{cov}\left(Z_n^{(1)},\ V_{n_1}\right) = -\mathrm{cov}\left(Z_n^{(2)},\ V_{n_1}\right) = \dfrac{\sqrt{\tau}}{2}\rho$, which can be directly derived from the definitions of $Z_n^{(1)}$, $Z_n^{(2)}$, and V_{n_1} (Homework 13.1).

The conditional distributions

$$S_{n_1} \mid T_n^{(1)} \sim N\left(\eta T_n^{(1)},\ 1 - \eta^2\right) \text{ and } S_{n_1} \mid T_n^{(2)} \sim N\left(-\eta T_n^{(1)},\ 1 - \eta^2\right)$$

follow from Equation (2.1) in Chapter 2 and Homework 4.2 in Chapter 4 (Homework 13.2). Hence, the first term of Equation (13.4) becomes

$$\Pr\left(T_n^{(1)} \le w - \Delta' - \delta_1',\ -S_{n_1} < -c' + \lambda\right)$$

$$= \int_{-\infty}^{w-\Delta'-\delta_1'} \Pr(-S_{n_1} < \lambda' \mid T_n^{(1)} = t)\phi(t)dt$$

$$= \int_{-\infty}^{w-\Delta'-\delta_1'} \Pr\left(\frac{-S_{n_1} + \eta t}{\sqrt{1-\eta^2}} < \frac{\lambda' + \eta t}{\sqrt{1-\eta^2}} \mid T_n^{(1)} = t\right)\phi(t)dt$$

$$= \int_{-\infty}^{w-\Delta'-\delta_1'} \Phi\left(\frac{\lambda' + \eta t}{\sqrt{1-\eta^2}}\right)\phi(t)dt \tag{13.5}$$

where $\lambda' = \lambda - c'$. The second term of (13.4) becomes

$$\Pr\left(T_n^{(2)} \le w - \Delta' - \delta_2', S_{n_1} < c' - \lambda\right)$$

$$= \int_{-\infty}^{w-\Delta'-\delta_2'} \Pr(S_{n_1} < -\lambda' \mid T_n^{(2)} = t)\,\phi(t)dt$$

$$= \int_{-\infty}^{w-\Delta'-\delta_2'} \Pr\left(\frac{S_{n_1} + \eta t}{\sqrt{1-\eta^2}} < \frac{-\lambda' + \eta t}{\sqrt{1-\eta^2}} \mid T_n^{(2)} = t\right)\phi(t)dt$$

$$= \int_{-\infty}^{w-\Delta'-\delta_2'} \Phi\left(\frac{-\lambda' + \eta t}{\sqrt{1-\eta^2}}\right)\phi(t)dt \tag{13.6}$$

Under H_0, Wang et al. (2017) extended the results from Shun et al. (2008) and showed that $\dfrac{W - \mu_0}{\sigma_0}$ can be approximated by a standard normal distribution, where

$$\mu_0 = \eta\sqrt{\frac{2}{\pi}} = \rho\sqrt{\frac{\tau}{2\pi}} \text{ and } \sigma_0^2 = 1 - \mu_0^2. \tag{13.7}$$

(More on the normal approximation is discussed in Section 13.2.) Therefore, for a one-sided α level, the critical value $w_\alpha = z_\alpha \sigma_0 + \mu_0$.

Notice that the critical value does not depend on the NI margin Δ, nor on the selection of the dose (which dose is selected, the constant c, or the winning probability p), but depends on the information time τ of the interim analysis and the correlation ρ between the interim and final endpoints via $\eta = \dfrac{\sqrt{\tau}}{2}\rho$. As long as (τ, ρ) gives the same η, the critical value is the same. Table 13.1 gives some critical values w_α for the test statistic W in Equation (13.2) as a function of $\eta = \dfrac{\sqrt{\tau}}{2}\rho$ for $\alpha = 0.025$.

TABLE 13.1

Critical Values w_α for the Test Statistic W as a Function of $\eta = \frac{\sqrt{\tau}}{2}\rho$ for $\alpha = 0.025$ Using the Normal Approximation Method

$\rho \backslash \tau$	0.25	0.33	0.50	0.60
0.00	1.96	1.96	1.96	1.96
0.40	2.033	2.043	2.060	2.069
0.50	2.050	2.062	2.081	2.091
0.65	2.073	2.087	2.110	2.121

We can see from Table 13.1 that the adjustment increases (compared to 1.96) as the correlation increases or the interim analysis time gets later. If the interim selection is performed at an earlier information time of the study, there will be less multiplicity, but more adaptability. In general, the earlier the interim selection is performed, the lesser the inflation in type I error rate (thus, less adjustment of the critical value) will be. If the interim selection is performed very close to the end of the study, the situation becomes one of conventional multiple comparisons with a "many-to-one" design: Each treatment dose group is compared with a common control. In this case, Dunnett (1955) developed a method to control the overall type I error rate. However, interim analysis should also have enough data to obtain reliable results. As for choosing a surrogate endpoint, we would like it to be well correlated with the primary endpoint. However, the larger the correlation, the more the multiplicity, leading to more correction for the critical value. When designing the study protocol, one can plan for the interim analysis time and assume a correlation value based on information from other studies. Simulation work will be helpful. The actual correlation can be estimated from the trial's data of the first stage, and the actual interim analysis time will be known at the end of the trial when the final sample size is realized.

Example 13.1:

A trial to treat age-related macular degeneration (AMD) is conducted using the seamless Phase II/III select-the-winner design. At the first phase of the trial, patients are randomized to the standard of care (SOC) active control, doses 1.0 or 1.5 mg of the test treatment. The primary efficacy endpoint is the best corrected visual activity (BCVA) measured by changes in Early Treatment Diabetic Retinopathy Study (ETDRS) letters (range from 0 to 100) at 52 weeks after baseline. The trial plans to conduct one interim analysis for Stage 1 using the changes of ETDRS letters at 16 weeks as a surrogate endpoint to select the winner between the two doses.

Assume that the interim analysis is performed at $\tau = 0.33$, and the correlation between the week 16 and week 52 changes of ETDRS letters is $\rho = 0.5$, then $\eta = \frac{\sqrt{\tau}}{2}\rho = 0.144, \mu_0 = \eta\sqrt{\frac{2}{\pi}} = 0.1146$, and $\sigma_0^2 = 1 - \mu_0^2 = 0.9869$. For

α = 0.025, the critical value is $w_{0.025} = z_{0.025}\sigma_0 + \mu_0 = 1.96*(0.9869)^{1/2}+0.1146$ = 2.062, by the following simple R code:

```
tau=0.33
rho=0.50
u0=(sqrt(tau)*rho/2)*sqrt(2/pi)
s2=1-u0**2
1.96*sqrt(s2)+u0
[1] 2.061677
```

This normal approximation is a convenient way to obtain the critical value and sheds the analytical insight as discussed above. The exact distribution of W, of course, is preferred for calculation of the critical value, which involves the numerical method given in the R code provided in Appendix 13.1 (with modification). The readers can compare the exact solution with the approximation shown in Table 13.1 (Homework 13.7).

13.2 Power and Sample Size Estimation

From (13.4), (13.5), and (13.6), at the significance level α, the power is

$$1-\beta = \Pr(W > w_\alpha) = 1 - F_W(w)$$

$$= 1 - \int_{-\infty}^{w_\alpha - \Delta' - \delta_1'} \Phi\left(\frac{\lambda' + \eta t}{\sqrt{1-\eta^2}}\right)\phi(t)dt - \int_{-\infty}^{w_\alpha - \Delta' - \delta_2'} \Phi\left(\frac{-\lambda' + \eta t}{\sqrt{1-\eta^2}}\right)\phi(t)dt$$

$$= 1 - \int_{-\infty}^{w_\alpha - \sqrt{\frac{n}{2\sigma_Y^2}}(\Delta+\delta_1)} \Phi\left(\frac{\sqrt{\frac{n\tau}{2\sigma_X^2}}(v_{12}-c)+\eta t}{\sqrt{1-\eta^2}}\right)\phi(t)dt$$

$$- \int_{-\infty}^{w_\alpha - \sqrt{\frac{n}{2\sigma_Y^2}}(\Delta+\delta_2)} \Phi\left(\frac{-\sqrt{\frac{n\tau}{2\sigma_X^2}}(v_{12}-c)+\eta t}{\sqrt{1-\eta^2}}\right)\phi(t)dt \qquad (13.8)$$

where the critical value w_α may be obtained by the exact method in Homework 13.7 or by the approximation method $w_\alpha = z_\alpha\sigma_0 + \mu_0$ from Equation (13.7).

The sample size n can be determined from (13.8) for given power, significance level, and other design parameters. Appendix 13.1 provides an R program to solve (13.8) for sample size n. Notice that, adding the sample size n_1 of the dose group that is not selected for expansion after the interim analysis, the total sample size of the trial is $2n + n_1$. Although this power is for testing the global hypothesis only, not yet including testing the individual hypothesis, the discussion in Section 13.3 shows that it is also the power including testing the individual hypotheses. When designing a trial, we advise to perform simulation studies with different assumptions and scenarios.

An alternative way is to use normal approximation as discussed below. The normal approximation worked well and provided the simple solution for the critical value as we saw in Section 13.1. Moreover, it also sheds some light on the comparison of sample size with the non-adaptive design as follows.

Wang et al. (2017) also extended the results of Shun et al. (2008) and showed that the distribution of W in (13.4) can well be approximated by a mixture of normal distributions. As a result, the power can be approximated by the following equation:

$$1-\beta \approx 1 - p\Phi\left(\frac{w_\alpha - (\delta_1 + \Delta)\sqrt{\frac{n}{2\sigma_Y^2}} - \mu_1}{\sigma_1}\right) - q\Phi\left(\frac{w_\alpha - (\delta_2 + \Delta)\sqrt{\frac{n}{2\sigma_Y^2}} - \mu_2}{\sigma_2}\right)$$

(13.9)

$$\equiv 1 - p\beta_1 - q\beta_2$$

where

$$p = \Phi(\lambda')$$

$$\mu_1 = \frac{\eta}{p\sqrt{2\pi}}e^{-\frac{\lambda'^2}{2}}$$

$$\mu_2 = \frac{\eta}{q\sqrt{2\pi}}e^{-\frac{\lambda'^2}{2}}$$

$$\sigma_1^2 = 1 - \lambda'\eta\mu_1 - \mu_1^2$$

$$\sigma_2^2 = 1 + \lambda'\eta\mu_2 - \mu_2^2$$

(13.10)

and $\lambda' = \lambda - c'$, $\eta = \frac{\sqrt{\tau}}{2}\rho$, and $\tau = n_1/n$ indicates the timing of the interim analysis.

We can determine the sample size per group n at the final stage by solving (13.9) for given type I error rate α, power $1 - \beta$, and other parameters. For the scenario that different endpoints are used for the interim and final analyses, we can calculate $\eta = \dfrac{\sqrt{\tau}}{2}\rho$, $\lambda = \sqrt{\dfrac{n_1}{2\sigma_X^2}}(v_1^X - v_2^X) = \sqrt{\dfrac{n\tau}{2\sigma_X^2}}v_{12}$. When the same endpoint is used for the interim and final analyses, $\eta = \dfrac{\sqrt{\tau}}{2}$, $\lambda = \sqrt{\dfrac{n\tau}{2\sigma_X^2}}(\delta_1 - \delta_2)$.

In either situation, $c' = c\sqrt{\dfrac{n\tau}{2\sigma_X^2}}$, $\lambda' = \lambda - c' = \sqrt{\dfrac{n\tau}{2\sigma_X^2}}(v_{12} - c)$, and $p = \Phi(\lambda')$ for given c, we plug these parameters into (13.7) and (13.10) to obtain μ_i and σ_i^2, $i = 0, 1, 2$. Then, for given α, and $1 - \beta$, we can solve for n, β_1, and β_2 in (13.9). Recursive calculation is required since λ' and c' also involve n, and μ_i and σ_i^2 involve λ'. For recursive calculations, we need to have an initial guess of the range of n. (This range is also needed in the R program in Appendix 13.1.) To find a reasonable range, we consider a special case below.

A special and common case of the situation with the same endpoint is $c = 0$, $\delta_1 = \delta_2 = \delta$ for the two dose groups. Then, $\lambda = 0$ and $p = 0.5$, $\mu_i = \eta\sqrt{\dfrac{2}{\pi}} = \sqrt{\dfrac{\tau}{2\pi}}$, $\sigma_i^2 = 1 - \dfrac{2\eta^2}{\pi} = 1 - \dfrac{\tau}{2\pi}$, for $i = 0, 1, 2$, and $\beta = \beta_1 = \beta_2$. With the critical value $w_\alpha = z_\alpha\sigma_0 + \mu_0$, we obtain from (13.9) the following:

$$z_\beta = \frac{(\delta + \Delta)\sqrt{\dfrac{n}{2\sigma_Y^2}} - z_\alpha\sigma_0}{\sigma_0}. \tag{13.11}$$

Hence,

$$n = 2\sigma_0^2(z_\alpha + z_\beta)^2\left(\frac{\sigma_Y}{\delta + \Delta}\right)^2 = 2\left(1 - \frac{\tau}{2\pi}\right)(z_\alpha + z_\beta)^2\left(\frac{\sigma_Y}{\delta + \Delta}\right)^2. \tag{13.12}$$

It is interesting to compare (13.12) to (4.26) for the non-adaptive two-group design case, and notice a sample size (per group) reduction by a factor of $\left(1 - \dfrac{\tau}{2\pi}\right)$ in (13.12). This indicates the efficiency gain for the Phase II/III seamless design compared the non-adaptive design. Either (13.12) or (4.26) may be the basis for setting the range of sample size in the recursive calculation for the R program in Appendix 13.1.

If there is a need to predetermine n_1 instead of τ, we replace τ by n_1/n in (13.12), then let $Q = (z_\alpha + z_\beta)^2\left(\dfrac{\sigma_Y}{\delta + \Delta}\right)^2$, and after some algebra, we obtain

$$n = 2\left(1 - \frac{n_1}{2n\pi}\right)Q$$

$$= Q + Q\left(1 - \frac{n_1}{\pi Q}\right)^{1/2} \tag{13.13}$$

Example 13.2:

Continue Example 13.1. The task is to find the sample size n to provide a power 80% or 90% for the global hypothesis. The NI margin is set to be $\Delta = 5$ letters. We assume that, on average, dose 1.0 mg (dose 1) is 2 letters better than the control (i.e., $\delta_1 = 2$), dose 1.5 mg (dose 2) is 3 letters better than the control (i.e., $\delta_2 = 3$) at week 52 as well as at week 16 (i.e., $v_{12} = v_1^X - v_2^X = 1$), and $\sigma_X = \sigma_Y = 15$ letters. The 1.0 mg dose (dose 1) will be chosen only if its sample mean is at least 5 letters better than that of the 1.5 mg dose group (i.e., $c = 5$). Suppose we adopt the approach of prespecifying $\tau = 0.33$ to conduct the interim analysis. From Example 13.1, $\eta = \frac{\sqrt{\tau}}{2} \rho = 0.144$, $\mu_0 = \eta\sqrt{\frac{2}{\pi}} = 0.1146$, $\sigma_0^2 = 1 - \mu_0^2 = 0.9869$, obtain the critical value $w_{0.025} = 2.062$ by the normal approximation method and assuming the correlation $\rho = 0.5$ between the surrogate week 16 endpoint and the week 52 primary endpoint. Now, before we utilize the R program in Appendix 13.1, we find a reasonable range for n, using (13.12) by letting $\delta = (\delta_1 + \delta_2)/2$

```
> 2*(1-0.5/(2*pi))*(qnorm(0.025)+qnorm(0.20))**2*(15/
(5+2.5))**2
[1]  57.79429
```

Hence, setting a range of 50 to 120, we use the R program in Appendix 13.1 and obtain the following:
   For 80% power, n = 71.

```
> find_sample_size_two_arm(50, 120, 0.80, 2.062, c=5,
0.33, 0.5, 1, 3, 2, 15, 15, 5)
[1]  70.5673
```

For 90% power, n = 97.

```
> find_sample_size_two_arm(50, 120, 0.90, 2.062, c=5,
0.33, 0.5, 1, 3, 2, 15, 15, 5)
[1]  96.2086
```

Operationally, for 80% power, the first stage (at $\tau = 0.33$) would randomize 24 * 3=72 patients with 24 in each group. The total sample size for the trial would be 2 * 72+24=168 patients. The probability of selecting the low dose is about 18%. For 90% power, the first stage would randomize 33 * 3 = 99 patients with 33 in each group. The total sample size for the trial would be 2 * 99 + 33 = 231 patients. The probability of selecting the low dose is about 14%.

Discussion

1. When planning the trial protocol for sample size and power calculation, there are two options: either fixing the timing τ of the interim analysis or specifying the probability p of selecting the correct winner. However, it is conceivable that when the mean effect difference between the dose groups is near the constant c, requiring selecting correct winner with probability different from 0.5 will be impossible. Hence, we usually would choose fixing the information time to estimate the sample size for given power.

2. It is sometimes difficult to find good prior data to estimate the correlation parameter at planning. We advise to carry out simulations with varying correlation and interim analysis timing assumptions to see the robustness of the design. The actual correlation between the surrogate endpoint and the primary endpoint can be estimated at the interim analysis using the Stage 1 data, and then it should be used for calculating the critical value of the final test.

3. Although we assume the observations are from normal distribution, what really matters is the sample means are normally distributed, which is a result of the Central Limit Theorem for reasonable sample sizes.

13.3 Test for Individual Hypothesis of Each Dose

As we alluded to before, when the global null hypothesis is rejected, we need to continue testing for the component of the global hypothesis regarding each dose at the same level α. For the dose that is selected, the associated test is the same final test as W, and since the critical value $w_\alpha = z_\alpha \sigma_0 + \mu_0 > z_\alpha$ from Equation (13.7), this individual null hypothesis is automatically rejected as well at level α. For the dose that is not selected, we simply (i.e., conservatively) do not reject its individual null hypothesis whether the case is "discontinued follow-up" or "complete follow-up." Therefore, the power we obtained in the previous section for the global hypothesis is also the power for the "global hypothesis plus the individual hypotheses." Specifically, for H_{01},

Pr(reject $H_{01} \mid H_{01}$)
   = Pr(dose 1 selected at Stage 1, reject H_{01} at final analysis $\mid H_{01}$)
      + Pr(dose 1 not selected at Stage 1, reject H_{01} at final analysis $\mid H_{01}$).

From Eq. (13.2), the first term follows:

$$\Pr\left(Z_n^{(1)} + \Delta' \geq w_\alpha, \ V_{n_1} > c' \mid H_{01}\right)$$

$$\leq \Pr\left(W \geq w_\alpha \mid H_{01}\right) = \alpha$$

The second term is zero per the procedure's definition, regardless of "discontinued follow-up design" or "complete follow-up design." Similarly, for H_{02},

Pr(reject H_{02} | H_{02})
= Pr(dose 2 selected at Stage 1, reject H_{02} at final analysis | H_{02})
+ Pr(dose 2 not selected at Stage 1, reject H_{02} at final analysis | H_{02}).

From Eq. (13.2), the first term follows:

$$\Pr\left(Z_n^{(2)} + \Delta' \geq w_\alpha, \ V_{n_1} < c' \big| H_{02}\right)$$

$$\leq \Pr\left(W \geq w_\alpha \ | \ H_{02}\right) = \alpha$$

The second term is zero likewise, regardless of "discontinued follow-up design" or "complete follow-up design."

Discussion
This procedure that simply does not reject the individual null hypothesis for the unselected dose is a conservative approach. For the "discontinued follow-up design" case, no data are collected for the unselected dose by design; thus, we are facing a missing data problem. Instead of simply not rejecting the null hypothesis of the unselected dose due to missing the final endpoint, we may use some regression method to impute the missing final endpoint. The topic of missing data is discussed in Chapter 15.

For "complete follow-up design" or when no surrogate endpoint is used (i.e., $X = Y$), we have the $Z_{n_1}^{(i)}$ values from the $2n_1$ patients entered in the first stage, how to utilize these data is also a research topic.

13.4 Test Based on Combination of Two-Stage P-Values

Friede et al. (2008, 2011) following the general concepts of Bretz et al. (2006) also developed a test procedure that controls the FWER in the strong sense through the application of the closed testing procedure together with the combination test method using stage-wise p-values. (Recall that we have discussed the method of combining stage-wise p-values in Appendix 8.3.2 of Chapter 8 in a different context, but the idea is the same.) Their method also adopts the conservative approach of not rejecting the null hypothesis of the unselected dose. The advantage of their method is that it can easily include more treatments or doses in the first selection stage as well as in the second extension stage. Their method is implemented with simulation capability in R package "ASD" (adaptive seamless design; Parsons et al. 2011). Furthermore, Kunz et al. (2015) did a comparison study with other methods, except that the comparison did not include the method we presented here. We leave the reading and perhaps a comparison study to the readers as a homework or research project.

Appendix 13.1: Seamless Phase II/III Select-the-Winner Design Sample Size R Program[1]

```
#===============================================================
gamma_w1w2 <- function(wa, c, n, tau, rho, nu12, delta1,
delta2, sigmaX,sigmaY, epsilon) {
# epsilon is the NI margin (triangle delta in text); delta1
and delta2 are the lower case delta in text.
n1<-n*tau
eta <- sqrt(tau)/2*rho
lambda <- sqrt(n1/2/sigmaX^2)*(nu12-c)
sOneEta2 <- sqrt(1-eta^2)
k0 <- lambda / sOneEta2
k <- eta / sOneEta2
w1<-sqrt(n/2/sigmaY^2)*delta1
w2<-sqrt(n/2/sigmaY^2)*delta2
niconst<-sqrt(n/2/sigmaY^2)*epsilon
#---------------------------------------------------------------
term1 <- integrate(function(z1e) {
        d1 <- dnorm(z1e)
        d3 <- pnorm(k0 + k*z1e)
        rvTerm1Function <- d1*d3
        return(rvTerm1Function)
        }
        , -Inf, wa-w1-niconst)$value
#---------------------------------------------------------------
term2 <- integrate(function(z1e) {
        d1 <- dnorm(z1e)
        d3 <- pnorm(-k0 + k*z1e)
        rvTerm2Function <- d1*d3
        return(rvTerm2Function)
        }, -Inf, wa-w2-niconst)$value
#---------------------------------------------------------------
return(1-term1-term2)
#---------------------------------------------------------------
}
#===============================================================
#Sample size estimation(surrogate endpoints are used)
#for two-stage winner design with two experimental treatments
and an active control.
#nu12=nu1-nu2 is the treatment effect difference of the
surrogate endpoint between the two experimental treatments
at the interim look.
```

[1] Written by Pin-Wen Wang with Slight Modifications

```
#c is the least difference for interim dose selection
comparing to nu12
#rho is the correlation between surrogate and primary
endpoints
#delta1 and delta2 are the target treatment effect of the
primary endpoint at the final analysis
#wa is the alpha-level critical value determined using a
separate code in the chapter text
#tau is the interim time fraction
#epsilon is the NI margin constant (=triangle delta in the
chapter text)
#===========================================================
find_sample_size_two_arm <- function(nBegin, nEnd, power, wa,
c, tau, rho, nu12,delta1,delta2,sigmaX, sigmaY, epsilon)
{ return(uniroot(function(n) { return(power - gamma_w1w2(wa, c,
n, tau,rho, nu12, delta1, delta2, sigmaX, sigmaY, epsilon))},
c(nBegin, nEnd))$root)
}


#Examples in Wang et al. (2017)
find_sample_size_two_arm(nBegin=50, nEnd=120, power=0.80,
wa=2.168, c=0, tau=0.5, rho=1, nu12=1, delta1=3, delta2=2,
sigmaX=15, sigmaY=15, epsilon=4)
[1] 75.80142
find_sample_size_two_arm(50, 120, 0.80, 2.168, 0, 0.5, 1, 1,
3, 2, 15, 15, 3)
[1] 105.0752

#Example 11.2 in the text
find_sample_size_two_arm(50, 120, 0.80, 2.062, c=5, 0.33, 0.5,
1, 3, 2, 15, 15, 5)

[1] 70.5673

find_sample_size_two_arm(50, 120, 0.90, 2.062, c=5, 0.33, 0.5,
1, 3, 2, 15, 15, 5)

[1] 96.2086
```

HOMEWORK 13.1

Derive the covariance $\eta = \text{cov}\left(Z_n^{(1)}, V_{n_1}\right) = -\text{cov}\left(Z_n^{(2)}, V_{n_1}\right) = \frac{\sqrt{\tau}}{2}\rho$ from the definitions of $Z_n^{(1)}$, $Z_n^{(1)}$, and V_{n_1}.

HOMEWORK 13.2

Work out the conditional distributions in Section 13.1: $S_{n_1} \mid T_n^{(1)}$
$N\left(\eta T_n^{(1)}, 1-\eta^2\right)$ and $S_{n_1} \mid T_n^{(2)} \sim N\left(-\eta T_n^{(1)}, 1-\eta^2\right)$

HOMEWORK 13.3

Follow Example 13.2, suppose the interim analysis is scheduled at
$\tau = 0.5$, and find the sample size for power 0.8 and 0.9. Discuss the timing impact on the sample size.

HOMEWORK 13.4

Follow Homework 13.3, suppose the correlation $\rho = 0.65$, and find the
sample size for power 0.8 and 0.9. Discuss the correlation impact on the
sample size.

HOMEWORK 13.5

Follow Homework 13.4, suppose the criterion value $c=2$ for dose selection at Stage 1, and find the sample size for power 0.8 and 0.9. Discuss
the impact of the selection criterion value c on the sample size.

HOMEWORK 13.6

Consider the situation with the same endpoint, and assume $\delta_1 = \delta_2 = \delta$
for the two dose groups. Compare the total sample size of two trials: Trial A is to use the traditional three-group parallel non-adaptive
design. Trial B is to use the Phase II/III select-the-winner design with
$\tau = 0.5$, and the selection criterion value is $c = 0$. The same power and
type I error rate of your choice are used for both trials.

HOMEWORK 13.7

Modify the R code in Appendix 13.1 for finding the critical values using
the exact distribution of W. Construct a display and compare it with
Table 13.1. How close is the normal approximation in Table 13.1 to the
exact solution?

HOMEWORK 13.8

1. Read the reference "Designing a seamless phase II/III clinical trial using early outcomes for treatment selection: an application in multiple sclerosis" (*Stat Med* 2011, 1528–1540 by Friede et al).

2. Use the R package "ASD" (see treatsel.sim: ASD simulation for treatment selection in asd: simulations for adaptive seamless designs (rdrr.io)) to carry out the design simulation in Homework 13.3–13.6 by the method of Friede et al. (2008, 2011).

References

Bardia A, Mayer IA, Vahdat LT, et al. (2019). Sacituzumab govitecan-hziy in refractory metastatic triplenegative breast cancer. *The New England Journal of Medicine*: 380: 741–751. DOI: 10.1056/NEJMoa1814213

Bretz F, Pinheiro J, and Bransosn M. (2005). Combining multiple comparisons and modeling techniques in dose-response studies. *Biometrics* 61: 738–748.

Bretz F, Schmidli S, Knig F, et al. (2006). Confirmatory seamless phase II/III clinical trials with hypotheses selection at interim: General concepts. *Biometrical Journal* 48, 623–634.

Dunnett C (1955). A multiple comparison procedure for comparing several treatments with a control. *Journal of the American Statistical Association* 50(272):1096–1121.

Fang F, Lin Y, Shih WJ, et al. (2013). Methods of designing two-stage winner trials with survival outcomes. *Statistics in Medicine* 33:1539–1563.

Friede T, Parsons N, Stallard N, et al. (2011). Designing a seamless phase II/III clinical trial using early outcomes for treatment selection: an application in multiple sclerosis. *Statistics in Medicine* 30: 1528–1540.

Friede T and Stallard N. (2008). A comparison of methods for adaptive treatment selection. *Biometrical Journal* 50: 767–781.

Ji Y, Liu P, Li Y, and Bekele BN. (2010). A modified toxicity probability interval method for dose-finding trials. *Clinical Trials*, 7: 653–663.

Kunz CU, Friede T, Parsons N, Todd S, and Stallard N. (2015). A comparison of methods for treatment selection in seamless phase II/III clinical trials incorporating information on short-term endpoints. *Journal of Biopharmaceutical Statistics* 25: 170–189.

Lin Y and Shih WJ. (2001). Statistical properties of the traditional algorithm-based designs for phase-I cancer clinical trials. *Biostatistics* 2: 203–215.

Liu S and Yuan Y. (2015). Bayesian optimal interval designs for phase I clinical trials. *Journal of the Royal Statistical Society: Series C (Applied Statistics)*, 64(3): 507–523.

sMarcus R, Peritz E, and Gabriel KR (1976). "On closed testing procedures with special reference to ordered analysis of variance". *Biometrika* 63: 655–660.

Merck Sharp and Dohme Corp. (2021). A study of the efficacy and safety of MK-5475 in participants with pulmonary arterial hypertension (INSIGNIA-PAH: Phase 2/3 Study of an Inhaled sGC Stimulator in PAH) (MK-5475-007). NCT04732221 https://clinicaltrials.gov/ct2/show/NCT04732221?term=NCT04732221&draw=2 &rank=1

Parsons N, Friede T, Todd S, and Stallard N. (2011). Software tools for implementing simulation studies in adaptive seamless designs: introducing R package ASD. Trials 2011 12(Suppl 1):A8.treatsel.sim: ASD simulation for treatment selection in asd: Simulations for Adaptive Seamless Designs (rdrr.io).

Shih WJ and Lin Y. (2006). Traditional and modified algorithm-based designs for phase I cancer clinical trials. In *Statistical Methods for Dose-Finding Studies,* Chevret S (Ed.), John Wiley.

Shun Z, Lan KKG, and Soo Y. (2008). Interim treatment selection using the normal approximation approach in clinical trials. *Statistics in Medicine.* 27:597–618.

Tao A, Lin Y, Pinheiro J, Shih WJ. (2015) Dose finding method in joint modeling of efficacy and safety endpoints in phase II studies. *International Journal of Statistics and Probability* 4(1): 33–48.

Wang PW, Lu SE, Lin Y, Shih WJ, and Lan KKG (2017). Two-stage winner designs for non-inferiority trials with pre-specified non-inferiority margin, *Journal of Statistical Planning and Inference*, 183:44–61.

14

Statistical Significance and p-Values

Understanding the meaning of p-values is a fundamental, interesting, yet broad and complex topic. It relates to how most scientists view the strength of an experiment, including its *repeatability* (or *replicability* or *reproducibility*; see Chapter 2, Section 2.3) and, in turn, creditability. However, there are many misunderstandings or misuses of p-values. The American Statistical Association (ASA) on March 7, 2016, has released a "Statement on Statistical Significance and p-Values" with six principles underlying the proper use and interpretation of the p-value. The intention was *"to improve the conduct and interpretation of quantitative science and inform the growing emphasis on reproducibility of science research."* (Wasserstein and Lazar 2016, with discussion). The statement's six principles are assertions (without elaboration). As we know, almost all clinical trials reported in medical journals use p-values as an indicator of evidence and summary of the results. Thus, appreciating what the p-value means and does not mean, and how it should be used and interpreted is an important subject for researchers and practitioners in clinical trials. In the following, we first highlight the ASA's six principles and then discuss more details so that these principles, as assertions, are understood and practiced better. The six principles are as follows:

1. P-values can indicate how incompatible the data are with a specified statistical model.
2. P-values do not measure the probability that the studied hypothesis is true, or the probability that the data were produced by random chance alone.
3. Scientific conclusions and business or policy decisions should not be based only on whether a p-value passes a specific threshold.
4. Proper inference requires full reporting and transparency.
5. A p-value, or statistical significance, does not measure the size of an effect or the importance of a result.
6. By itself, a p-value does not provide a good measure of evidence regarding a model or hypothesis.

14.1 Stimulating Questions

Principle 1 is the only assertion for what the p-value can do. Principle 4 is to point out the credibility of a study relies on its process more than its result. Relating to Principles 2, 3, 5, and 6, we start with some questions to stimulate further discussion. A general (questionable) regard for the p-value is that it measures the null hypothesis (H_0): the smaller the p-value, the lesser the support for H_0 by the data. Conversely, the bigger the p-value, the more the support for H_0. To those who hold this regard, consider the follow-up thought-provoking questions: If so, does the same p-value represent the same level of support or nonsupport to H_0? If there are two trials, one with 100 patients and the other with 200 patients, and both get the same p-value, is the trial of small or large sample size more convincing, or do the two provide the same level of evidence support for H_0? What is the relationship between p-values and sample size? For repeatability or replicability of an experiment, does a trial with a smaller p-value mean that the results are more credible or more replicable? If so, how small should the p-value be to indicate that the result may be repeated?

14.2 Distinguish p-Value and Neyman–Pearson Binary Decision

Using the classical N-P (Neyman–Pearson) hypothesis testing frame, we design and parse an experiment. We consider controlling the type I and type II error rates. As used in the previous chapters, let the maximum allowable type I error rate (also known as the "critical level") be α, and let β be the desirable type II error rate. These are design parameters that are determined before the experiment. In the frame of N–P, the decision is binary: reject or not reject H_0. When the probability of making a false-positive conclusion (*probability of false positive*) is less than or equal to α, we reject H_0; otherwise, we do not reject H_0. The result associated with not rejecting H_0 is the so-called "nonsignificant" result, and the other is "significant" result. We have discussed multiplicity and controlling the familywise error rate (FWER) in Chapter 10. The overall type I error rate α is generally set at either 0.05 (two-sided) or 0.025 (one-sided). This die-hard convention has been in practice for many generations although it may be changed in certain situations. Another approach is to calculate the p-value, which is the probability of a false-positive conclusion, i.e., $\Pr(\text{data to reject } H_0 | H_0)$, also known as *observed significance level* or *significance probability*. It would be reasonable from intuition to think that the p-value should provide evidence more directly than the simplified binary approach in the N-P frame. This is not completely so.

In fact, the questions raised about p-value in Section 14.1 indicates this intuition encounters some problems.

We know that p-value is Pr(data to reject $H_0 | H_0$), not $Pr(H_0 | data)$. But the latter is what scientists often think of and is what they often want to know. However, p-values do not directly address the researchers' interest. Differentiating what is of interest and what is presented is a first step toward the proper understanding and use of p-values. The next step is to distinguish between the score of p-value and the N-P binary decision. Let us use a simple and frequent framework to formally explain.

14.3 Probability That a Replicate May Yield Another "Significant" Result

We follow the notation of Chapter 4.2 where a randomized trial is conducted to compare two treatment groups: $Y_i \sim N(\mu_i, \sigma^2)$; i=1, 2, and σ^2 is assumed known for simplicity. We are to test $H_0 : \delta = \mu_1 - \mu_2 = 0$ versus $H_A : \delta > 0$. The experimental design is fixed sample size using the z-test and meeting the requirement of given power of $1 - \beta$ at level α to detect a clinically meaningful δ^*. Let n be the per group sample size, $\hat{\delta} = \bar{Y}_1 - \bar{Y}_2$. The z-test statistic is

$$T = \sqrt{\frac{n}{2}} \frac{\hat{\delta}}{\sigma} \sim N\left(\sqrt{\frac{n}{2}} \frac{\delta}{\sigma}, 1\right) \tag{14.1}$$

Suppose the trial shows a "significant" result based on T; i.e., the p-value of T is less than α or, equivalently, $T > z_\alpha = \Phi^{-1}(1 - \alpha)$. We ask the following questions: (a) If we replicate this trial under the same experimental condition with the same investigators using the same sample size, what is the probability we get the same directional "significant" result in the next trial? (b) If we change the sample size, how the above probability will change accordingly?

Be mindful when answering the Question (a) above that this is a conditional probability calculation about the next trial given the result of the current trial. We must clearly define what we know from the current trial. Let us contemplate the following different considerations:

1. We do not know the true value of δ, and if we do not make any supposition, then we do not know the expected value of T, so we cannot calculate $Pr(T > z_\alpha) = \Phi\left(\delta\sqrt{\frac{n}{2\sigma^2}} - z_\alpha\right)$ for the next trial.

2. Although we do not know the true value of δ, we do know the result of the current experiment is "significant" and $H_0 : \delta = 0$ is rejected.

If we only accept $\delta > 0$ as the conclusion, then all we can say is $\Pr(T > z_\alpha \mid \delta > 0) > \alpha$.

3. Further, if we are willing to assume $\delta = \delta^*$ as the current trial was designed, we of course get the same power $\Pr(T > z_\alpha \mid \delta = \delta^*) = 1 - \beta$ with the same sample size for the replicate.

4. However, we not only obtain a binary "significance," but also the p-value. We may use it to assume δ. That is, $T = \sqrt{\dfrac{n}{2}}\,\dfrac{\hat{\delta}}{\sigma} = z_p$, which leads to $\hat{\delta} = z_p \sigma \sqrt{\dfrac{2}{n}}$. We then calculate

$$\Pr\left(T > z_\alpha \mid \delta = z_p \sigma \sqrt{\frac{2}{n}}\right) = \Phi(z_p - z_\alpha). \tag{14.2}$$

Notice that the second and third bullet points are based on the N-P binary framework: "significant" (reject H_0) or "not significant" (not reject H_0). The last bullet point (4) uses the p-value itself. For the same Question (a) above, we have very different answers. For the commonly referenced one-sided $\alpha = 0.025$, Table 14.1 displays a few calculations based on (14.2) for different scenarios of p-value of the first trial.

In general, the probability of getting a same directional "significant" result in a replicate trial is surprisingly low. For example, if the first trial's p-value is 0.025 (right on the nose of being significant), then the replicate has only the probability of $\Phi(z_p - z_\alpha) = \Phi(1.96 - 1.96) = 0.50$ to be "significant." Only when the first trial reaches p-value of 0.0025 can the replicate trial have a probability of $\Phi(z_p - z_\alpha) = \Phi(2.81 - 1.96) = 0.80$ to be "significant." Wonder why this does not quite agree with our intuition? Perhaps that is because our

TABLE 14.1

Relationship between the p-Value of the Current Trial and Probability of Replicate Trial Being Significant

	Probability of replicate trial being significant by using the p-value of the first trial for $\delta = z_p \sigma \sqrt{\dfrac{2}{n}}$	
$\alpha = 0.025$ (one-sided)	Formula (14.2)	
P-value of the first trial	Same sample size	Replicate doubles the sample size
0.025	0.50	0.79
0.005	0.73	0.95
0.0025	0.80	0.98
0.0005	0.91	0.99

intuition is somehow based on the N-P hypothesis testing framework, i.e., bullet point (3).

Of course, we cannot be so sure about assuming $\delta = \hat{\delta} = z_p \sigma \sqrt{\dfrac{2}{n}}$ exactly, unless n is quite large in the current trial. We may add some uncertainty, perhaps adopting a Bayesian prior distribution on δ. If so, then when the first trial reaches p=0.0025, the probability of the replicate to have the same directional significance would be even less than 0.80. The exercise is left to Homework 14.1.

Thus, it makes sense for many government health authorities, such as the US FDA, to require at least two pivotal clinical trials, unless the number of patients in a single pivotal trial is large and the p-value is "highly significant."

14.4 P-value and Estimated Treatment Effect

The comparison between bullet points (2) and (4) in the last section is also interesting. When we obtain a statistic, $T = \sqrt{\dfrac{n}{2}}\,\dfrac{\hat{\delta}}{\sigma} = z_p$, we should also report estimate of the treatment effect $\hat{\delta} = z_p \sigma \sqrt{\dfrac{2}{n}}$ in addition to hypothesis test. Substituting $n = 2(z_\alpha + z_\beta)^2 \left(\dfrac{\sigma}{\delta^*}\right)^2$, we have

$$\hat{\delta} = \left(\frac{z_p}{z_\alpha + z_\beta}\right)\delta^* \qquad (14.3)$$

For example, for $\alpha = 0.025$ (one-sided) and $1 - \beta = 0.80$, if p = 0.025, then

$$\hat{\delta} = \left(\frac{1.96}{1.96 + 0.84}\right)\delta^* = (0.7)\delta^*.\ \text{If p} = 0.005, \text{then } \hat{\delta} = \left(\frac{2.58}{1.96 + 0.84}\right)\delta^* = (0.92)\delta^*.$$

Thus, $\hat{\delta}$ is usually smaller than δ^*, the value assumed in the alternative hypothesis. No wonder the probability (14.2) in point (4) is smaller than the power in (3). Here, we are also led to a seemingly awkward situation: If the original δ^* is a clinically meaningful amount of effectiveness, but $(0.7)\delta^*$ or $(0.92)\delta^*$ may not necessarily be meaningful, then how should we regard this statistically called "significant" result? Of course, the key is on understanding the meaning of the so-called "statistical significance." Since the null hypothesis is $H_0 : \delta = 0$, when the result is statistically called "significant," it simply means that $\delta = 0$ is excluded. So, it is not surprising that $\hat{\delta} = (0.7)\delta^*$ is large enough to exclude $\delta = 0$.

As for the question of estimating the effect size, it would be much clear to report the confidence interval of δ based on $\hat{\delta}$, not to just report the p-value. For example, when $\hat{\delta} = (0.7)\delta^*$, report the treatment effect estimated by the 95% confidence interval $(0, 1.4\delta^*)$. Fortunately, reporting confidence intervals has already been a common practice in most medical literature now.

14.5 Replicate with a Different Sample Size

It is now easy to answer the Question (b) posted previously under Eq. (14.1): If we change the sample size of the replicate, how will the above probability change accordingly? Let the sample size per group be n for the first trial and m for the replicate. From the first trial, we obtain $\hat{\delta}(n) = z_p \sigma \sqrt{\dfrac{2}{n}}$. The z-test statistic of the replicate $T(m) = \sqrt{\dfrac{m}{2}} \dfrac{\hat{\delta}(m)}{\sigma} \sim N\left(\sqrt{\dfrac{m}{2}} \dfrac{\delta}{\sigma}, 1\right)$. Hence,

$$\Pr\left(T(m) > z_\alpha \mid \delta = \hat{\delta}(n) = z_p \sigma \sqrt{\dfrac{2}{n}}\right) = \Phi\left(\sqrt{\dfrac{m}{n}} z_p - z_\alpha\right) \qquad (14.4)$$

Table 14.1 shows some results for m = 2n. Doubling the sample size for the replicate trial will of course increase the chance of reaching the same significance level as the current trial. There is another application for (14.4): If the first trial is a Phase II trial, we can use the same idea to help design the sample size for a Phase III trial.

14.6 The Distribution of p-Value

The discussions in the above sections attempt to explore some meaning of p-value from the perspective of answering the questions regarding its relationship to "evidence" or "replicability" of a trial. In this section, we study the distribution of p-value to understand its statistical properties. After all, p-value is a random variable. Properties of the p-value can be understood directly from its distribution.

Continuing the same setup, the z-test statistic T is given in (14.1). Let $\phi(\cdot)$ denote the probability density function (pdf) of the standard normal distribution. For fixed δ and n, the pdf of T is $f(t \mid \delta, n) = \phi\left(t - \sqrt{\dfrac{n}{2}} \dfrac{\delta}{\sigma}\right)$. The p-value is a one-to-one mapping of T: $p = \Pr(T > t \mid H_0) = 1 - \Phi(t) = \Phi(-t)$. $t = z_p$. Or, in the form of random variables, $P = 1 - \Phi(T)$. Thus, $dp = -\phi(t)dt$. For fixed δ and n, let the pdf of P be $g(p \mid \delta, n)$, and we obtain

$$g(p \mid \delta, n) = f(t \mid \delta) \mid dt/dp \mid = \phi\left(t - \sqrt{\frac{n}{2}}\frac{\delta}{\sigma}\right) / \phi(t)$$

$$= \phi\left(z_p - \sqrt{\frac{n}{2}}\frac{\delta}{\sigma}\right) / \phi(z_p) \tag{14.5}$$

This shows the probability distribution of P depends on the sample size and the true treatment effect.

The expected value of P is as follows:

$$E(P \mid \delta, n) = \int_0^1 p\phi\left(z_p - \sqrt{\frac{n}{2}}\frac{\delta}{\sigma}\right) / \phi(z_p)dp$$

$$= \int_{-\infty}^{\infty}\left[\Phi(-t)\phi\left(t - \sqrt{\frac{n}{2}}\frac{\delta}{\sigma}\right) / \phi(t)\right][\phi(t)]dt$$

$$= \int_{-\infty}^{\infty}\Phi(-t)\phi\left(t - \sqrt{\frac{n}{2}}\frac{\delta}{\sigma}\right)dt \tag{14.6}$$

The second moment and variance can also be obtained similarly (Homework 14.2).

The cumulative distribution function (cdf) of the p-value can be obtained as follows:

$$G(p \mid \delta, n) = \Pr(P \le p \mid \delta, n) = \int_0^p g(x \mid \delta, n)dx = \int_0^p \frac{\phi\left(z_x - \sqrt{\frac{n}{2}}\frac{\delta}{\sigma}\right)}{\phi(z_x)}dx$$

We make the following transformation in the above expression: Let $y = z_x = \Phi^{-1}(1-x)$, and then $\Phi(y) = 1 - x$ and $dx = -\phi(y)dy$. The above expression becomes

$$G(p \mid \delta, n) = \int_{z_p}^{\infty}\phi\left(y - \sqrt{\frac{n}{2}}\frac{\delta}{\sigma}\right)dy$$

$$= 1 - \Phi\left(z_p - \sqrt{\frac{n}{2}}\frac{\delta}{\sigma}\right)$$

$$= \Phi\left(\sqrt{\frac{n}{2}} \frac{\delta}{\sigma} - z_p\right) \qquad (14.7)$$

Thus, if $n_1 < n_2$, $G(p \mid \delta, n_1) < G(p \mid \delta, n_2)$. This is what we are familiar with: Fixing δ/σ, when the sample size is larger, the chance is greater to obtain a smaller p-value. Let $\delta/\sigma = 0.40$, and we graph $G(p \mid \delta, n)$ versus p-value for $n = 60$ (solid line) or 100 (dashed line) in Figure 14.1.

Let us examine some special cases for (14.7): Under the null hypothesis, $\delta = 0$, $G(p \mid \delta, n) = p$. This is the uniform distribution $U(0,1)$, which we are familiar with (see Appendix 11.1 in Chapter 11). If we set $\delta = \delta^*$, $n = 2(z_\alpha + z_\beta)^2 \left(\frac{\sigma}{\delta^*}\right)^2$, then

$$G\left(p \mid \delta = \delta^*, n = 2(z_\alpha + z_\beta)^2 \left(\frac{\sigma}{\delta^*}\right)^2\right) = \Phi\left(z_\alpha + z_\beta - z_p\right)$$

Thus,

$$\Pr\left(P \leq \alpha \mid \delta = \delta^*, n = 2(z_\alpha + z_\beta)^2 \left(\frac{\sigma}{\delta^*}\right)^2\right)$$

$$= G\left(\alpha \mid \delta = \delta^*, n = 2(z_\alpha + z_\beta)^2 \left(\frac{\sigma}{\delta^*}\right)^2\right)$$

$$= \Phi\left(z_\beta\right) = 1 - \beta.$$

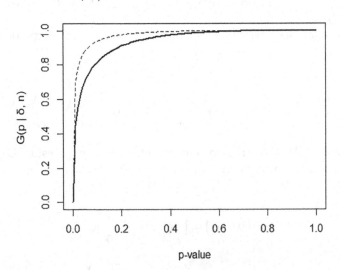

FIGURE 14.1
$G(p \mid \delta, n)$ versus p-value for $n = 60$ (solid line) or 100 (dotted line); $\delta/\sigma = 0.40$.

This is what we asserted in bullet point (3) previously. Further, when $\delta = \hat{\delta} = z_p\sigma\sqrt{\dfrac{2}{n}}$, $T = z_p = \sqrt{\dfrac{n}{2}}\dfrac{\hat{\delta}}{\sigma}$, we have $\Pr(P \le \alpha) = G(\alpha \mid \delta = \hat{\delta}) = \Phi(z_p - z_\alpha)$. This is what we obtained in (14.2) for bullet point (4).

Consider two trials designed to test the same true underlying treatment effect $\delta/\sigma = 0.40$ with the same $\alpha = 0.025$ (one-sided). One trial enrolls n = 60 per group (yielding power=0.60), and the other enrolls n = 150 per group (yielding power=0.93). Suppose both observe p = 0.005, i.e., $T = z_{0.005} = 2.58$. Since

$$E(P \mid \delta/\sigma = 0.40,\ n = 60) = 0.06;\ \text{Var}(P \mid \delta/\sigma = 0.40,\ n = 60) = 0.0124\ ;$$

$$E(P \mid \delta/\sigma = 0.40,\ n = 150) = 0.0072;\ \text{Var}(P \mid \delta/\sigma = 0.40,\ n = 150) = 0.00076,$$

we see that the p-value, as a random variable, its expected value and variance of the first trial with n=60 are quite different from that of the second trial with n=150. Furthermore,

$$\Pr(P < 0.005 \mid \delta/\sigma = 0.40,\ n = 60) = G(0.005 \mid \delta/\sigma = 0.40,\ n = 60)$$

$$= \Phi\left(\sqrt{\frac{n}{2}}\frac{\delta}{\sigma} - z_p\right) = \Phi(0.4\sqrt{30} - 2.58) = 0.35\ ;$$

$$\Pr(P < 0.005 \mid \delta/\sigma = 0.40,\ n = 150) = G(0.005 \mid \delta/\sigma = 0.40,\ n = 150)$$

$$= \Phi(0.4\sqrt{75} - 2.58) = 0.81.$$

We can see that the p-value=0.005 is the 35-th percentile of the first trial (n=60), while the same value is the 81-st percentile of the second trial (n=150).

14.7 Evidence to Measure H_0

From the above, it is debatable whether the p-value fits as an evidence summary to measure H_0 to the extent that its magnitude may indicate supportive or not supportive for H_0. Some may think that a root cause for the dispute is that p-value does not directly address the $\Pr(H_0 \mid \text{Data})$ interest. In fact, even on the topic of $\Pr(H_0 \mid \text{Data})$, the so-called "Data" also need clarification. Many statisticians advocate to look at $\Pr(H_0 \mid \text{Data})$ to $\Pr(H_A \mid \text{Data})$ contrast. Let us examine this quantity as well. From Bayes theorem (see Chapter 7.1.3), $\Pr(H \mid \text{Data}) = \Pr(\text{Data} \mid H)\,\Pr(H)\,/\,\Pr(\text{Data})$. Thus,

$$\frac{\Pr(H_0 \mid \text{Data})}{\Pr(H_A \mid \text{Data})} = \frac{\Pr(\text{Data} \mid H_0)}{\Pr(\text{Data} \mid H_A)} \frac{\Pr(H_0)}{\Pr(H_A)}$$

If "Data" is the result of the N-P significance test, then

$$\frac{\Pr(H_0 \mid \text{Data})}{\Pr(H_A \mid \text{Data})} = \frac{\alpha}{1 - \beta} \frac{\Pr(H_0)}{\Pr(H_A)} \tag{14.8}$$

Consider again the above example of two trials testing for the same true underlying treatment effect $\delta/\sigma = 0.40$ with the same $\alpha = 0.025$ (one-sided). One trial enrolls $n = 60$ per group (yielding power = 0.60), and the other enrolls $n = 150$ per group (yielding power = 0.93). Suppose both observe "significant" result: $T > 1.96$. Then,

for the trial with $n = 60$: $\dfrac{\Pr(H_0 \mid \text{Significant})}{\Pr(H_A \mid \text{Significant})} = \dfrac{0.025}{0.60} \dfrac{\Pr(H_0)}{\Pr(H_A)}$

and for the trial with $n = 150$: $\dfrac{\Pr(H_0 \mid \text{Significant})}{\Pr(H_A \mid \text{Significant})} = \dfrac{0.025}{0.93} \dfrac{\Pr(H_0)}{\Pr(H_A)}$

If both trials have the same "prior belief" $\Pr(H_0)/\Pr(H_A)$, obviously, it is more convincing for the larger trial to support H_A against H_0, since the larger trial provides greater power for the significance test.

If "Data" is the observed p-value, then

$$\frac{\Pr(H_0 \mid \text{Data})}{\Pr(H_A \mid \text{Data})} = \frac{g(p \mid H_0)}{g(p \mid H_A)} \frac{\Pr(H_0)}{\Pr(H_A)} \tag{14.9}$$

Substitute (14.5) for $g(p \mid \delta, n) = \phi\left(z_p - \sqrt{\dfrac{n}{2}} \dfrac{\delta}{\sigma}\right) / \phi(z_p)$. Notice that $g(p \mid H_0) = g(p \mid \delta = 0, n) = 1$. If both trials obtain p-value = 0.005 (i.e., $T = z_{0.005} = 2.58$), we have the following:

For the trial with $n = 60$: $\dfrac{\Pr(H_0 \mid p = 0.005)}{\Pr(H_A \mid p = 0.005)} = \dfrac{\phi(2.58)}{\phi(2.58 - 0.4\sqrt{30})} \dfrac{\Pr(H_0)}{\Pr(H_A)}$

$$= \frac{0.014}{0.370} \frac{\Pr(H_0)}{\Pr(H_A)} = 0.0378 \frac{\Pr(H_0)}{\Pr(H_A)}$$

And for the trial with $n = 150$: $\dfrac{\Pr(H_0 \mid p = 0.005)}{\Pr(H_A \mid p = 0.005)} = \dfrac{\phi(2.58)}{\phi(2.58 - 0.4\sqrt{75})} \dfrac{\Pr(H_0)}{\Pr(H_A)}$

$$= \frac{0.014}{0.270} \frac{\Pr(H_0)}{\Pr(H_A)} = 0.052 \frac{\Pr(H_0)}{\Pr(H_A)}$$

If both trials have the same "prior belief" $\Pr(H_0) / \Pr(H_A)$, this time it is more convincing for the smaller trial to support H_A against H_0. While this result is surprising, let us check the following third trial with a middle size of $n=84$:

$$\text{For the trial with } n=84: \frac{\Pr(H_0 \mid p = 0.005)}{\Pr(H_A \mid p = 0.005)} = \frac{\phi(2.58)}{\phi(2.58 - 0.4\sqrt{42})} \frac{\Pr(H_0)}{\Pr(H_A)}$$

$$= \frac{0.014}{0.399} \frac{\Pr(H_0)}{\Pr(H_A)} = 0.036 \frac{\Pr(H_0)}{\Pr(H_A)}$$

Thus, the larger trial with $n = 84$ is now more convincing to support H_A against H_0, compared to the small trial with $n = 60$. The explanation of this phenomenon is as follows: Define

$$v(n,p) \equiv \frac{\Pr(H_0 \mid p,n)}{\Pr(H_A \mid p,n)} = \frac{g(p \mid H_0,n)}{g(p \mid H_A,n)} \frac{\Pr(H_0)}{\Pr(H_A)}$$

$$\propto \frac{1}{g(p \mid \delta, n)}$$

$$\propto \frac{1}{\phi\left(z_p - \sqrt{\dfrac{n}{2}} \dfrac{\delta}{\sigma}\right)}$$

$$\propto \exp\left[\frac{1}{2}\left(z_p - \sqrt{\frac{n}{2}} \frac{\delta}{\sigma}\right)^2\right]$$

Taking natural logarithm on both sides, $\log v(n,p) \propto \left(z_p - \sqrt{\dfrac{n}{2}} \dfrac{\delta}{\sigma}\right)^2$. Hence, $v(n,p)$ is a decreasing function of n when $n < 2\left(z_p \dfrac{\sigma}{\delta}\right)^2$, but an increasing function of n when $n > 2\left(z_p \dfrac{\sigma}{\delta}\right)^2$. In the above example, the turning point of n is $2\left(z_p \dfrac{\sigma}{\delta}\right)^2 = 2(2.58/0.4)^2 = 83.2$. Therefore, when $n \geq 84$, for the same p-value, it is more convincing for a smaller trial to support H_A. On the contrary, when $n < 84$, for the same p-value, it is then more convincing for a larger trial to support H_A. See Figure 14.2 for the plot.

The above exploration demonstrates that the expression of $\dfrac{\Pr(H_0 \mid \text{Data})}{\Pr(H_A \mid \text{Data})}$ (i.e., the so-called *Bayes Factor*) adds more convolution and controversy to the p-values.

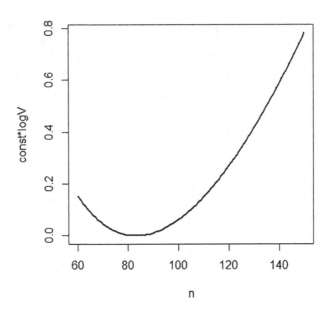

FIGURE 14.2
v(n, p) versus n for p=0.005 and δ/σ =0.40.

14.8 Conclusions

On the framework of the classical N-P hypothesis testing, we only ask whether
the test statistic falls in the rejection region of H_0, and there is no need to know at
where it exactly is in the rejection region. Therefore, the p-value does not play a
role with this framework. But, since the rejection region is defined by the alpha-
critical level, which is somewhat arbitrary, many researchers report the test's
p-value and render the judgement and decision on the H_0 to the readers. Many
authors have discussed about p-values; see a few interesting papers listed in the
references. In this chapter, we discussed some controversial issues encountered
by using p-values. To those who are interested in the statistical theory, we have
raised and explored some challenging thinking. For practitioners in clinical trials, in addition to explaining the principles asserted in the ASA's statement, we
offer the following pieces of advice for the proper use of the p-values:

- Do not use the p-value by itself. When sample size is large, p-value
  is generally small, leading to rejecting H_0 easily even when H_A is
  near H_0 since the power is high. Conversely, when the sample size
  is small, p-value is generally large, leading to accept H_0 easily even
  when H_0 is far from H_A since the power is low. Therefore, pay attention to the sample size/power and (H_0, H_A) when using p-values. For
  example, as we cautioned in Chapter 8, for safety analyses of specified laboratory data, it is usually inappropriate to perform t-tests and

report p-values or significance/nonsignificance for those continuous urine or serum measurements since the tests are often overpowered. Instead, to be clinically meaningful, we should use the normal ranges for these laboratory tests and conduct categorical data analyses.

- While reading and writing study reports, pay attention to the confidence interval as well as the p-value.

- Restrict the p-value obtained within the trial itself; do not compare p-values across trials. The former is easier to comprehend, while the latter invites confusion.

Appendix 14.1: The R Code for Figure 14.1

```
##  G(p|δ,n) versus p-value for n = 60 (black solid line) or
100 (red dotted line); δ/σ =0.40
pvalue=seq(0,1,by=0.01)
zp=qnorm(1-pvalue)
n=60
gpn=pnorm(0.4*sqrt(n/2)-zp)
plot(pvalue, gpn, type="l", xlab="p-value", ylab="G(p, n)",
lwd=2)
n=100
gpn=pnorm(0.4*sqrt(n/2)-zp)
lines(pvalue, gpn, type="l", xlab="p-value", ylab="G(p, n)",
lwd=1, lty = "dashed")
```

Appendix 14.2: The R Code for Figure 14.2

```
n=seq(60,150,by=1)
v=(2.58-0.4*sqrt(n/2))**2
plot(n, v, type="l", xlab="n", ylab="logV", lwd=2)
```

Appendix 14.3: The R Code for Simulating the Estimate of Probability of a Replicate Trial of the Same Sample Size Being Significant by Placing Prior Distribution on δ/σ

```
p=0.0025
nn=50
zp=qnorm(1-p)
mm=zp*sqrt(2/nn)
v=mm/3
dsig=rnorm(n=10000, mean = mm, sd = sqrt(v))
test=dsig*sqrt(nn/2)
summary(test>1.96)
mean(test>1.96)
```

HOMEWORK 14.1

Referring to the comment made in discussion of Table 14.1 based on formula (14.2), we now add some uncertainty on the estimate of the treatment effect by placing a prior distribution for δ/σ by assuming

$\delta/\sigma \sim N\left(\hat{\delta}/\sigma = z_p\sqrt{\dfrac{2}{n}},\ V\right)$. Let $V = \dfrac{\hat{\delta}}{3\sigma}$. Follow Appendix 14.3 to generate 10,000 samples of δ/σ from this prior distribution for $p = 0.0025$ and $n = 50$. What is the proportion of $T = \sqrt{\dfrac{m}{2}}\dfrac{\hat{\delta}}{\sigma}$ (for the next 10,000 trials with the same sample size $m = n$) that exceeds 1.96? Verify that the proportion is lower than 0.80. How about the sample size of the replicate is $m = 2n$?

HOMEWORK 14.2

From the distribution function of the p-value given in Eq. (14.5), derive the second moment and variance of P.

HOMEWORK 14.3

Read the discussion of the ASA statement on p-values from the link to the article: https://doi.org/10.1080/00031305.2016.1154108

References

Berger JO and Delampady M. (1987). Testing precise hypotheses. (With discussion). *Statistical Science* 2:317–351.

Gibbons JD and Pratt JW. (1975). P-value: Interpretation and methodology. *The American Statistician* 29:20–25.

Goodman SN. (1992). A comment on replication, P-values and evidence. *Statistics in Medicine* 11:875–879.

Hung HMJ, O'Neill RT, Bauer P, and Kohne K. (1997). The behavior of the P-value when the alternative hypothesis is true. *Biometrics* 50:11–22.

Royall RM. (1987). The effect of sample size on the meaning of significance tests. *The American Statistician* 40:313–315 1986. (Discussions: The Am Stat, 41, 245–247, 1987).

Schervish MJ. (1996). P values: What they are and what they are not. *The American Statistician* 50:203–206.

Wasserstein RL and Lazar NA. (2016). The ASA Statement on p-Values: Context, Process, and Purpose. *The American Statistician* 70:129–133

15

Estimand, Intercurrent Events, and Missing Data

In the beginning of Chapter 5, we pointed out that all data analyses must be tied to the study design, even more fundamentally, to the study objective, and subsequently also to the interpretation of the results. This statement is especially true when a clinical trial is facing the ubiquitous problem of missing data. In fact, not just missing data, the International Conference on Harmonization (ICH) recently finalized an important addendum for its E9 guidance (E9-R1, November 2019) to expand the discussion of missing data to the so-called "intercurrent events" (ICEs) in relation to the study objective and design. It reinforced the concept of "estimand" discussed in the report by National Research Council (NRC 2010) and provided further recommendations regarding the study design, conduct, and analysis to minimize possible patient withdrawal and impact of missing data. In other words, we should take a holistic approach to the conventional "missing data" problem. In this chapter, we first review these concepts and recommendations. Methods of analysis ("estimators") focusing on main and sensitivity analyses then follow in the later part of this chapter.

Some key points regarding missing data are highlighted below:

- Missing data, especially when a substantial amount appears in a randomized trial, diminish the merits of the randomization and can invalidate as well as cause loss of efficiency of the trial. Hence, we should use proper design and conduct and monitor trials responsibly to limit possible occurrence and impact of missing data (Little et al. 2012a, b).

- We should distinguish *withdrawal from the study treatment* and *withdrawal from the study follow-up*. For ethical reasons, patients are allowed to withdraw from the study treatment at will at any time and investigators have the obligation to withdraw the study treatment when injury to the patient seems likely (see Chapter 1). However, it is important to keep the patient in the trial by providing follow-up visits and collecting key data from patients who have discontinued the study treatment. This continuing follow-up is beneficial to patients as well as for furthering the knowledge of the experimental treatment; it should be explained to all patients in their informed consent before randomization. In fact, we should let the patient discontinue

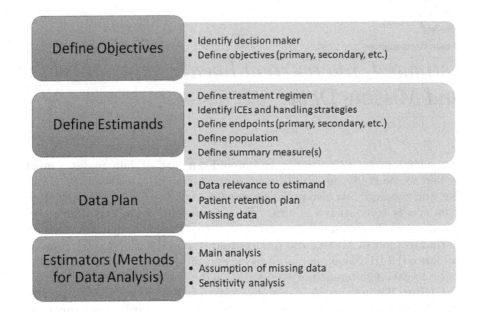

FIGURE 15.1
Study and data development process flowchart.

the study follow-up only when the patient either withdraws from the consent or is deceased.

- No single analytical method can recover the information lost in the missing data. Hence, when considering methods of handling missing data, both NRC report and the ICH guidance emphasize the importance of performing sensitivity analyses to achieve a robust conclusion when data are incomplete.

The discussions in the following sections will follow a flowchart similar to that given in the ICH guidance (2019) and elaborated in Ratitch et al. (2019); see Figure 15.1.

15.1 Study Objective and Decision Maker

On top of Figure 15.1, we start with the study objective development. All randomized clinical trials have a common, broad objective: to assess treatment effects. However, under this broad objective, we should ask: what are the "treatment effects" this trial is to assess or to compare with and about? First, does the "treatment" refer to the initial randomized study treatment only, or the "treatment regimen" including also the concomitant therapies that are planned in the study protocol, such as medications that treat certain side effects, in case, occurring, or rescue therapies that according to standard medical practice should be provided to patients when ethically necessary? Second, what are the "effects" and the time point of outcome measurements to assess or compare on? Different decision makers—the patient and healthcare provider, the insurance payer, the drug maker, and the regulatory authority—would argue for their different interests in defining "treatment" and "effects," whether on the individual or population level, and whether with or without "cost" in consideration. Often, they are multiple objectives. We need to understand and express the study objectives clearly and orderly so that the study design may address them properly with priorities.

15.2 Intercurrent Events and Estimand

When the "effect" is on a population level, as often is for the interest of the regulatory authority, drug maker, or insurance payer, we usually refer to the effect as population average effect. Then, we need to articulate the following question: "What is the target population to average?" Considering beyond the population that is defined by the eligibility (inclusion/exclusion) criteria in the study protocol, is it the "compliant" population only, or the mixture of compliant and noncompliant populations together? If noncompliant patients are also included in the target population, as often is the case for late-phase trials, is there a degree of noncompliance, or a kind of noncompliance that makes them different from other noncompliance, such as allowed versus not allowed rescue medication? Would the endpoints be different for this mixture of compliant and noncompliant populations? For example, compliant patients reflect the effect of a full treatment duration, while the noncompliant patients reflect only partial duration. The answer to these questions will obviously lead to different data plans and analyses.

The term *estimand* is simply "the target of estimation of the treatment effect." As discussed above, there may be several estimands of interest in a trial. We need to define at least the primary estimand in terms of the attributes we just alluded to: "treatment," "effect," "population," and "endpoint." The pivot of these attributes is the "intercurrent events" (ICEs) as discussed in the following. See Figure 15.2.

In a perfect situation, which seldom exists in clinical trials, all patients fully adhere to the data collection process—taking the randomized medicine as prescribed to the full course and never missing a visit during the trial. In reality, some "intercurrent events" almost always occur after randomization that alter the course of the randomized treatment during the intended study treatment period and may (or may not) render subsequent outcome

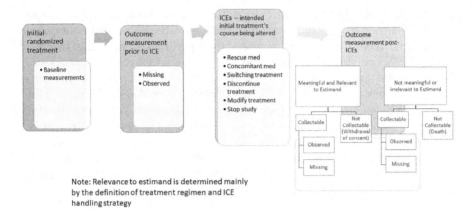

Note: Relevance to estimand is determined mainly by the definition of treatment regimen and ICE handling strategy

FIGURE 15.2
Intercurrent events and outcome data process flowchart.

measurements irrelevant. Some ICEs are anticipated, which should be discussed in the protocol as they may play a role in defining the estimand of interest, such as taking certain allowable rescue or concomitant medications, or dose modification for the initial study treatment. Rescue medication in the event of disease worsening is related to the lack of efficacy of the initial study treatment. Concomitant medication and study treatment dose modification could be for alleviating adverse reaction or related to patient's other background disorders. Some ICEs may not be foreseeable in the protocol. Then the ground rule of handling them should be defined before unblinding the treatment code. The "treatment regimen" should be clearly defined with the study treatment and these treatment alterations.

ICH E9-R1 provides five strategies for identifying and handling ICEs that are a break from the planned treatment. Ratitch et al. (2019, 2020) further elaborate their interpretations with enlightening examples. At the study planning stage, the choice of strategy or combination of strategies depends on the clinical question of interest (i.e., objective of the study) and leads to defining the estimand(s). Outcome data after the occurrence of ICEs may or may not be meaningful (e.g., after organ transplant or death), or relevant to the estimand. If relevant, are they collectable or not collectable? Why not collectable? We also need to consider, if outcome measurements are not relevant to the main estimand after ICE, may they be relevant to other (secondary or supportive) estimands and thus should still be collected? If collectable, during data analysis, we then examine observed and missing data.

1. Treatment policy strategy. In this strategy, ICE marks a change in study treatment course, but is taken to be part of the treatment regimen of interest. The treatment effect targeted by the estimand is a combined effect of the initial study treatment and treatment modified as a result of the ICE. With this strategy, the measurements

collected after the rescue medication, for example, are relevant. The conventional "intention-to-treat" (ITT) principle takes this strategy. Since this strategy includes all kinds of ICEs and treatments, outcome measurements after ICE are relevant and the imputation of missing data, when appearing after ICE occurrence, needs to be specific to the type of ICE of the patient. For example, missing data after rescue medication should be imputed from those patients who took the rescue medication and continued rather than those who continued with the initial study treatment. For overall survival, censoring time is the last followup day, regardless of ICE, for ITT.

2. Hypothetical strategies. In this strategy, ICE is a confounding factor for inference about the treatment regimen of interest. The scientific question of interest is "what would the treatment effect be if patients withdrew from the treatment group switched to a specific hypothetical scenario?" The "specific hypothetical scenario" has the flexibility of covering a wide range of different possible hypothetical (counterfactual) situations. It is important to precisely describe the hypothetical conditions reflecting the scientific question of interest in the context of the specific trial, since there could be many possible hypothetical scenarios. For example, (1) one might ask what outcomes would be for the initially randomized treatment (or treatment regimen) if relevant ICEs had not occurred and patient continued to receive the initial treatment (or treatment regimen); or (2) what outcomes would be if the withdrawal patients were offered another reference drug, i.e., an active control or rescue medication; or (3) what outcomes would be if the withdrawal patients were not taking any medication effect (alias switching to placebo, implying the treatment effect prior to ICE would gradually vanish). Scenario (1) is often an interest in early-phase (proof-of-concept) trials, not for late-phase pivotal trials in the regulatory setting. In some literature (e.g., Carpenter and Kenward 2013; Permutt 2016), this is called *"de jour estimand"* in contrast to the *"de facto"* scenarios (2) and (3).

3. Composite variable strategies: In this strategy, ICE itself, possibly with outcome(s) before it, provides all necessary information about the effect of treatment. Data after the ICE provide no additional information. ICEs that can be accounted for by a composite strategy are usually important clinical outcomes that are considered to lead to an immediate conclusion about success or failure of treatment. With this strategy, the data after taking the rescue medication, for example, would be rendered irrelevant to the estimand. Terminal events, such as death or organ transplant, are perhaps the most salient examples of the need for the composite strategy, where organ function is the outcome measurement and organ transplant or death is the ICE. Combination of events is also taking such a strategy: MACEs (major

adverse cardiovascular events) in heart disease trial are a composite endpoint that measures the treatment effect on a combination of events such as cardiac death, nonfatal myocardial infarction (MI), nonfatal stroke, and hospitalization for heart failure (HF). Another example is progression-free survival (PFS) in oncology trials, which measures the treatment effect on a combination of tumor growth and survival. With this strategy, the estimand may mix the efficacy and safety to indicate the "effectiveness" of the treatment regimen.

4. While-on-treatment strategy: This strategy is used when the outcomes up to the time of occurrence of ICE provide all necessary information about the effect of treatment rather than the landmark time point. Different from the survival time in the composite variable strategy, the actual duration of treatment in this case is not important or is taken into account for determining treatment benefits. Outcome of recurrent events assuming constant event rate within a unit time period often adopts this strategy. An example is the annualized exacerbations in asthma or COPD (chronic obstructive pulmonary disease) trials. If used, the usual "last observation carried forward" (LOCF) analysis has a new interpretation for the associated estimand under this strategy.

    Note that, like the composite variable strategy, the while-on-treatment strategy can be thought of as impacting the definition of the endpoint, in this case by restricting the observation time of interest to the time before the intercurrent event. In these two strategies, particular care is required if the occurrence of the ICE differs between the treatments being compared. The differential occurrence of ICE between the treatment groups implies that the ICE is also treatment related.

5. Principal stratum strategies. In this strategy, ICE means the potential ICE. The target population might be taken to be the "principal stratum" in which a potential ICE would occur or would not occur. For example, the clinical interest is treatment effect in patients who can tolerate the therapy, or who do not need rescue medication. However, correctly identifying strata prior to randomization is generally not possible because the occurrence of ICEs is difficult to predict. Using a run-in period before randomization and "randomized withdrawal" are designs that can help in attaining such stratum of patients to some extent. In a parallel-group design, membership in a principal stratum must usually be inferred from covariates. It is important to distinguish "principal stratification," which is based on potential ICEs (for example, subjects who would discontinue therapy if assigned to the test/control product), from "subsetting based on actual ICEs" (subjects who discontinue therapy on their assigned treatment). The subset of subjects who experience an ICE on the test

treatment will often be a different subset from those who experience the same ICE on control. Treatment effects defined by comparing outcomes in these subsets confound the effects of the different treatments with the differences in outcomes possibly due to the differing characteristics of the subjects. This strategy often requires complex assumptions in practice.

15.3 Missing Data Fundamentals: Patterns and Mechanisms

Proper imputation remains to be the most useful method to deal with the missing data problem for the estimands targeted by the treatment policy, hypothetical, and while-on-treatment strategies. When imputation of missing data is employed (see Section 15.4), we need to understand the process that causes the missing data. Let us first contrast the situations of complete data and incomplete data. Let $Y = \{y_{ij}\}$ denote the complete-data matrix of the outcome measurement, possibly observed incompletely. We can write it as $Y = (Y_{obs}, Y_{mis})$, where Y_{obs} is the observed part and Y_{mis} is the missing part. Furthermore, let $M = \{m_{ij}\}$ denote the missing data indicator matrix that identifies whether Y_{ij} is observed or missing. M is usually called the *missing data pattern* (Rubin 1976). A key to the analysis of missing data is to be aware that M is part of the random variables that need to be considered, in addition to Y, when missing data are present. The observed "dataset" is $V = (Y_{obs}, M)$, not Y_{obs} alone. This is similar to the censoring indicator variable for the survival data analysis. (In fact, missing data and censored data both belong to the larger class of incomplete data.) In addition, the underlying reason for the missing data is also an important part of the information that should be considered in the analysis. For some approaches, as we shall see later, M incorporates the cause and/or time of the missing data.

For simplicity, we use the bracket [Y; θ] to denote the distribution of a random variable Y with parameter θ. Because the *missing data pattern* M is a part of the data, we need to consider the joint distribution of Y and M, [Y, M]. We may add in the randomized treatment assignment Z with other predefined baseline covariates, and the post-randomization ICE occurrence X. (Note that there may be some potential ambiguity of the notation here in Z and X: Suppose Z is the initial randomized study treatment group ID; the treatment regimen includes Z and the concomitant and potential rescue medications even though the latter are not randomized. Imputation of missing data needs to incorporate X as it may well be ICE-specific, as seen for the treatment policy strategy. For the composite variable and while-on-treatment strategies, there is a change of the endpoint in the outcome measurement Y with occurrence of X.) Because the focus here is on missing outcomes, Z and X are assumed to be always observed. Conditioning on Z and X, the parameter θ in $[Y|X, Z; \theta]$ is the covariate-adjusted treatment (regimen) effect, which is the parameter of primary interest. The "estimand" is mathematically represented in a condensed way by this θ. In the following, we first omit X and Z for simplicity, but all essential results are still applicable when X and Z are conditioned on.

The joint distribution $[Y, M]$ can be factored into the conditional and marginal distributions as

$$[Y, M] = [M \mid Y; \varphi] \, [Y; \theta] \tag{15.1}$$

or

$$[Y, M] = [Y \mid M; \theta_M] \, [M] \tag{15.2}$$

Analysis methods with the first type of factorization are said to use the *selection model approach*, and analysis methods with the second type of factorization are said to use the *pattern-mixture model* (PMM) *approach* (Little 1995). In the first factorization, the conditional distribution $[M|Y; \varphi]$ with parameter φ characterizes how the missing data depend on the outcome measure Y and is called the *missing data process* or *missing data mechanism* (MDM). In the second factorization, the conditional distribution $[Y|M; \theta_M]$ is the conditional distribution given the missing data pattern, with parameter θ_M. Note that we write explicitly the associated parameters for clear inference and interpretation in each approach. With the selection model approach, one must specify an explicit model for the MDM $[M|Y; \varphi]$ to make an appropriate inference for θ. It is a useful research tool for performing simulation studies with missing data, but it is difficult to apply to a real data analysis because $[M|Y; \varphi]$ may involve the missing data Y_{mis}. The example in the next section gives a simple illustration for θ and φ. Shih (1992) and Diggle and Shih (1993) contain a more advanced example of $[Y; \theta]$ and $[M|Y; \varphi]$ (Homework 15.2). The PMM approach, on the other hand, has no such concern in $[M]$. However, the parameter of $[Y|M; \theta_M]$ is conditioning on the missing data pattern. Except for the principal stratum estimand, we need to combine θ_M over all the patterns M to obtain the parameter θ of the marginal $[Y]$; see Equation 15.13 for an illustration.

15.4 Ignorability and Nonignorability of Missing Data

All estimands but the principal stratum estimand discussed in Section 15.2 make inferences about θ. The inference should be based on the entire observed data $V = (Y_{obs}, M)$, not on Y_{obs} alone. However, because it is generally simpler and easier to ignore M and to make the inference based on Y_{obs} alone, a fundamental question is, when is it appropriate to ignore M and base the analysis on Y_{obs} alone? The first type of factorization (Equation 15.1) is useful in answering the above question: whether the missing data are ignorable or not. Actually, to be precise we should say, whether or not the mechanism or the process producing the missing data is ignorable in making the inference regarding the parameter/estimand θ. The exact answer to this question involves the definitions of *missing completely at random* (MCAR), *missing at random* (MAR), and *distinct parameters* (DP) given by Rubin (1976). Details are given in Appendices 15.1 and 15.2 of this chapter. In brief:

If the MDM is not related to the observed or potential outcome of the patient, then MCAR may be assumed. Using the notation in Equation 15.1, [M|Y]=[M] represents MCAR. Examples include patients moving away, the study ending, and late enrollment of patients being administratively "censored." When MCAR is applicable, the inference on θ based on Y_{obs} alone is appropriate. The usual two-sample t-test based on the sample means and the method of *generalized estimating equations* (GEEs) for unbalanced clustered data including repeated measures (Liang and Zeger 1986) requires the assumption of MCAR because these methods are based on sampling distributions.

MAR may be assumed if the missing data depend on the observed data, but not the current unobserved or future potential outcomes. Using the notation in Equation 15.1, [M|Y]=[M|Y_{obs}]. More appropriately, see (15.4) below. MAR is reasonable for missing data under the hypothetical strategy, scenarios (1) and (2) that ask what "outcome would be for the initial treatment or treatment regimen if relevant ICEs had not occurred and patient continued to receive the initial treatment or treatment regimen." When MAR is applicable, the likelihood-based inference based on Y_{obs} alone is appropriate, provided that the parameter of interest, θ, and the missing data process parameter, φ, are distinct. The method of *weighted estimation equations* (Robins, Rotnitzky, and Zhao 1995; Paik 1997), the mixed-effect models (Laird and Ware 1982) in SAS PROC MIXED, and the multiple imputation method (Rubin 1998) in SAS PROC MI (Yuan 2001) all require the MAR assumption.

At this point, let us be more explicit on the expressions involving X and Z. In general, corresponding to (15.1):

$$[Y, M \mid X, Z] = [M \mid Y, X, Z; \varphi]\,[Y \mid X, Z; \theta] \qquad (15.3)$$

Corresponding to [M | Y]=[M | Y_{obs}], MAR is

$$[M \mid Y, X, Z; \varphi] = [M \mid Y_{obs}, X, Z; \varphi] \qquad (15.4)$$

That is, the MDM only depends on the observed information including Y_{obs}, the strategy of handling the ICE (X), and the defined treatment regimen (Z). The requirement of "distinct parameters" (DP) means that φ of the MDM should be irrelevant to (alias, containing no information about) the estimand

θ of [Y | X, Z;θ]. Since the strategies of handling ICE and defining treatment regimen pretty much determine the relevance of the data after the ICE occurrence, MAR and DP conditions are reasonable assumptions in most cases.

"Not missing at random" (NMAR), or "missing not at random" (MNAR), is when the missing data process is dependent on the current unobserved or future potential outcomes. Using the notation of Equation 15.1, we cannot reduce [M|Y]=[M|Y_{obs}, Y_{mis}]. The MDM is nonignorable under MNAR or when the DP condition is violated. Since MAR is not testable from the observed data, sensitivity analysis to MAR assumption is necessary for obtaining robust conclusions. More discussion is given later in the sequel. Now, we provide a simple example from Choi and Lu (1995) to illustrate the concept of NMAR and show how bias can occur under NMAR if the MDM is ignored.

Example 15.1

Consider the case of comparing two randomized treatment groups, X and Y, with respect to a binary endpoint, with 1 being response and 0 being non-response. Let the response rate of treatment group X be p_x and that of treatment group Y be p_y. In notation, $p_x=E(X)=Pr(X=1)$; the same is true for p_y. We are interested in $\theta=p_x-p_y$. Suppose that there is a mechanism that will cause the outcome to go missing, depending on whether the outcome is a response or a non-response. The MDM is indexed by the parameters (φ_0, φ_1), where $\varphi_0=Pr$(missing X|X=0)=Pr(missing Y|Y=0), and $\varphi_1=Pr$(missing X|X=1)=Pr(missing Y|Y=1). Note that, for simplicity, the MDM is assumed to be the same for both treatment groups. In this setting, $|\varphi_0-\varphi_1|$ is an indication of the degree of NMAR, compared to MAR/MCAR, where $\varphi_0=\varphi_1$. We now examine what the bias would be if the MDM were ignored by using the difference of the sample proportions, $\hat{p}_x-\hat{p}_y$.

Suppose X_i, i=1, ..., n_x, and Y_j, j=1, ..., n_y are observed. (n_x and n_y are also random variables.) Note that Pr(X is observed)=1−Pr(X is missing)

$$= 1-\left[Pr(X \text{ is missing} \mid X = 0)Pr(X = 0)+Pr(X \text{ is missing} \mid X = 1)Pr(X = 1)\right]$$

$$= 1-\left[\varphi_0(1-p_x)+\varphi_1 p_x\right]$$

$$\equiv \pi_x$$

Likewise, Pr(Y is observed)=1 − [φ_0(1 − p_y)+$\varphi_1 p_y$]=π_y.
The expected value of $\hat{p}_x$ is obtained as follows:

$$E(\hat{p}_x) = E\left(n_x^{-1}\sum_{i=1}^{n_x}X_i\right)$$

$$= E\left\{E\left(n_x^{-1}\sum_{i=1}^{n_x}X_i \mid n_x\right)\right\}$$

$$= E\left\{n_x^{-1}\, E\left(\sum_{i=1}^{n_x} X_i \mid n_x\right)\right\}$$

$$= E\left\{n_x^{-1} \sum_{i=1}^{n_x} E\left(X_i \mid n_x\right)\right\} \tag{15.5}$$

In Equation 15.5, $E(X_i \mid n_x) = Pr(X_i = 1 \mid X_i \text{ is observed})$

$$= \frac{Pr\left(X_i \text{ is observed} \mid X_i = 1\right) Pr\left(X_i = 1\right)}{Pr\left(X_i \text{ is observed}\right)}$$

$$= \frac{\left(1 - \varphi_1\right) p_x}{\pi_x}$$

Plug this into Equation 15.5 to obtain $E(\hat{p}_x) = \dfrac{\left(1 - \varphi_1\right) p_x}{\pi_x}$. Likewise,
$E(\hat{p}_y) = \dfrac{\left(1 - \varphi_1\right) p_y}{\pi_y}$.

Hence,

$$E\left(\hat{p}_x - \hat{p}_y\right) = \frac{\left(1 - \varphi_1\right) p_x}{\pi_x} - \frac{\left(1 - \varphi_1\right) p_y}{\pi_y}$$

$$= \frac{\pi_y \left(1 - \varphi_1\right) p_x - \pi_x \left(1 - \varphi_1\right) p_y}{\pi_x \pi_y}$$

$$= \frac{\left(1 - \varphi_0\right)\left(1 - \varphi_1\right)\left(p_x - p_y\right)}{\pi_x \pi_y} \tag{15.6}$$

Equation 15.6 shows a bias multiplier factor $\dfrac{\left(1 - \varphi_0\right)\left(1 - \varphi_1\right)}{\pi_x \pi_y}$. The sample mean difference $(\hat{p}_x - \hat{p}_y)$ is an unbiased estimator of $\theta = p_x - p_y$ if $\varphi_0 = \varphi_1$ (MCAR, the multiplier factor equals 1), or if $\theta = 0$ (no treatment effect).

15.5 Analysis under the MAR Assumption by Multiple Imputation

By "proper imputation" (mentioned in last section), we meant to exclude the method of "assigning the worst rank to treatment failures" for the composite variable strategy, and the method of LOCF (last observation carried forward) or BOCF (baseline observation carried forward) in the while-on-treatment strategy or some scenario under the hypothetical strategy. Proper imputation is the method of *multiple imputation* (MI). It is perhaps the most useful technique to provide a main estimator when the MAR assumption is attainable, as well as for sensitivity analyses with a range of plausible models of NMAR. The MI method, in general, is carried out in three steps: (a) Select a multivariate model and sample from this model to impute (fill in) the missing values G times to obtain G complete datasets; (b) for each of the G complete datasets, perform the proper analysis for complete data (such as the mixed-effect model for repeated measures or MMRM), obtaining the mean and within-imputation and between-imputation variances of the summary outcome measure; and (c) combine the G means by incorporating the within-imputation and between-imputation variances. For example, let $\hat{\theta}_j$ be the estimate of the treatment effect θ and v_j be the estimate of the variance of $\hat{\theta}_j$ from the j-th imputation. Then, the combined estimate is $\bar{\theta} = \sum_{j=1}^{G} \hat{\theta}_j / G$, and the (total) variance is

$$\sum_{j=1}^{G} v_j / G + \left(1 + G^{-1}\right) B$$

where the first term is the average within-imputation variance, $B = \dfrac{1}{G-1} \sum_{j=1}^{G} \left(\hat{\theta}_j - \bar{\theta}\right)^2$ is the between-imputation variance, and the multiplier $(1+G^{-1})$ is a finite number correction.

For analyses with the MAR assumption, steps (a) and (c) are directly implemented in SAS PROC MI and PROC MIANALYZE. Details can be found in the SAS documentation. For analyses with a particular NMAR assumption, the imputation step (a) in SAS needs to be augmented by a specific NMAR model (Section 15.7).

Sometimes in practice, the assumption of MAR may be in doubt. However, according to Schafer (1997) and Rubin (1998), the plausibility of the MAR assumption will be enhanced when there are sufficient covariates in the imputation model of step (a). We have also argued previously that when conditioning on the planned ICEs and treatment regimen, the MAR assumption seems reasonably attainable for many estimands. The model in step (a) is called the "imputer's model," which can have a larger set of covariates than the complete-data analysis model in step (b) after the missing values have been imputed. The subset of covariates used for the complete-data analysis is called the "analyst's model."

15.6 Analysis of Longitudinal Data with Monotone Pattern Missing Values under MAR

For longitudinal data with missing data caused by "dropouts," as is commonly the case in clinical trials, a monotone pattern is formed naturally. Specifically, consider a study with T scheduled post-baseline visits. Let Y_k denote the outcome at visit k, k=0, 1, 2, ..., T, where k=0 is the baseline visit. Under the monotone missing data pattern, if the subject's (relevant) outcome Y_k is missing at visit k, then the (relevant) outcomes Y_j at the future visits j>k are also missing. For this discrete time model, let L be the follow-up time, that is, the last visit that a subject has a measurement observed. The monotone missing data pattern M is then characterized by L=0, 1, ..., T, where L=T is when the subject completes the study visits. The baseline values are assumed to always be observed. A feasible analysis in this situation is based on the factorization in Equation 15.2, that is, the PMM approach. We discuss the approach with the case where T=4, as illustrated in Table 15.1.

With the PMM approach, the MAR condition $[M|Y]=[M|Y_{obs}]$ is equivalent to $[Y_{mis}|Y_{obs}, M]=[Y_{mis}|Y_{obs}]$. That is, the conditional distributions of the variables with missing data given observed variables are the same across the missing data pattern (see Appendix 15.4 for proof of the equivalence). For example, Table 15.1 illustrates the imputation using the pattern-mixture MAR condition $[Y_{mis}|Y_{obs}, M]=[Y_{mis}|Y_{obs}]$. This imputation is also called "as assigned treatment" (AAT) estimand.

Let us see how the $[Y_{mis} | Y_{obs}, M]=[Y_{mis} | Y_{obs}]$ condition identifies all the joint distributions for each pattern. For the observations with the pattern L=0, only Y_0 (baseline) is observed and all other follow-up values Y_1 to Y_4 need to be imputed. Using the MAR with PMM approach

TABLE 15.1

Monotone Missing Data for T=4 and Missing at Random Conditions with PMM

	Y_k				
	k=0	k=1	k=2	k=3	k=4
L=0	x	?=$[Y_1\|Y_0, L>0]$	?=$[Y_2\|Y_0, Y_1, L>1]$	?=$[Y_3\|Y_0, Y_1, Y_2, L>2]$	?=$[Y_4\|Y_0, Y_1, Y_2, Y_3, L>3]$
L=1	x	$[Y_1\|Y_0, L=1]$	?=$[Y_2\|Y_0, Y_1, L>1]$	?=$[Y_3\|Y_0, Y_1, Y_2, L>2]$	?=$[Y_4\|Y_0, Y_1, Y_2, Y_3, L>3]$
L=2	x	$[Y_1\|Y_0, L=2]$	$[Y_2\|Y_0, Y_1, L=2]$	?=$[Y_3\|Y_0, Y_1, Y_2, L>2]$	?=$[Y_4\|Y_0, Y_1, Y_2, Y_3, L>3]$
L=3	x	$[Y_1\|Y_0, L=3]$	$[Y_2\|Y_0, Y_3 L=3]$	$[Y_3\|Y_0, Y_1, Y_2, L=3]$	?=$[Y_4\|Y_0, Y_1, Y_2, Y_3, L>3]$
L=4	x	$[Y_1\|Y_0, L=4]$	$[Y_2\|Y_0, Y_1, L=4]$	$[Y_3\|Y_0, Y_1, Y_2, L=4]$	$[Y_4\|Y_0, Y_1, Y_2, Y_3, L=4]$

Note: k=study visit; L=last study visit with observed measure, describing the missing data pattern. Each row may represent one or more subjects. x denotes the observed data; ? denotes the missing data and is identified by the specified distribution.

$$\left[Y_1,\ Y_2,\ Y_3, Y_4 \mid Y_0,\ L = 0\right]$$

$$= \left[Y_1, Y_2, Y_3, Y_4 \mid Y_0\right]$$

$$= \left[Y_4 \mid Y_0, Y_1, Y_2, Y_3\right]\left[Y_1, Y_2, Y_3 \mid Y_0\right]$$

$$= \left[Y_4 \mid Y_0, Y_1, Y_2, Y_3,\ L = 4\right]\left[Y_3 \mid Y_0, Y_1, Y_2\right]\left[Y_1, Y_2 \mid Y_0\right]$$

$$= \left[Y_4 \mid Y_0, Y_1, Y_2, Y_3,\ L = 4\right]\left[Y_3 \mid Y_0, Y_1, Y_2,\ L \geq 3\right]\left[Y_2 \mid Y_0, Y_1\right]\left[Y_1 \mid Y_0\right]$$

$$= \left[Y_4 \mid Y_0, Y_1, Y_2, Y_3,\ L = 4\right]\left[Y_3 \mid Y_0, Y_1, Y_2,\ L \geq 3\right]\left[Y_2 \mid Y_0, Y_1\ L \geq 2\right]\left[Y_1 \mid Y_0\ L \geq 1\right]$$

$$\tag{15.7}$$

Hence, the joint distribution of $[Y_1,\ Y_2,\ Y_3,\ Y_4|Y_0,\ L=0]$ can be estimated because all the factors on the right-hand side of Equation 15.7 can be identified from the observed data. The same factorization and application of the MAR to the variables with missing values are performed for patterns $L=1, 2, 3$. (There are no missing data in $L=4$.) Missing values are sampled from the predictive/conditional distributions. This is the basis for the MI method. The derivations of Equation 15.7 suggest that the imputation can be done sequentially from $[Y_1|Y_0]=[Y_1|Y_0,\ L\geq1]$ to $[Y_4|Y_0,\ Y_1,\ Y_2,\ Y_3]=[Y_4|Y_0,\ Y_1,\ Y_2,\ Y_3,\ L=4]$, conditioning on the previous responses, as follows:

$$\left[Y_1 \mid Y_0,\ L = 0\right] = \left[Y_1 \middle|\ Y_0,\ L > 0\right]$$

$$\left[Y_2 \mid Y_0, Y_1,\ L = 1\right] = \left[Y_2 \middle|\ Y_0,\ Y_1,\ L > 1\right]$$

$$\left[Y_3 \mid Y_0, Y_1, Y_2,\ L = 2\right] = \left[Y_3 \middle|\ Y_0,\ Y_1,\ Y_2,\ L > 2\right]$$

$$\left[Y_4 \mid Y_0, Y_1, Y_2, Y_3,\ L = 3\right] = \left[Y_4 \middle|\ Y_0,\ Y_1,\ Y_2,\ Y_3,\ L > 3\right]$$

$$\tag{15.8}$$

In the above, for the pattern $L=j$, the predictive/conditional distribution at the right-hand side can be obtained from the observed data in the pattern $L>j$. Missing values Y_{j+1} in the pattern $L=j$ (left-hand side) are sampled from the predictive/conditional distribution of the right-hand side, as performed by the MI procedures in SAS. In PROC MI, the sequential imputations can be carried out in one command (Homework 15.2).

In a situation where the data have some cases with intermittent missing values (e.g., missing before ICE occurrence; see Figure 15.2), SAS PROC MI has an option to first create a monotone pattern from the intermittent missing values using the Markov Chain Monte Carlo (MCMC) method before proceeding with the analysis with a monotone pattern.

The following are SAS codes to carry out MI under MAR. Assume we have a dataset called "datain," which has an arbitrary missing data pattern. The covariates are age, sex, race, and treatment group (trt). Age is continuous, and other covariates are categorical variables. First, we generate the monotone missing pattern:

```
proc mi data = datain out = outmono nimpute = 2 seed = 1234;
mcmc impute = monotone;
var age sex racel race2 race3 trt Y0 Y1 Y2 Y3 Y4;
run;
```

Note that we created a design matrix (with dummy variables) for race in the above procedure (without showing the previous step of creation racel to race3) because the MCMC procedure that is used to fill in intermittent missing values assumes multivariate normality in SAS; therefore, it cannot take categorical variables directly by the CLASS statement when mcmc is used. This step outputs the monotone pattern data "outmono." There are two copies made for "outmono" through the option "nimute=2."

Next, perform MI on each of the copies of the "outmono" dataset using the regression (conditional expectation) method.

```
proc mi data = outmono out = miout nimpute = 5 seed = 1234;
monotone method = REG;
var age sex racel race2 race3 trt y0 y1 y2 y3 y4;
run;
```

The imputation by regression is carried out sequentially in the order specified in the var statement above. The conditional expectation starts from the first variable that has missing data and fills in the missing data with regression, which conditions on all the preceding variables as factors. It is not necessary to separate the sequential imputation with multiple steps. However, when we need to augment the conditional expectation (from MAR) with additional restrictions, as in NMAR, some strategy may require separation of the sequential steps.

15.7 Sensitivity Analysis under NMAR-NFD Model by MI

When the assumption of MCAR or MAR cannot be made, one cannot simply "ignore M." Hence, the likelihood-based analysis based on the factorization in Equation 15.1, that is, the selection model approach, requires modeling the MDM $[M|Y_{obs}, Y_{mis}; \varphi]$. Because there are infinitely many such models and none can be verified from the observed data, no general computing program is available. A prudent strategy is to perform "sensitivity analyses" with various models. A useful subclass of NMAR, called *nonfuture dependence* (NFD) *missingness*, introduced by Kenward, Molenberghs, and Thijs (2003) is given in Appendix 15.5. We discuss the specific analysis under NFD missingness in this section (Homework 15.3).

15.7.1 NFD with Mean-Shift Adjustment

The NFD can be formulated so that MAR is a special case of NFD. We continue the PMM approach to the analysis of data with a monotone pattern in order to make a connection between the NFD missingness and the MAR model. Continuing with the example described in Table 15.1 with T=4, for MAR, we illustrate in Table 15.2 the NFD missingness conditions given in Appendix 15.5, Equation 15A.11.

Contrasting Tables 15.1 (MAR) and 15.2, we see that the NMAR-NFD (Table 15.2 and Equation 15A.11) is not a comprehensive set of conditions. That is, there are missing data distributions left unidentified (denoted by a double question mark in Table 15.2). In order to further identify those missing data denoted as double question marks (??) in Table 15.2, we need a further assumption that can link to Equation 15.8 under MAR as follows.

A simple way to describe the departure from MAR is by a model with a shift in the conditional means of Equation 15.8. This *mean-shift model* assumption cannot be verified from the data itself. The justification for this choice is based mainly on interpretability: Place a penalty on the imputed value for missing data due to unfavorable reasons such as lack of efficacy or AE. It works as follows. First, assume linear regression (i.e., conditional mean) models for the observed (right-hand side of Equation 15.8), which can and should be checked with the observed data:

$$E\left(Y_1 \mid Y_0, L > 0\right) = \alpha_1 + \beta_1 Y_0$$

$$E\left(Y_2 \mid Y_0, Y_1, L > 1\right) = \alpha_2 + \beta_{20} Y_0 + \beta_{21} Y_1$$

TABLE 15.2

Monotone Missing Data for T=4 and Nonfuture Dependence Not Missing at Random Conditions with PMM

	Y_k				
	k = 0	k = 1	k = 2	k = 3	k = 4
L = 0	x	??	? = [Y_2 | Y_0, Y_1, L≥1]	? = [Y_3 | Y_0, Y_1, Y_2, L≥2]	? = [Y_4 | Y_0, Y_1, Y_2, Y_3, L≥3]
L = 1	x	[Y_1 | Y_0, L=1]	??	? = [Y_3 | Y_0, Y_1, Y_2, L≥2]	? = [Y_4 | Y_0, Y_1, Y_2, Y_3, L≥3]
L = 2	x	[Y_1 | Y_0, L=2]	[Y_2 | Y_0, Y_1, L=2]	??	? = [Y_4 | Y_0, Y_1, Y_2, Y_3, L≥3]
L = 3	x	[Y_1 | Y_0, L=3]	[Y_2 | Y_0, Y_1, L=3]	[Y_3 | Y_0, Y_1, Y_2, L=3]	??
L = 4	x	[Y_1 | Y_0, L=4]	[Y_2 | Y_0, Y_1, L=4]	[Y_3 | Y_0, Y_1, Y_2, L=4]	[Y_4 | Y_0, Y_1, Y_2, Y_3, L=4]

Note: k=study visit; L=last study visit with observed measure, describing the missing data pattern; each row may represent one or more subjects; x denotes the observed data; ? denotes the missing data and is identified by the specified distribution; and ?? denotes the missing data and unidentified distributions (which implies that we need more assumptions, and will relate to sensitivity analysis).

$$E\left(Y_3 \mid Y_0, Y_1, Y_2, L > 2\right) = \alpha_3 + \beta_{30} Y_0 + \beta_{31} Y_1 + \beta_{32} Y_2$$

$$E\left(Y_4 \mid Y_0, Y_1, Y_2, Y_3, L > 3\right) = \alpha_4 + \beta_{40} Y_0 + \beta_{41} Y_1 + \beta_{42} Y_2 + \beta_{43} Y_3 \quad (15.9)$$

All the intercept and slope coefficients can be estimated from the observed data. Next, to embed the MAR specification in this larger class of NMAR models, the NMAR class will be indexed by shifts in linking the dropouts with the observed conditional means. Third, assume that the shift is in the intercept, not in the slopes or the residual variances (Daniels and Hogan 2007, page 240; NRC 2010, page 100). That is,

$$E\left(Y_1 \mid Y_0, L=0\right) = (\alpha_1 + \Delta_1) + \beta_1 Y_0$$

$$= E\left(Y_1 \mid Y_0, L > 0\right) + \Delta_1 \text{ for all } Y_0$$

$$E\left(Y_2 \mid Y_0, Y_1, L = j\right) = \left(\alpha_2 + \Delta_{2j}\right) + \beta_{20} Y_0 + \beta_{21} Y_1$$

$$= E\left(Y_2 \mid Y_0, Y_1, L > 1\right) + \Delta_{2j} \text{ for } j = 0, 1 \text{ and all } Y_0, Y_1$$

$$E\left(Y_3 \mid Y_0, Y_1, Y_2, L = j\right) = \left(\alpha_3 + \Delta_{3j}\right) + \beta_{30} Y_0 + \beta_{31} Y_1 + \beta_{32} Y_2$$

$$= E\left(Y_3 \mid Y_0, Y_1, Y_2, L > 2\right) = \Delta_{3j} \text{ for } j = 0, 1, 2$$

$$\text{and all } Y_0, Y_1, Y_2$$

$$E\left(Y_4 \mid Y_0, Y_1, Y_2, Y_3, L = j\right) = \left(\alpha_4 + \Delta_{4j}\right) + \beta_{40} Y_0 + \beta_{41} Y_1 + \beta_{42} Y_2 + \beta_{43} Y_3$$

$$= E\left(Y_4 \mid Y_0, Y_1, Y_2, Y_3, L > 3\right) + \Delta_{4j} \text{ for } j = 0, 1, 2, 3$$

$$\text{and all } Y_0, Y_1, Y_2, Y_3 \quad (15.10)$$

Furthermore, an additional simplification is that $\Delta_{2j} = \Delta_2$ for $j=0, 1$; $\Delta_{3j} = \Delta_3$ for $j=0, 1, 2$; and $\Delta_{4j} = \Delta_4$ for $j=0, 1, 2, 3$. That is, the shift is the same across patterns for each visit with missing data. This is derived from the characteristic of the NFD missingness (Kenward, Molenberghs, and Thijs 2003); see Appendix 15.5 for more details.

Because the regression parameters can all be estimated, the left-hand side of Equation 15.10 can also be estimated when the shift parameters $\Delta = (\Delta_1, \Delta_2, \Delta_3, \Delta_4)$ are specified. The missing data in pattern $L=j$ will be filled in sequentially with the conditional mean in Equation 15.10. Computationally, because Equation 15.10 (for NFD missing) is only a shift of Equation 15.9 (for MAR), we can utilize the MI procedure based on MAR and apply shifts to the imputed values obtained from PROC MI. Note that the shift parameters $\Delta = (\Delta_1, \Delta_2, \Delta_3, \Delta_4)$ are applied together after the process of filling in the missing data under MAR is completed through MIs. They are not involved in the process of MI with MAR. It is a nonrecursive procedure. A recursive procedure is presented by Ratitch, O'Kelly, and Tosielloc (2013), which applies the shift parameters sequentially from time point to time point while conducting the imputation. That is, perform MI for the first time point with missing data under MAR, then apply Δ_1 to the imputed values in each of the imputations. Treating these Δ_1-adjusted values as observed, perform imputation for the second time point with missing data under MAR, and then apply Δ_2 to the imputed values of the second time point. Treating these Δ_2-adjusted values as observed, perform imputation for the third time point with missing data under MAR, etc. Note that, to avoid compounding MIs when there are many time points with missing data, sometimes it is necessary to limit imputations to only the first time point, and then for each of these imputations, a single imputation is performed for all subsequent time points. This is called single adjustment algorithm. Peng (2015) examines these algorithms (nonsequential, sequential, and single adjustment) and concludes that nonsequential and single adjustment work better than the sequential algorithm. A homework exercise is to compare these three procedures (Homework 15.3(2)).

Analytically, we can show how to obtain the marginal means of the outcome at each visit in each pattern and the marginal mean at the final visit over the patterns. Denote $\mu_k^{(j)} = E(Y_k \mid L = j)$. It follows from Equation 15.10 that for each follow-up visit post-baseline, we can sequentially obtain the pattern-specific marginal means:

$$\mu_1^{(0)} = E(Y_1 \mid L = 0) = (\alpha_1 + \Delta_1) + \beta_1 \, \mu_0^{(0)} \qquad (15.11)$$

where $\mu_0^{(0)}$ is estimated directly from the pattern-specific observed data.

$$\mu_2^{(j)} = E(Y_2 \mid L = j) = (\alpha_2 + \Delta_2) + \beta_{20} \, \mu_0^{(j)} + \beta_{21} \, \mu_1^{(j)} \text{ for } j = 0, 1 \qquad (15.12)$$

where $\mu_0^{(0)}, \mu_0^{(1)}, \mu_1^{(1)}$ are estimated directly from the observed data and $\mu_1^{(0)}$ is obtained from Equation 15.11.

$$\mu_3^{(j)} = E(Y_3 \mid L = j) = (\alpha_3 + \Delta_3) + \beta_{30} \, \mu_0^{(j)} + \beta_{31} \, \mu_1^{(j)} + \beta_{32} \, \mu_2^{(j)} \text{ for } j = 0, 1, 2 \quad (15.13)$$

where $\mu_0^{(0)}, \mu_0^{(1)}, \mu_0^{(2)}, \mu_1^{(1)}, \mu_1^{(2)}, \mu_2^{(2)}$ are estimated directly from the observed data, $\mu_1^{(0)}$ is obtained from Equation 15.11, and $\mu_2^{(0)}, \mu_2^{(1)}$ are obtained from Equation 15.12.

$$\mu_4^{(j)} = E(Y_4 \mid L = j) = (\alpha_4 + \Delta_4) + \beta_{40} \, \mu_0^{(j)} + \beta_{41} \, \mu_1^{(j)}$$

$$+\beta_{42} \, \mu_2^{(j)} + \beta_{43} \, \mu_3^{(j)} \text{ for } j = 0, 1, 2, 3 \qquad (15.14)$$

where $\mu_0^{(0)}, \mu_0^{(1)}, \mu_0^{(2)}, \mu_0^{(3)}, \mu_1^{(1)}, \mu_1^{(2)}, \mu_1^{(3)}, \mu_2^{(2)}, \mu_2^{(3)}, \mu_3^{(3)}$ are estimated directly from the observed data, while $\mu_1^{(0)}$ is obtained from Equation 15.11, $\mu_2^{(0)}, \mu_2^{(1)}$ are obtained from Equation 15.12, and $\mu_3^{(0)}, \mu_3^{(1)}, \mu_3^{(2)}$ are obtained from Equation 15.13. Using the notation of Equation 15.2, $\theta_M = \left\{ \mu_4^{(j)}, j = 0, 1, 2, 3 \right\}$.

In many clinical trials, the primary interest is on the marginal mean of the final visit at the last time point T. For the illustration of T=4,

$$\theta = E(Y_4) = \sum_{j=0}^{4} \omega_j E(Y_4 \mid L = j) = \sum_{j=0}^{4} \omega_j \mu_4^{(j)} \tag{15.15}$$

where $\omega_j = Pr(L=j)$ is estimated by the proportion of subjects in the pattern L=j.

The shift parameters $\Delta = (\Delta_1, \Delta_2, \Delta_3, \Delta_4)$ can be varied over a space of Δ, $D(\Delta)$, to perform sensitivity analysis to see how the result changes from the MAR case where $\Delta = (0, 0, 0, 0)$. The scale of departure from MAR can be determined in different ways. One metric is to use the residual standard deviation of Y_k given $(Y_0, ..., Y_{k-1})$, RSD_k, which can be obtained from the imputed complete data under MAR before engaging the NMAR model. For example, we may set the maximum range of departure from MAR at visit k equal to a factor f_k of RSD_k. If prior belief about the value of Δ_k is confined to being within $f_k \times RSD_k$, then $D(\Delta) = (f_1 \times RSD_1, ..., f_4 \times RSD_4)$. Each missing value at visit k is then replaced with $E(Y_k|Y_0, ..., Y_{k-1}, L> k-1) + Unif \times f_k \times RSD_k$, where $E(Y_k|Y_0, ..., Y_{k-1}, L>k-1)$ is estimated from the imputation steps under MAR and Unif is a random value from the uniform (0, 1) distribution. For example, Daniels and Hogan (2007) used $f_k = 1$ for all k=1, ..., T. It is conceivable that $RSD_k \geq RSD_{k'}$ for $k<k'$, because fewer Y's are included in the regression model at earlier time points. This also indicates that greater penalties are more likely to be placed on the earlier dropouts than the later ones, which is reasonable. Another metric is to use the STD_K (pooled standard deviation at time point k). STD_k would be increasing over time, contrary to RSD_k. It is also reasonable to add more "penalty" to missing data because the treatment effect would be wearing off more and more as time goes on after withdrawal. Peng (2015) also examines the sensitivity analysis using the two different metrics and recommends RSD over STD (Homework 15.3(2)).

For simplicity, Tables 15.1 and 15.2 and all illustrations above are performed without regard to the treatment group. In practice, we would include the treatment group as a covariate in the regression model instead of performing the MI separately for each treatment group.

When the missing values are multiply imputed by the NMAR model, other restrictions may also be considered. For example, for a pain score that ranges from 0 to 10, the imputed value should also be restricted in this range. Suppose that a clinical interpretation of withdrawal due to ineffective therapy means that the missing value should not be better than the baseline value; the imputed value should then also adopt this restriction.

15.7.2 NFD with Mean-Shift Adjustment Using Type of ICE or Reason for Initial Treatment Discontinuation and Follow-Up Time to Form the Missing Data Pattern

The above illustration uses T=4; thus, the monotone pattern is L=0, 1, ..., 4, which can easily be generalized. The pattern can also be set up to incorporate other factors than just using the discrete follow-up time L, the last visit with observation. For example, it is very reasonable to use the type of ICE or reason of initial treatment discontinuation as one factor in addition to L. In this case, we can use the same *shifting factor* f_k across visits, but vary them for different types of ICE or reasons for treatment discontinuation. It is conceivable that for analyzing the efficacy outcome, we apply a larger shifting factor value for ICE that relates to, or treatment discontinuation due to, lack of efficacy ($f_1 = f_2 = ... = f_T = f_{LOE}$), and a distinct or smaller shifting factor value for the ICE or withdrawal due to adverse event ($f_1 = f_2 = ... = f_T = f_{AE}$). $f_{LOE} = f_{AE}$ is a special case. For loss to follow-up that is truly neutral to efficacy or safety, we may set the *shifting factor* ($f_1 = f_2 = ... = f_T = f_{NEU}$) equal to 0, which reduces to the MAR case. The effect of the NMAR data on the treatment comparison will naturally be dependent on the proportion of missing data in each pattern when performing the data analysis, which is the ω_j in Equation 15.15. These *shifting factors* (f_{LOE}, f_{AE}, and f_{NEU}), which control the shift parameters Δ, are the *sensitivity parameters*. The parameters Δ and the baseline restriction for LOE (and/or AE) represent the presumption that a missing value due to LOE or AE would have a bad outcome if it were observed. This is especially true for, say, a pain score or blood pressure when the missing data are from a patient who discontinued the study treatment or took a rescue medication.

After all the MI steps under the NFD missingness are done, the usual statistical method for complete longitudinal data analysis can then be performed for each imputed set, and the results are integrated, for example, as performed by PROC MIANALYZE in SAS.

It is also a useful practice to display the sensitivity analysis by the summary of the efficacy results with different levels of the shifting factors. Table 15.3 illustrates a hypothetical example, using the p-values as the summary of efficacy results for different values of the sensitivity parameters (f_{LOE}, f_{AE}) with $f_{NEU} = 0$ and $f_{NEU} = 0.5$. If the conclusions are consistent within a reasonable range of the shifting parameters, then one can comfortably accept the result under the assumed model. Otherwise, the result will be subject to more scrutiny by skeptical reviewers.

TABLE 15.3

Summary of Sensitivity Analyses: A Hypothetical Example Using
p-Values as the Summary of Efficacy Results for Different Values of the
Sensitivity Parameters (f_{LOE}, f_{AE}, and f_{NEU})

p-Value	f_{LOE}				
$f_{NEU}=0$					
f_{AE}	*0*	*0.5*	*0.75*	*1.0*	*1.2*
0	*0.005*	0.007	0.012	0.024	0.035
0.5	0.006	0.008	0.014	0.030	0.037
0.75	0.009	0.012	0.023	0.033	0.041
1.0	0.013	0.022	0.030	0.042	0.049
1.2	0.023	0.027	0.033	0.044	0.053
$f_{NEU}=0.5$					
f_{AE}		*0.5*	*0.75*	*1.0*	*1.2*
0.5		0.010	0.016	0.032	0.039
0.75		0.014	0.025	0.035	0.043
1.0		0.024	0.032	0.044	0.051
1.2		0.029	0.035	0.046	0.055

15.8 Sensitivity Analyses under Other MNAR Models

15.8.1 Reference-Based Imputation (RBI)

An extensive amount of literature also exists on other NMAR models to perform sensitivity analyses (to the main analysis based on the MAR assumption).
For example, a large class of methods is called reference-based imputation
(RBI) or "as control treatment" (ACT) estimand, following some scenarios of
the hypothetical strategy (Section 15.2) that is adopted to target the estimand
toward the scientific question: What outcomes would be for patients who
discontinued initial treatment if they have taken "reference" medication. The
reference medication could be an active rescue or no-treatment placebo that
was not included in the trial or that was included but not all patients adhered
to. One variant of reference-based imputation, termed *jump to reference* (J2R),
is implemented such that imputed values for patients in the experimental
arm take on the attributes of the reference arm (placebo) immediately after
ICEs. In a second approach, called *copy reference* (CR), the imputations result
in a treatment effect that gradually diminishes toward the reference arm
after ICEs in accordance with the correlation structure implied by the imputation model. The third approach, called *copy increment from reference* (CIR),
assumes that the slopes, or differences in imputed values, across visits are
similar to those in the reference group. In all the three approaches, since the

treatment effect difference is sought, it is assumed that missing data in the reference arm are MAR and we borrow from the reference arm mean treatment effect information to impute active arm missing values. Details are found in Carpenter et al. (2013), Lu (2014a, b), Liu and Pang (2016, 2017), Mehrotra et al. (2017), and Sheng (2019). RBI analyses are gaining popularity with the regulatory agencies in superiority trials because they are conservative, that is, they tend to shrink toward no treatment difference.

For overall survival (OS), popular methods corresponding to RBI to handle treatment crossover ICE include *rank-preserving structure failure time* (RPSFT) (see, for example, Korhonen et al. 2012) and *inverse probability of censoring weighting* (IPCW) (see, for example, Robins and Finkelstein 2000; Latimer et al. 2019). Unlike ITT, the censoring occurs at the time of the treatment switching for these methods.

15.8.2 Shared Parameter or Random-Coefficient-Dependent Models

Another large class of NMAR is a special kind of random effects model where the missing data are assumed to depend on the underlying (unobserved) random effects, or latent variables. Sometimes, this class of NMAR is called *shared parameter* or *random-coefficient-dependent models*; see Molenberghs and Kenward (2007). Shih, Quan, and Chang (1994) illustrated the univariate case based on the simple random effect model introduced in Section 4.5. They assumed that the MDM depends on the unobserved true value of the endpoint, instead of the potentially observed endpoint itself (Homework 15.6). In a sequence of papers, Wu and Bailey (1988, 1989), Wu and Carroll (1988), Schluchter (1992), Mori, Woodworth, and Woolson (1992), and Wu, Hunsberger, and Zucker (1994) developed methods of analyzing longitudinal data by using the rate of change (slope) as the estimand. The missing data due to dropouts are assumed to depend on the true (unobserved) underlying slope of the individual. For example, individuals with a gradual decrease in blood pressure tend to remain in the study, while those with an increase would drop out of the study prematurely. In this context, the term *informative right-censoring* or *informative missing* data was used to mean that the MDM is not ignorable. The hazard of dropout in a shared parameter model will generally imply or directly result in a dependence of the missing data on future observations, even after conditioning on the past and current observations. These models can be very useful for complex data structures, but because many layers of assumptions are needed for the model to fit the data, they have not been widely used in a regulatory setting. The sensitivity analysis in this class of NMAR models is an active and open research area.

Appendix 15.1: Sampling Distribution Inference

The inference is based on some (sufficient) statistic, say S(V). To "ignore" the missing data usually means to fix M=m, the observed missing data pattern, and to compare the observed value of S(V) to the distribution of S(V) found from $S(V)=S(Y_{obs}, M=m)=S(Y_{obs})$, that is, from the marginal distribution of Y_{obs} alone: $[Y_{obs}] = \int [Y]dY_{mis}$. However, the correct reference distribution should be the conditional distribution of Y_{obs} given M:

$$[Y_{obs} \mid M] = \frac{\int [Y, M]dY_{mis}}{[M]} = \frac{\int [M \mid Y][Y]dY_{mis}}{\int [M \mid Y][Y]dY} \qquad (15A.1)$$

When [M|Y] does not depend on Y, then we simplify the right-hand side of Equation 15A.1 and find $[Y_{obs} \mid M] = \int [Y]dY_{mis,} = [Y_{obs}]$; in other words, "ignoring" the missing data is appropriate. The above condition "[M|Y] does not depend on Y" is termed MCAR in the literature.

From the above discussion, we can see that a more precise way of saying "ignoring the missing data" should really be "ignoring the process that causes the missing data," because it is the [M|Y] that is being ignored in Equation 15A.1.

In a clinical trial, if the cause of the missing data is not related to the observed or potential outcome of the patients, then MCAR may be assumed. Examples include patients who have moved away, the study ending, and late entry of patients being administratively "censored."

Appendix 15.2: Likelihood Inference

The inference is based on the likelihood function L(θ; V). When "ignoring" the missing data, we usually mean that $L(\theta; V) \propto [Y_{obs}]$ for $\theta \in \Omega_\theta$ (the parameter space of θ), that is,

$$L(\theta; V) \propto I(\theta \in \Omega_\theta) \int [Y]dY_{mis} \qquad (15A.2)$$

where I(·) is the indicator function.

However, the correct likelihood should be based on the joint distribution, that is, $L(\theta; V) \propto [Y_{obs}, M]$ for $(\theta, \varphi) \in \Omega_{\theta,\varphi}$ (the joint parameter space of θ and φ). Thus,

$$L(\theta; V) \propto I((\theta, \varphi) \in \Omega_{\theta,\varphi}) \int [M \mid Y][Y]dY_{mis} \qquad (15A.3)$$

If (a) $\Omega_{\theta,\varphi} = \Omega_\theta \times \Omega_\varphi$ and (b) $[M \mid Y] = [M \mid Y_{obs}]$, then Equation 15A.3 reduces to Equation 15A.2, and ignoring the missing data process is appropriate. Condition (a) above is termed *distinct parameters* (DP), and condition (b) is termed *missing at random* (MAR) in the literature. See discussion in Shih (1992).

In a longitudinal clinical trial, MAR may be assumed if the patient withdrawal from the study is due to the observed outcome in the past, not the current unobserved or future potential outcomes.

Appendix 15.3: Bayesian Inference

The discussion is similar to that in Appendix 15.2 with an extra prior distribution on the parameter space, $\Omega_{\theta,\varphi}$. The conditions for an ignorable missing data process are the same (a) and (b) as in Appendix 15.2.

The above "ignorability" discussion is naturally applicable to each treatment group, if we consider the conditional distribution $[Y|Z_1]$ throughout the discussion, where Z_1 denotes the treatment group and it can also be extended to conditioning on all predefined baseline covariates Z. Second, the "ignorability" conditions given in the previous section are *sufficient conditions*. There may be other conditions by which the missing data process could also be ignorable. This is especially true when considering *testing* between treatment groups as opposed to the estimation within each treatment group's parameters. The example in Section 15.4 illustrated a case where, under the null hypothesis that $\theta=0$ (no treatment effect), the inference based on the observed data is unbiased. A discussion of sufficient conditions for *stratified testing* can be found in Shih and Quan (1998).

Appendix 15.4: Equivalence between Selection Model and Pattern-Mixture Model for MCAR and MAR

1. Rubin's (1976) definition of MCAR is based on the selection model factorization of the joint distribution of Y and M:

$$[Y, M] = [M \mid Y][Y] = [M][Y] \tag{15A.4}$$

when [M] does not depend on Y.

The PMM, on the other hand, is based on a different factorization of the joint distribution of Y and M:

$$[Y, M] = [Y \mid M][M] \tag{15A.5}$$

For Equation 15A.4 = 15A.5, it follows that

$$[Y] = [Y \mid M] \tag{15A.6}$$

This is the MCAR under the PMM; that is, the marginal distribution of Y is the same regardless of the pattern M. The reverse direction from Equation 15A.6 to implying [M|Y]=[M] is straightforward to show.

2. Rubin's (1976) definition of MAR is based on the selection model factorization of the joint distribution of Y and M:

$$[Y, M] = [M \mid Y][Y] = [M \mid Y_{obs}, Y_{mis}][Y] = [M \mid Y_{obs}][Y] \qquad (15A.7)$$

when $[M \mid Y_{obs}, Y_{mis}] = [M \mid Y_{obs}]$, which is the selection model's condition of MAR.

Under this condition, Equation 15A.7 is written as

$$
\begin{aligned}
[Y_{obs}, Y_{mis}, M] &= [M \mid Y_{obs}][Y_{obs}, Y_{mis}] \\
&= \frac{[Y_{obs} \mid M][M]}{[Y_{obs}]}[Y_{obs}, Y_{mis}] \\
&= [Y_{obs} \mid M][M]\frac{[Y_{obs}, Y_{mis}]}{[Y_{obs}]} \\
&= [Y_{obs}, M][Y_{mis} \mid Y_{obs}]
\end{aligned} \qquad (15A.8)
$$

However, $[Y_{obs}, Y_{mis}, M] = [Y_{obs}, M] [Y_{mis} \mid Y_{obs}, M]$. Equating this to Equation 15A.8, we obtain

$$[Y_{mis} \mid Y_{obs}, M] = [Y_{mis} \mid Y_{obs}] \qquad (15A.9)$$

Equation 15A.9 is the conditional of MAR with the PMM approach. It says that the conditional distribution of Y_{mis} given Y_{obs} is independent of the pattern.

Conversely, starting from the PMM approach, we factor

$$[Y, M] = [Y_{obs}, Y_{mis}, M] = [Y_{obs}, M][Y_{mis} \mid Y_{obs}, M]$$

Under the condition of Equation 15A.9,

$$
\begin{aligned}
[Y, M] &= [Y_{obs}, M][Y_{mis} \mid Y_{obs}] \\
&= [Y_{obs} \mid M][M]\frac{[Y_{mis}, Y_{obs}]}{[Y_{obs}]} \\
&= \frac{[Y_{obs} \mid M][M]}{[Y_{obs}]}[Y_{obs}, Y_{mis}] \\
&= [M \mid Y_{obs}][Y_{obs}, Y_{mis}] \\
&= [M \mid Y_{obs}][Y]
\end{aligned}
$$

We arrive at Equation 15A.7.

The equivalence of $[M|Y_{obs}, Y_{mis}]=[M|Y_{obs}]$ (MAR under the selection model approach) and $[Y_{mis}|Y_{obs}, M]=[Y_{mis}|Y_{obs}]$ (MAR under the PMM approach) has far-reaching implications. The selection model approach is useful for simulation studies to generate missing data with known mechanisms. The PMM approach is useful for data analysis, where we can use the observed data to fit a predictive model of Y_{mis} given Y_{obs} (and other covariates and/or prior distribution of the parameters), from which the Y_{mis} can then be sampled. This is the foundation of the MI method.

Appendix 15.5: NFD Missingness Mechanism as a Subclass of NMAR for Longitudinal Data with Monotone Missing Data Pattern

With the selection model setting, we factor $[Y, M]=[M|Y][Y]=[M \mid Y_{obs}, Y_{mis}][Y]$. When the MDM $[M|Y]=[M|Y_{obs}, Y_{mis}]$ depends not only on Y_{obs} (as for MAR), but also on the missing data Y_{mis}, it is called NMAR or MNAR. As there are infinitely many different ways M can depend on Y_{mis}, we shall further subclass the NMAR models. For longitudinal data with Y_k, k=0, 1, 2, ... T, where k=0 is the baseline visit, following the monotone missing data pattern characterized by L=0, 1, ..., T, as described in Section 15.7, the above selection model factorization is then written as

$$\left[Y_0, Y_1, ..., Y_j, ..., Y_T, L = j \right] = \left[L = j | Y_0, Y_1, ..., Y_j, ..., Y_T \right]$$

$$\times \left[Y_0, Y_1, ..., Y_j, ..., Y_T \right]$$

Recall that L is the last visit during which a subject has a measurement observed. If the MDM is such that

$$\left[L = j | Y_0, Y_1, ..., Y_j, ..., Y_T \right] = \left[L = j | Y_0, Y_1, ..., Y_j, Y_{j+1} \right] \qquad (15A.10)$$

it is then called NFD missingness; in other words, the current unobserved outcome Y_{j+1} (for the pattern L=j) depends on the past observed outcomes $(Y_1, ..., Y_j)$ as well as the presently missing outcome Y_{j+1} (itself), but not on the future outcomes $(Y_{j+2}, ..., Y_T)$ (Kenward, Molenberghs, and Thijs 2003).

This NFD missingness is a subclass of the NMAR. NFD missingness includes MAR as a special case, because it adds one more restriction on the missing mechanism in addition to that for MAR.

This definition of NFD missingness, expressed by the MDM (Equation 15A.10), is with the selection model framework and is very intuitive.

However, for analyzing data, it is more convenient to use the PMM approach (see Equation 15A.13). With the pattern-mixture framework, NFD missingness has another form, defined by Kenward, Molenberghs, and Thijs (2003) as follows.

Assume that the baseline value Y_0 is always observed, and that the first missing data occur at the first follow-up visit. (If the first missing data occur at a visit beyond the first follow-up visit, then we can let Y_0 be a vector of observed visits, for easier notation.) The NFD missingness is such that, for all follow-up visits $k \geq 2$ and all patterns $j < k-1$,

$$\left[Y_k \mid Y_0, Y_1, \ldots, Y_{k-1}, L = j\right] = \left[Y_k \mid Y_0, Y_1, \ldots, Y_{k-1}, L \geq k - 1\right] \quad (15A.11)$$

It can be shown that the condition in Equation 15A.11 is equivalent to

$$\left[Y_k \mid Y_0, Y_1, \ldots, Y_{k-1}, L = j\right] = \left[Y_k \mid Y_0, Y_1, \ldots, Y_{k-1}\right] \quad (15A.12)$$

The proof uses similar steps as in Appendix 15.4(2) and is assigned as a homework problem (Homework 15.4).

Another homework assignment is to show the equivalence between Equations 15A.10 and 15A.12; see Appendix 15.6.

Note that with the NFD missing data condition (Equation 15A.11), the distribution $[Y_k \mid Y_0, Y_1, \ldots, Y_{k-1}, L = k-1]$ was left unspecified for $k = 1, \ldots, T$. We need to make an assumption for this unidentified model to proceed. As in the MAR case, we link it with the $L > k$ patterns where Y_{k+1} is observed. One such an assumption is the mean-shift model as a simple departure from MAR, as discussed in Section 15.7. This assumption is not verifiable from the observed data and requires sensitivity analyses for varying shift values.

Specifically, we write the whole joint distribution with the pattern-mixture factorization

$$\left[Y_0, Y_1, \ldots, Y_j, \ldots, Y_T, L = j\right] = \left[Y_0, Y_1, \ldots, Y_j, \ldots, Y_T \mid L = j\right]\left[L = j\right] \quad (15A.13)$$

The pattern-specific joint distribution $[Y_0, Y_1, \ldots, Y_j, \ldots, Y_T \mid L=j]$ can be written as

$$\left[Y_0, Y_1, \ldots, Y_j, \ldots, Y_T \mid L = j\right] = \left[Y_0, Y_1, \ldots, Y_j \mid L = j\right]\left[Y_{j+1} \mid Y_0, Y_1, \ldots, Y_j, L = j\right]$$

$$\times \prod_{k=j+2}^{T}\left[Y_k \mid Y_0, Y_1, \ldots, Y_{k-1}, L = j\right] \quad (15A.14)$$

The first factor of Equation 15A.14 is clearly identifiable from the observed data. The second and beyond are not identified due to the missing data and require additional assumptions. The second factor could be identified by linking it to the observed $[Y_{j+1}|Y_0, Y_1, ..., Y_j, L \geq j+1]$ with an additional assumption. (The special shift parameter model is a simple yet useful way to link.) The third and beyond factors could be identified with the help of the NFD condition (Equation 15A.11) together with the same link as for the second factor as follows: Using Equation 15A.11, for $k \geq j+2$,

$$\left[Y_k \mid Y_0, Y_1, ..., Y_{k-1}, L = j\right] = \left[Y_k \mid Y_0, Y_1, ..., Y_{k-1}, L \geq k-1\right]$$

Furthermore, the right-hand side $[Y_k|Y_0, Y_1, ..., Y_{k-1}, L \geq k-1]$

$$= \sum_{s=k-1}^{T} \frac{[Y_0, Y_1, ..., Y_{k-1}, L=s]}{[Y_0, Y_1, ..., Y_{k-1}, L \geq k-1]} [Y_k \mid Y_0, Y_1, ..., Y_{k-1}, L=s] \quad (15A.15)$$

and

$$\frac{[Y_0, Y_1, ..., Y_{k-1}, L=s]}{[Y_0, Y_1, ..., Y_{k-1}, L \geq k-1]} = \frac{P(L=s)[Y_0, Y_1, ..., Y_{k-1} \mid L=s]}{\sum_{s=k-1}^{T} P(L=s)[Y_0, Y_1, ..., Y_{k-1} \mid L=s]}$$

Note that $[Y_0, Y_1, ..., Y_{k-1}|L=s]$ can be identified from the observed data for $s \geq k-1$. $[Y_k|Y_0, Y_1, ..., Y_{k-1}, L=s]$ can be identified from the observed data for $s \geq k$. The unidentified $[Y_k|Y_0, Y_1, ..., Y_{k-1}, L=k-1]$ is linked to $[Y_k|Y_0, Y_1, ..., Y_{k-1}, L \geq k]$ by the same shift model as for the second factor. Thus, all factors in Equation 15A.14 can be identified. The mean-shift model as a simple yet useful way to describe the departure from MAR is expressed as

$$E\left[Y_k \mid Y_0, Y_1, ..., Y_{k-1}, L = k-1\right] = E\left[Y_k \mid Y_0, Y_1, ..., Y_{k-1}, L \geq k\right] + \Delta_k$$

An example for T=4 is given in Section 15.7 for illustration.

Appendix 15.6: Equivalence between the Selection Model NFD Missingness Condition (Equation 15A.10) and the Pattern-Mixture Model NFD Missingness Condition (Equation 15A.12)

The proof is given in the study by Peng (2015) (Homework 15.5).

HOMEWORK 15.1

Read the reference "Defining efficacy estimands in clinical trials: examples illustrating ICH E9 (R1) guidelines" by Ratitch et al. (Ther Innov Regul Sci 2020, 54: 370–384), and discuss the example trials regarding the strategies of handling ICEs and the corresponding estimands.

HOMEWORK 15.2

Generate a longitudinal dataset with MAR missing values by the selection model specification and analyze the trend.

1. Consider the following model. First, the complete data are a sequence $\{Y_t : t=1, \ldots, 10\}$ from a multivariate normal distribution with $E(Y_t)=\alpha_0+\alpha_1 t$ and covariance matrix $(1-\rho)I+\rho J$; that is, variances=1 at each t and the correlation between Y_s and Y_t equals ρ for all $t \neq s$. (See the parameter values below.) Second, the monotone missing pattern and the MDM are defined as follows. Let L be the last time point t at which Y_t is observed. Let $Pr(L=j+1 \mid Y_1, \ldots, Y_j, L \geq j+1)=p(Y_j \mid L \geq j+1)$, and set $\log[p(y)/(1 - p(y))]=\beta_0+\beta_1 y$. That is, we assume a logistic regression model for the monotone MDM that the chance of missing or observing at $t=j+1$ depends only on the last observed value at $t=j$. Finally, generate a set of $n=100$ realizations of the above process by assuming the correlation $\rho=0.9$, $\alpha_0=1$, $\alpha_1=0$ (i.e., no trend), $\beta_0=-1$, and $\beta_1=-2$. Let the missing value occur when the probability of missing is greater than 0.6. Note that, using the notation of the selection model factorization (Equation 15.1), $\theta=(\alpha_0, \alpha_1, \rho)$ and $\varphi=(\beta_0, \beta_1)$. This model satisfies both MAR and DP conditions. Plot the generated data. As a sampling-distribution-based inference (see Appendix 15.1), connect the sample mean values at each time point $t=1, \ldots, 10$. Comment on and explain what you see about the empirical trend.

2. As a likelihood-based inference (see Appendix 15.2), use PROC MIXED and use PROC MI and PROC ANALYZE to analyze the data generated above and estimate the true trend α_1. Comment

62   *Statistical Design, Monitoring, and Analysis*

on your estimates (one from single imputation PROC MIXED and another from multiple imputation PROC MI) in contrast to the empirical trend in (1).
3. Do the same as above, but change to $\rho=0$. Again, compare the estimated trend with the empirical trend.

HOMEWORK 15.3

Generate a longitudinal dataset with NMAR-NFD missing values, and analyze the data.

1. The complete-data model and the monotone pattern are the same as above, but use the following MDM model: $\Pr(L=j+1 \mid Y_1, ..., Y_j, L \geq j+1) = p(Y_{j+1} \mid L \geq j+1)$, and $\log[p(y)/(1-p(y))] = \beta_0 + \beta_1 y$. That is, the chance of missing or observing at $t=j+1$ depends on only the current value at $t=j+1$. Use the same parameter values for $\rho=0.9$, $\alpha_0=1$, $\alpha_1=0$, $\beta_0=-1$, and $\beta_1=-2$. Let the missing value occur when the probability of missing is greater than 0.6. Plot the realization set of data for $n=100$.
2. Conduct the PMM approach with Δ_k shift set to be within one RSD of Y_t given $Y_1, ..., Y_{t-1}$ (estimated from the imputed complete data under MAR), as described in Section 15.7.1. Use the single adjustment, nonrecursive/nonsequential, and recursive/sequential procedures to estimate the marginal means $E(Y_t)$ at each time point $t=1$ to 10 and compare their results.

HOMEWORK 15.4

Derive Equation 15A.12 from Equation 15A.11. (Hint: Use the similar steps as in Appendix 15.4.2.)

HOMEWORK 15.5

Prove the assertion in Appendix 15.6. (Hint: Use induction.)

HOMEWORK 15.6

Consider a two-stage random effect model for $Y = \{y_i, i=1, ..., N\}$

$$y_i \mid \mu_i \sim N\left(\mu_i, \sigma^2\right)$$

$$\mu_i \mid \mu \sim N\left(\mu, \tau^2\right)$$

where y_i is the response (e.g., change from baseline), μ_i is the true (unobserved) response of the i-th subject, σ^2 is the within-subject variance, and τ^2 is the between-subject variance. Note that this is related to the model (Equation 4.21) in Section 4.5. Our interest is to estimate μ, the group mean response. Suppose $Y_{obs} = [y_1, ..., y_n]$ are observed, and the rest $Y_{mis} = \{y_{n+1}, ..., y_N\}$ are missing. Use a question mark to denote missing values. We assume the MDM to follow $Pr(y_i = ? \mid \mu_i) = I(\mu_i < c)$ for some constant c, where I(.) is the indicator function. That is, when the true change is less than c, then the response is not observed. Note that μ_i is always unobservable.

1. Corresponding to Y, let $M = \{m_i, i=1, ..., N\}$ be the missing data pattern for Y; $m_i = 1$ when y_i is observed and 0 otherwise. The MDM can be written as $g(m_i \mid y_i, \mu_i) = I\{I(\mu_i > c) - m_i = 0\}$. Argue that this MDM is a nonignorable case.

2. If one ignores the (nonignorable) MDM and uses the sample mean $\bar{Y}_n$ to estimate μ, show that when N increases, but n/N remains constant, the asymptotic bias of $\bar{Y}_n$ is

$$\bar{Y}_n - \mu = \frac{N\tau}{n\sqrt{2\pi}} \exp\left\{ -\frac{1}{2}\left[\Phi^{-1}\left(\frac{N-n}{N} \right) \right]^2 \right\} > 0$$

where Φ^{-1} is the inverse of the cdf of the standard normal distribution.

References

CDER (US Department of Health and Human Services, Food and Drug Administration, Center for Drug Evaluation and Research). (2014). *Guidance for Industry—Analgesic Indications Developing Drug and Biological Products (Draft Guidance)*. http://www.fda.gov/Drugs/GuidanceComplianceRegulatoryInformation/Guidances/default.htm (accessed on March 31, 2014).

Carpenter JR, Roger JH, Kenward MG. (2013). Analysis of longitudinal trials with protocol deviation a framework for relevant, accessible assumptions, and inference via multiple imputation. *Journal of Biopharmaceutical Statistics* 23: 1352–1371.

Choi SC and Lu IL. (1995). Effect of non-random missing data mechanisms in clinical trials. *Statistics in Medicine* 14: 2675–2684. doi:10.1002/sim.4780142407.

Daniels MJ and Hogan JW. (2007). *Missing Data in Longitudinal Studies Strategies for Bayesian Modeling and Sensitivity Analysis*. Boca Raton, FL: Chapman & Hall/ CRC Press.

Diggle PJ and Shih WJ. (1993). On informative and random dropouts in longitudinal studies. *Biometrics* 49: 947–949.

EMEA (European Medicines Evaluation Agency). (1998). *Statistical Principles for Clinical Trials; Step 5 Note for Guidance on Statistical Principles for Clinical Trials.* International Conference on Harmonisation (ICH) Topic E9. http://www. ema.europa.eu/docs/en_GB/document_library/Scientific_guideline/2009/09/ WC500002928.pdf (accessed on April 21, 2015).

International Council for Harmonisation of Technical Requirements for Pharmaceuticals for Human use. (2019). Addendum on Estimands and Sensitivity Analysis in Clinical Trials to the Guideline on Statistical Principles for Clinical Trials E9(R1). Final version Adopted on 20 November 2019.

Finkelstein D and Schoenfeld D. (1999). Combining mortality and longitudinal measures in clinical trials. *Statistics in Medicine* 18: 1341–1354.

Kenward MG, Molenberghs G, and Thijs H. (2003). Pattern-mixture models with proper time dependence. *Biometrika* 90 53–71.

Kenward M. (2013). The handling of missing data in clinical trials. *Clinical Investigation* 2013; 3(3):241–250.

Korhonen P, Zuber E, Branson M. et al. (2012). Correcting overall survival for the impact of crossover via a rank-preserving structural failure time (RPSFT) model in the RECORD-1 trial of everolimus in metastatic renal-cell carcinoma. *Journal of Biopharmaceutical Statistics* 22: 1258–1271.

Laird NM and Ware JH. (1982). Random-effects models for longitudinal data. *Biometrics* 38: 963–74.

Latimer NR, Abrams KR, Siebert U. (2019). Two-stage estimation to adjust for treatment switching in randomised trials: a simulation study investigating the use of inverse probability weighting instead of re-censoring. *BMC Med Res Methodol.* 19(1):69.

Liang KY and Zeger SL. (1986). Longitudinal data analysis using generalized linear models. *Biometrika* 73: 13–22.

Little RJA. (1993). Pattern-mixture models for multivariate incomplete data. *Journal of the American Statistical Association* 88: 125–134.

Little RJA. (1995). Modeling the drop-out mechanism in repeated-measures studies. *Journal of the American Statistical Association* 90: 1112–1121.

Little RJA and Yao L. (1998). Statistical techniques for analyzing data from prevention trials treatment of no-shows using Rubin's causal model. *Psychological Methods* 3: 147–159.

Little RJA, Cohen ML, Dickersin K, Emerson SS, Farrar JT, Neaton JD, Shih WJ, et al. (2012a). The design and conduct of clinical trials to limit missing data. *Statistics in Medicine* July 2012. doi:10.1002/sim.5519.

Little RJA, Cohen ML, Dickersin K, Emerson SS, Farrar JT, Neaton JD, Shih, WJ, et al. (2012b). The prevention and treatment of missing data in clinical trials. *New England Journal of Medicine* 367:1355–1360. October 4, 2012. doi:10.1056/NE/Msrl203730.

Liu GF and Lei Pang L. (2016). On analysis of longitudinal clinical trials with missing data using reference-based imputation. *Journal of Biopharmaceutical Statistics* 26(5):924–936.

Liu GF and Pang L. (2017). Control-based imputation and delta-adjustment stress test for missing data analysis in longitudinal clinical trials. *Statistics in Biopharmaceutical Research* 9(2):186–194.

Lu K. (2014a). An analytic method for the placebo-based pattern-mixture model. *Statistics in Medicine* 33(7): 1134–1145.

Lu K. (2014b). An extension of the placebo-based pattern-mixture model. *Pharmaceutical Statistics* 13(2): 103–109.

Mallinckrodt CH, Bell J, Liu G. et al. (2020). Aligning estimators with estimands in clinical trials putting the ICH E9(R1) guidelines into practice. *Therapeutic Innovation & Regulatory Science*. 54(2): 353–364.

Mehrotra D, Liu F, Permutt T. (2017). Missing data in clinical trials control-based mean imputation and sensitivity analyses. *Pharmaceutical Statistics* 16:378–392.

Molenberghs G and Kenward MG. (2007). *Missing Data in Clinical Studies*. Chichester, UK Wiley.

Mori M, Woodworth G, and Woolson RF. (1992). Application of empirical Bayes methodology to estimation of changes in the presence of informative right censoring. *Statistics in Medicine* 11: 621–631.

Morris TP, Kahan BC, and White IR. (2014). Choosing sensitivity analyses for randomised trials principles. *BMC Medical Research Methodology* 14: 11 doi:10.1186/1471-2288-14-ll.

NRC (National Research Council). (2010). *The Prevention and Treatment of Missing Data in Clinical Trials*. Panel on Handling Missing Data in Clinical Trials. Committee on National Statistics, Division of Behavioral and Social Sciences and Education. Washington, DC: The National Academies Press.

Paik MC. (1997). The generalized estimating equation approach when data are not missing completely at random. *Journal of the American Statistical Association* 92: 1320–1329.

Peng L. (2015). Design of Primary and Sensitivity Analysis of Non-Future Dependence Missing Data in Clinical Trials with an Emphasis on the Type-I Error Rate Using Multiple Imputation and Pattern Mixture Model Approach. Ph.D. Dissertation, Department of Biostatistics, Rutgers School of Public Health, Rutgers University, The State University of New Jersey.

Permutt T for the FDA CDER Missing Data Working Group. (2016). Taxonomy of estimands for regulatory clinical trials with discontinuation. *Statistics in Medicine* 35(17): 2865–2875.

Ratitch B, O'Kelly M. (2011). Implementation of pattern-mixture models using standard SAS/STAT procedures. PharmaSUG 2011. http://pharmasug.org/proceedings/2011/SP/PharmaSUG-2011-SP04.pdf (accessed March 14, 2020).

Ratitch B, O'Kelly M, and Tosielloc R. (2013). Missing data in clinical trials from clinical assumptions to statistical analysis using pattern mixture models. *Pharmaceutical Statistics* (wileyonlinelibrary.com) doi:10.1002/pst.1549.

Ratitch B, Bell J, Mallinckrodt C, et al. (2019). Choosing estimands in clinical trials putting the ICH E9(R1) into practice. *Therapeutic Innovation & Regulatory Science*. doi:10.1177/2168479019838827.

Ratitch B, Goel N, Mallinckrodt C. et al. (2020). Defining efficacy estimands in clinical trials examples illustrating ICH E9(R1) Guidelines. *Therapeutic Innovation & Regulatory Science* 54: 370–384 (2020). doi:10.1007/s43441-019-00065-7.

Robins JM and Finkelstein DM. (2000). Correcting for noncompliance and dependent censoring in an aids clinical trial with inverse probability of censoring weighted (ipcw) log-rank tests. *Biometrics* 56: 779–788.

Robins JM, Rotnitzky A, and Zhao LP. (1995). Analysis of semiparametric regression models for repeated outcomes in the presence of missing data. *Journal of the American Statistical Association* 90 106–121.

Rubin DB. (1976). Inference and missing data. *Biometrika* 63: 581–592.

Rubin DB. (1998). *Multiple imputation for nonresponse in surveys.* New York: Wiley.

SAS® Institute. SAS/STAT® procedure release 9.2, PROC MIXED, PROC MI, PROC MIANALYZE.

Schafer JL. (1997). *Analysis of Incomplete Multivariate Data.* New York Chapman and Hall.

Schluchter MD. (1992). Methods for the analysis of informatively censoring longitudinal data. *Statistics in Medicine* 11: 1861–1870.

Sheng T. (2019). *Decay Model for Handling Missing Data due to Intercurrent Events in Clinical Trials.* A dissertation submitted to the School of Graduate Studies, Rutgers, The State University of New Jersey in partial fulfillment of the requirements for the degree of Doctor of Philosophy Graduate Program in Public Health.

Shih WJ. (1992). On informative and random dropouts in longitudinal studies. *Biometrics* 48: 970–972.

Shih WJ, Quan H, and Chang MN. (1994). Estimation of the mean when data contain non-ignorable missing values from a random effects model. *Statistics & Probability Letters* 19: 249–257.

Shih WJ and Quan H. (1998). Stratified testing for treatment effects with missing data. *Biometrics* 54: 782–787.

Yuan YC. (2001). Multiple Imputation for Missing Data Concepts and New Development SAS/STAT® 8.2. [http://www.sas.com/statistics]. Cary, NC SAS Institute.

Wu MC and Bailey KR. (1988). Analyzing changes in the presence of informative right censoring caused by death and withdrawal. *Statistics in Medicine* 7: 337–346.

Wu MC and Carroll RJ. (1988). Estimation and comparison of changes in the presence of informative right censoring by modeling the censoring process. *Biometrics* 44: 175–188.

Wu MC and Bailey KR. (1989). Estimation and comparison of changes in the presence of informative right censoring conditional linear model. *Biometrics* 45: 939–955.

Wu MC, Hunsberger S, and Zucker D. (1994). Testing differences in changes in the presence of censoring parametric and nonparametric methods. *Statistics in Medicine* 13: 635–646.

Index

Note: **Bold** page numbers refer to tables and *italic* page numbers refer to figures.

Printed in the United States
by Baker & Taylor Publisher Services